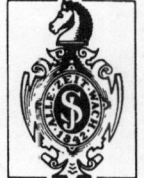

John A. Cosh · John V. Lever

Rheumatic Diseases and the Heart

With 112 Figures

Springer-Verlag
London Berlin Heidelberg New York
Paris Tokyo

John A Cosh, MA MD (Cantab), FRCP
Honorary Consultant Physician, Royal National Hospital for
Rheumatic Diseases, Upper Borough Walls, Bath BA1 1RL and
Royal United Hospital, Combe Park, Bath BA1 3NG, UK

John V Lever, BSc MBChB, FRCPath
Consultant Pathologist, Royal National Hospital for Rheumatic
Diseases, Upper Borough Walls, Bath BA1 1RL and Royal United
Hospital, Combe Park, Bath BA1 3NG, UK

ISBN-13:978-1-4471-1645-5   e-ISBN-13:978-1-4471-1643-1
DOI: 10.1007/978-1-4471-1643-1

British Library Cataloguing in Publication Data
Cosh, John A. (John Arthur), *1915*–
Rheumatic diseases and the heart. 1. Man. Heart. Rheumatic diseases I. Title
II. Lever, John V. (John Vernon), *1938*– 616.1'27
ISBN-13:978-1-4471-1645-5

Library of Congress Cataloging-in-Publication Data
Cosh, John A.
Rheumatic diseases and the heart. Includes bibliographies and index. 1. Heart—
Diseases. 2. Rheumatism—Complications and sequelae. I. Lever, John V. (John
Vernon), 1938–. II. Title. [DNLM: 1. Heart Diseases—complications. 2. Rheumatic
Heart Diseases—complications. 3. Rheumatism—complications. WG 200 C834r]
RC682.C69 1988   616.7'23   88–24848
ISBN-13:978-1-4471-1645-5

© Springer-Verlag Berlin Heidelberg 1988
Softcover reprint of the hardcover 1st edition 1988

The use of registered names, trademarks etc. in this publication does not imply, even
in the absence of a specific statement, that such names are exempt from the relevant
laws and regulations and therefore free from general use.

Product Liability: The publisher can give no guarantee for information about drug
dosage and application thereof contained in this book. In every individual case the
respective user must check its accuracy by consulting other pharmaceutical literature.

Filmset by Wilmaset, Birkenhead, Wirral

2128/3916–543210—Printed on acid-free paper.

Foreword

What medicine lacks in an increasingly specialised world is the medical polymath (or should it be medical bimath?) – the man who is an acknowledged expert in more than one field of medicine. Superspecialisation in the professional sense is an attempt to know more and more about less and less. It can be the microscopist's view of reality and such a microcosm can become also a refuge from realities. One reality difficult for the very specialised doctor to accept is that diseases don't exist. Only people with diseases exist and people do not always conform to convenient categories and compartments. It would be nice if they did but somehow they never do.

A cherished medical tradition in Britain is that specialists are not hatched straight from medical schools. Indeed, young doctors are actively discouraged from taking too narrow an interest but are plunged for at least four years into the unspecific pool of general medicine until they have developed a broad awareness of the totality of human disease. Before this they are not allowed to narrow their sights on one particular target.

In this metamorphosis one or two gifted individuals somehow manage to retain not just their general background but also a world class reputation in more than one speciality. The late Philip Ellman was a respiratory physician in one hospital and a rheumatologist in another. What more natural than that he would make *the* major contribution to the concept of rheumatoid lung and establish the idea of rheumatoid *disease*. And there are many other examples. Just such a bimath in the Ellman tradition is John Cosh, cardiologist in one hospital, rheumatologist in another. His unique and perhaps unrepeatable experience is the basis of this work. It is a double distillation of a lifetime's work in two fields of medicine.

Cardiac manifestations of disease are only too often a cause of death. But this has allowed John Lever, as pathologist, the opportunity to view and illustrate what actually happens to the heart and its surroundings as a result of these diseases.

Readers will find a dozen conditions described here in which patients may present both cardiac and rheumatic problems. Some are rare manifestations of common conditions such as rheumatoid arthritis. Some are curious associations like hyperlaxity of joints associated with a prolapsing or floppy mitral valve. The classical association of cardiac and joint disease, namely rheumatic fever with rheumatic heart disease, is now happily rare. The virtual disappearance of rheumatic fever and rheumatic heart disease from affluent countries gives one hope that some day the other painful and sometimes lethal conditions described in this book will also be banished from the earth.

Bath   Allan St. J. Dixon
1988

Preface

For many years rheumatology has been one of the growing areas in medicine. Our insight into the nature of the rheumatic diseases has developed rapidly in the last three decades. As knowledge of their immunological basis expands, our understanding has grown of their pathology, their clinical manifestations and their epidemiology, even though their ultimate causes still elude us.

We have come to see many of the rheumatic diseases as systemic disorders whose effects are by no means confined to the joints and musculo-skeletal system. Among their systemic effects there are often important lesions of the heart and sometimes of the great vessels. It is with these lesions that our text is concerned.

For nearly two centuries it could be said that rheumatic fever was the only rheumatic disease known to involve the heart. Its importance lay in its frequency and in its often devastating effects on the heart, rather than in its transient effects on the joints. But as rheumatic fever has now almost vanished in western countries, and its legacy of subsequent heart disease lessens, a greater relative importance begins to attach to the cardiac lesions of the chronic rheumatic diseases – rheumatoid arthritis, systemic lupus, ankylosing spondylitis and others. Such lesions are, of course, overshadowed in number by the commoner forms of heart disease, by coronary disease in particular. Indeed, if a patient with, say, rheumatoid arthritis is found to have a heart lesion, this may well have a separate cause, unrelated to rheumatoid arthritis, arising by coincidence.

Unfortunately, in many parts of the world rheumatic fever and the cardiac lesions that follow it continue tó be of major importance today. For this reason we have dealt fully with these topics. Moreover, the account given of the haemodynamic disturbances caused by a rheumatic heart valve lesion applies equally to similar lesions with a different underlying pathology.

The cardiac lesions caused by the different rheumatic diseases may seem superficially alike: they may involve the pericardium, myocardium or valves or combinations of these. But closer study of the pathology shows that there are specific features in each type, and that the morbid and histological changes in the heart reflect the special features of the underlying disease itself.

Our aim therefore in this book is to introduce the general features of each main rheumatic disease, and some uncommon ones, followed by a description of the cardiac lesions found in that disease. Where appropriate we seek to show how the cardiac pathology in each disease is characteristic of the pathology of that disease as a whole.

The rheumatologist, in his concern for his patient's physical problems may not always pay due attention to the heart. It is important for him to appreciate that heart disease may arise as an integral part of the rheumatic disease process, and that sometimes the cardiovascular problems may have to take precedence over those of the rheumatism.

This book is written for the general medical reader and assumes no special knowledge of cardiology or of rheumatology. But we hope that it will be of use to the cardiologist who may have little experience of rheumatology as well as to the rheumatologist who may have little experience of cardiology. We apologise therefore if some sections seem unduly elementary to some readers.

Bath   John Cosh
1988   John Lever

Acknowledgements

We wish to express our thanks to Mrs. Gina Machin and Mrs. Sally Jenner of the Medical Photographic Department at the Royal United Hospital, Bath, for their help with photographs and illustrations, and to Mrs. Kate Clark, Medical Librarian, Royal United Hospital and her staff.

We have been greatly helped by many of our collegues at the Royal National Hospital for Rheumatic Diseases, particularly Professor Allan Dixon and Professor Paul Bacon, now of Birmingham, and Professor Peter Maddison, Dr. Tony Clarke and Dr. David Scott. Also Drs. Ronald Bishton and Elizabeth Hall, pathologists, Dr. Edgar Moore, radiologist and Dr. RD Thomas, cardiologist, of the Royal United Hospital.

We also wish to thank Dr. Frank Ross, radiologist, of Bristol Royal Hospital for echocardiograms and cine-angiograms, and Professor JWB Bradfield for the use of material from the Pathology Department, University of Bristol.

Finally, we thank Dr. Richard Jacoby for his help in reviewing the text of the manuscript.

Contents

Chapter 1

Rheumatic Fever

Introduction: Rheumatic Fever and Chorea

Rheumatic fever is a systemic illness resulting from a delayed reaction to infection by a Group A haemolytic streptococcus in a susceptible host. The arthritis that it causes is painful but transient and leaves no permanent damage. But it can give rise to a pancarditis whose active phase may be prolonged for weeks or months with serious and lasting sequelae affecting the myocardium and heart valves. Without adequate prophylaxis there may be equally damaging recurrences of carditis after subsequent streptococcal infections.

Chorea is a manifestation of rheumatic fever, also following a streptococcal infection, though after a longer interval often in a subject who previously has had or may later have rheumatic fever. Chorea too may initiate an identical carditis with a sequel of permanent damage to the heart.

History

For two centuries or more rheumatic fever was the only rheumatic disease known to affect the heart. The best early description of the disease was that of Thomas Sydenham (1624–1689) whose name is still today associated with chorea. Although he clearly distinguished rheumatic fever from other rheumatic diseases, Sydenham did not appreciate its effect upon the heart. This was first described by David Pitcairn of St. Bartholomew's Hospital in 1788 and by Edward Jenner, the exponent of vaccination, in 1789. More detailed recognition of rheumatic pericarditis and valve lesions came from Jean Bouillaud in Paris (1836).

Aetiology

Rheumatic fever follows infection with the Group A beta-haemolytic streptococcus because that organism carries antigens which cross-react with antigens in

cardiac tissue. The development of a significant rise in titre of antibody is an
essential precursor to rheumatic fever (Fig. 1.1). Subjects whose infection only
causes a slight antibody rise or who are symptomless carriers of the
streptococcus do not suffer from the disease. The time interval for this antibody
rise to become effective explains the latent period between the onset of the
throat infection and the onset of rheumatic fever. This interval is usually
described as 14 days but in fact it can be some days shorter or many days longer.

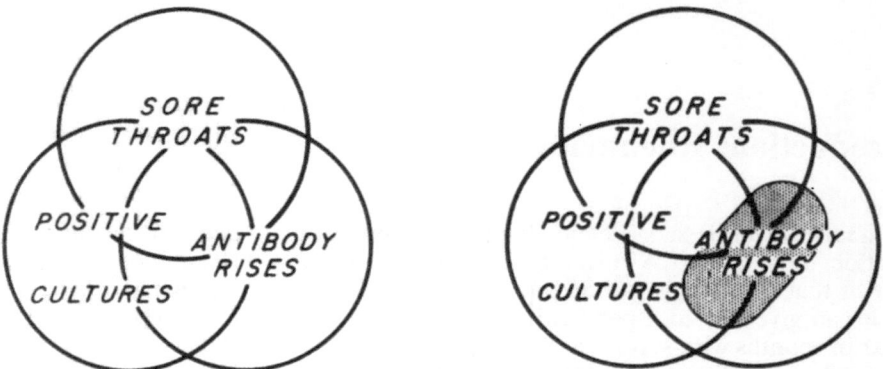

Fig. 1.1. Rheumatic fever. Venn diagrams showing (*L*) the spectrum of patients with sore throats,
positive cultures for streptococci and rising antibody titres. Rheumatic fever develops only among
those (*R*) who have rising antibody titres, whether or not they have sore throats or positive cultures.
(Feinstein 1966: by courtesy of the *Bulletin of Rheumatic Diseases*).

The site of the streptococcal infection is also significant. Infection with the
organism at sites other than the throat, e.g. in the skin as cellulitis or pyoderma,
rarely appears to give rise to rheumatic fever. The situation is different with
glomerulonephritis: although this is a comparable post-streptococcal illness,
groups other than A infecting sites other than the throat may initiate nephritis.

Patients of almost any age may develop rheumatic fever, but the commonest
age is 5 to 15 years, particularly for first attacks, with second and subsequent
attacks at older ages.

The sexes are equally affected by classical rheumatic fever and carditis, but
this is not true of chorea, which affects girls two or three times as often as boys.
Also with chorea the latent period after streptococcal infection is much longer,
up to six months. Consequently the antibody titre may have fallen by the time
that chorea develops and so cannot be used as a guide to diagnosis.

Individuals who have suffered one attack of rheumatic fever have an increased
susceptibility to subsequent attacks if a streptococcal infection recurs. Consequently secondary prophylaxis is of great importance, i.e. the protection of the
patient against further attacks by the use of long-term antibiotic cover. There is
no clear end-point at which this increased susceptibility ceases so that
prophylaxis is usually maintained for an arbitrary period such as 5 years and
sometimes longer.

There is a familial susceptibility to rheumatic fever quite apart from any increased environmental risk due to cross-infection with streptococci between members of a family. It has been found that the risk of rheumatic fever in both of a pair of monozygotic twins is three times that in a pair of dizygotic twins, in whom the risk is the same as that in ordinary siblings.

Incidence and Epidemiology

Rheumatic fever and rheumatic heart disease are found world-wide, in all climates and in all races. Their true incidence is difficult to determine without notification of the disease or screening studies of a population. Where differences of incidence are found between different populations the explanation is likely to lie in environmental circumstances, particularly socio-economic, rather than in any racial differences in susceptibility.

The incidence of rheumatic fever in the populations of the Western world has fallen almost to vanishing point in the last 50 years, but in much of the rest of the world it remains a major problem. However, in some countries, such as India, there are signs that the pattern of declining incidence and severity has started (Gotsman 1984; Editorial (*Lancet*) 1985).

The decline in chronic rheumatic heart disease has not kept pace with the fall in the incidence of rheumatic fever, even allowing for a time lag of several years between the acute illness and the subsequent heart lesions. This suggests that mild forms of rheumatic fever, or carditis without arthritis, are occurring without being recognised. The finding of established rheumatic heart lesions in patients who have never been known to have rheumatic fever is not uncommon, probably in as many as one-third, and this proportion may well be increasing.

In nineteenth and early twentieth century Britain rheumatic fever was one of the commonest reasons for hospital admission in children and young adults. It was then severe enough to have a considerable mortality. In Bristol Carey Coombs (1920) reported a death rate of 5% within the first year of developing rheumatic fever, and over 20% in 10 years. Surveys showed a far higher incidence of rheumatic fever and chronic rheumatic heart disease in those parts of the city where poverty and overcrowding were greatest (Perry and Roberts 1937).

Since the start of the twentieth century the mortality rate has fallen steadily; e.g. among London schoolchildren falling from 67 per million in 1900 to 2 per million in 1965 and virtually to zero today. Similarly, in the USA, figures from Boston showed a decline in the mortality and the severity of rheumatic fever in the period 1920–1950 (Table 1.1). The decline in the severity of the disease in Bristol schoolchildren by the 1960s is well shown by Perry's figures (Fig. 1.2). Although the proportion of children having signs of carditis with rheumatic fever was still significant (55%) in 1955–62 the carditis was evidently milder as shown by the higher proportion of children apparently making a full recovery and showing no signs of cardiac damage on follow-up (82%). Moreover the recurrence rate had fallen markedly.

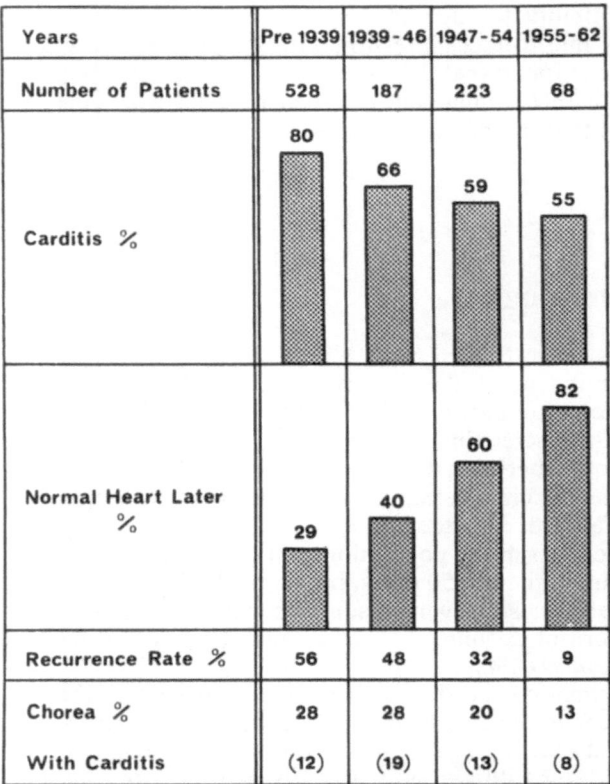

Years	Pre 1939	1939-46	1947-54	1955-62
Number of Patients	528	187	223	68
Carditis %	80	66	59	55
Normal Heart Later %	29	40	60	82
Recurrence Rate %	56	48	32	9
Chorea %	28	28	20	13
With Carditis	(12)	(19)	(13)	(8)

Fig. 1.2. Rheumatic fever and carditis in Bristol schoolchildren over successive 8-year periods. The numbers of children with rheumatic fever fell dramatically. The proportion suffering carditis declined, as did the proportion having recurrences of rheumatic fever, while many more were left with normal hearts subsequently. (Based on figures from Perry 1969).

Table 1.1. Declining severity of rheumatic fever over four decades. The figures are based on the first 100 patients admitted to the House of the Good Samaritan, Boston, in each of the specified years with first attacks of rheumatic fever. Approximately two-thirds of each group were children under 10 years of age (Bland 1960)

	1921	1930	1940	1950
Percentage with:				
Heart murmurs	75	65	58	60
Enlarged hearts	30	23	14	14
Subsequent return to normal heart size	20	20	38	45
Mortality	8	7	4	1

Antibiotic therapy and prophylaxis have certainly accounted for much of this change. However, reports from many different sources indicate that the severity of rheumatic fever began to diminish before the introduction of antibiotics. The most likely explanation is a general improvement in health and nutrition coupled with better living standards. An additional factor may well be a reduction in the virulence of the causative streptococci (Besterman 1970).

Although rheumatic fever is a vanishing disease in Western nations, its association with adverse economic circumstances may still be seen. A recent survey in Tennessee revealed a prevalence among black children living in inner cities that was eight times as high as the prevalence among white children living in suburban or rural areas (Land and Bisno 1983).

Exceptions to this trend, however, are the recent reports of outbreaks of rheumatic fever in both children and adults in the USA (Congeni et al. 1987; Giardina 1987; Veasy et al. 1987). Veasy et al. describe an outbreak in Utah in 1985–6, when 74 children were affected. They were predominantly white middle-class children from good homes and with ready access to medical care. There had not been any noticeable increase in previous streptococcal infections. The total incidence of carditis was 91% and chorea was a presenting feature in 31%. Two children developed mitral incompetence severe enough to require surgical valve replacement. One feature of this study was the use of Doppler echocardiography to detect mitral regurgitation that could not be appreciated by ordinary auscultation; on this basis mitral incompetence was diagnosed in 14 patients, in addition to the 53 in whom it was diagnosed by auscultation. Rheumatic fever evidently remains a potential threat in the Western world.

Rheumatic Fever in the Third World

In his "Global view of rheumatic fever today" Stollerman (1976) says: "The virtual disappearance of acute rheumatic fever among relatively affluent populations in N. America and Europe especially in cities with few if any slums, and optimal housing conditions, is one of the dramatic events of recent medical history".

The situation is very different in other parts of the world, such as Turkey, Egypt, Central and South America, India, the Phillipines, Hong Kong and Singapore. There the incidence of rheumatic fever remains high and is associated with overcrowding, large families, poverty and malnutrition (Taranta and Markowitz 1981). That this is not simply a matter of climate is shown by the virtual freedom from rheumatic fever of the wealthier residents in these areas.

Economically the association of rheumatic fever and rheumatic heart disease with poverty and a low standard of living is shown by the inverse relationship between the gross national product of a country and the prevalence of these diseases in its children (Table 1.2).

Table 1.2. Gross national product (GNP) and prevalence of rheumatic fever and rheumatic heart disease. The prevalence of rheumatic fever and rheumatic heart disease is greatest in countries with the lowest gross national product (Agarwal 1981)

Country	GNP in $US per head	Prevalence of rheumatic fever and rheumatic heart disease in schoolchildren (%)
India	150	0.56
Pakistan	170	0.7
Egypt	280	0.1
China	410	0.15
Algeria	990	0.15
UK	4020	0.01
USA	7890	0.07 to 0.16

Surveys in India show that rheumatic fever accounts for only two or three of every 1000 hospital admissions, but that rheumatic heart disease makes up one-third of all heart disease treated in hospital. The low figure for hospital admission with rheumatic fever indicates that the disease continues to occur in mild or unrecognised form. Rheumatic carditis certainly continues to be serious, giving rise to the phenomenon of "juvenile mitral stenosis" in India and the Far East, virtually unknown in the West. In India a quarter of all patients with mitral stenosis are under the age of 20 years and half of these cases are severe enough to require surgery. In Singapore one-fifth are under the age of 20 years, but in Japan the proportion has fallen in recent years to 6% (South East Asia Conference 1975).

Strasser (1978) reviewed the decline in rheumatic fever beginning to be seen in some of the less affluent countries in the world, where the pattern already experienced in the West is now being echoed. The drive against rheumatic fever in these countries must be based mainly on social and economic improvements coupled with an effective secondary prophylaxis programme. The experience of WHO has been that such programmes will only endure and succeed if they form part of a general health care organisation and should not be mounted as an ad hoc attack on rheumatic fever in isolation.

Immunopathology

Infection by Group A streptococci induces the production by the host of a number of specific antibodies, the most important of which is anti-streptolysin O. Virtually every patient with rheumatic fever can be shown to have rising titres of this or other streptococcal antibodies at the onset of the illness (Feinstein 1966).

Evidence for cross-reactivity between antigens in heart tissue and antigens in streptococci was put forward by Kaplan (1969). Antisera produced in rabbits by inoculation with Group A streptococci were shown to react with human heart tissue by the techniques of immunofluorescent staining and complement fixation. The responsible streptococcal antigen was found to originate in the bacterial cell wall and to be closely associated with, if not identical to, the M protein, the "virulence factor" of the Group A streptococcus.

Studies on sera from patients with rheumatic fever showed that these sera react with the same components of cardiac tissue that were identified in the rabbit experiments viz. sarcolemma of myocardial muscle fibre and smooth muscle in blood vessel wall and endocardium. This immunological reaction was found more often in patients with active carditis than in those with inactive rheumatic heart disease, and little or no reaction was obtained with normal human sera.

In the hearts of children dying with rheumatic carditis and heart failure widespread deposits of gammaglobulin and complement were seen in cardiac muscle indicating the sites of antibody attachment in vivo.

The inference that this state of immunological reactivity is induced by streptococcal infection is impressive though indirect. Thus, sera from patients with active rheumatic fever lost their ability to react against cardiac tissue after the sera were absorbed with extracts from streptococcal cell walls. Alternatively, these sera lost their ability to form precipitates in agar diffusion plates against streptococcal cell wall antigens if the sera had been previously absorbed with homogenates of cardiac muscle. With such techniques Kaplan (1976) was able to show the presence of cross-reactive antibodies in the sera of patients with rheumatic fever – a reaction rarely present in control sera or sera from patients with rheumatoid arthritis or systemic lupus.

Significant titres of such cross-reacting antibodies persist during the attack of rheumatic fever but decline in 1–2 years and are no longer detectable after 5 years. However, a fresh streptococcal infection may quickly evoke a rise in titre and it is likely that if this rise is sufficiently high the patient may suffer a recurrence of rheumatic fever (Zabriskie 1976).

A possible explanation for the predominance of mitral and aortic valve lesions comes from an observation by Gelfand et al. (1981). Fresh normal human heart valves obtained at autopsy were exposed to sensitised sheep red cells carrying bound IgG. Attachment of the Fc fragment of the IgG was found on the surfaces of the mitral, aortic, tricuspid and pulmonary valves in descending order of frequency. The reason for this preferential attachment is not clear but if attachment of streptococcal antibody followed the same pattern it would have a bearing on the relative frequencies of the different valve lesions in rheumatic heart disease.

Antibodies reactive with components of cardiac tissue may also be found in the sera of patients who have recently undergone cardiac surgery or suffered myocardial infarction. These probably form the basis for the inflammatory response seen in the post-cardiotomy and post-myocardial infarction syndromes. However, these antibodies do not exhibit cross-reactivity with streptococcal antigens and are not capable of initiating rheumatic fever.

Morbid Anatomy

All layers of the heart are involved i.e. there is a pancarditis.

Both the visceral and the parietal layers of the *pericardium* become covered by granulation tissue and exude abundant fibrin. At autopsy the two layers are separated with difficulty to reveal two ragged yellow surfaces, with an appearance known as the "bread and butter heart" (Fig. 1.3).

In the fibrous septa of the *myocardium* are the small granulomas known as Aschoff bodies, often closely associated with blood vessels (Fig. 1.4). They are barely visible to the naked eye although discernible with a hand lens. On microscopy they are seen to have a characteristic structure, appearing as foci of mucoid or fibrinoid degeneration of collagen diffusely infiltrated by lymphocytes and macrophages. Some of the latter have large hyperchromatic nuclei, often multiple (Aschoff cells) while others have a dense central nucleolus giving an "owl eye" appearance (Anitschoff cells). The hyperchromatic nuclei and eosinophilic cytoplasm of some of the cells in Aschoff bodies have led some pathologists to consider that they are derived from muscle cells. However, histochemical and electron microscopic studies favour an origin from histiocytes (Wagner and Siew 1970). Gross and Ehrlich (1934) described the progressive

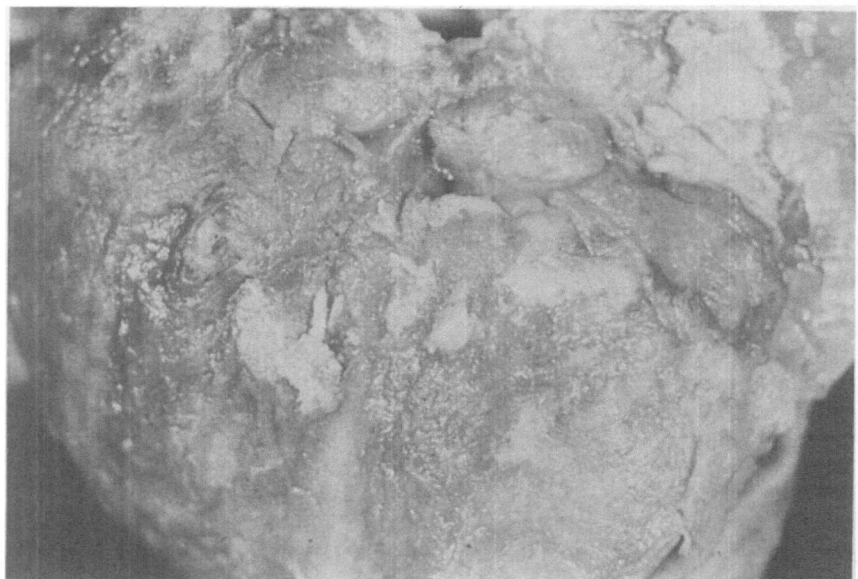

Fig. 1.3. Rheumatic pericarditis. The heart at autopsy from a 12-year-old girl who died from rheumatic carditis, showing the florid acute pericarditis ("bread and butter pericardium").

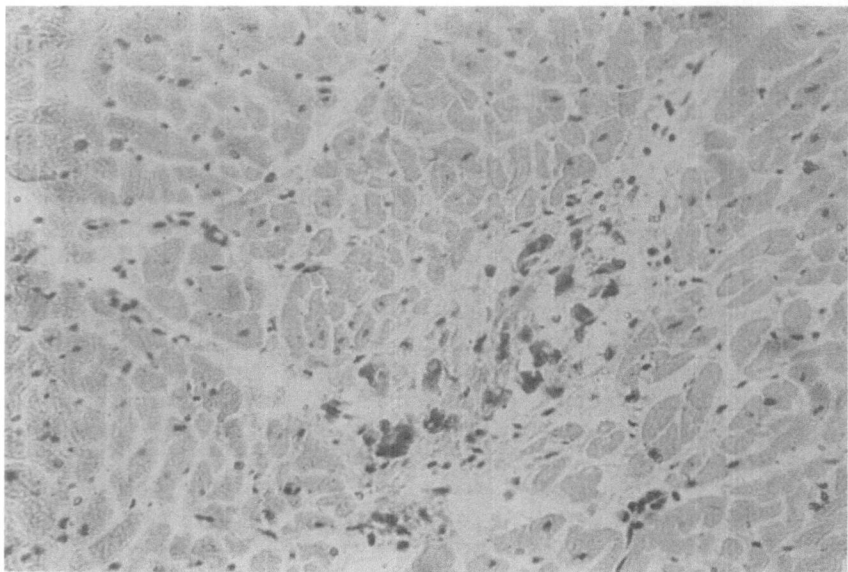

Fig. 1.4. Rheumatic carditis. The myocardium of the same patient as Fig. 1.3 showing an Aschoff body in a fibrous septum (× 225).

change in appearance of Aschoff bodies from an initial highly cellular structure ultimately to a fibrous scar in the course of time.

The *endocardium* of all four chambers of the heart may contain Aschoff bodies, not only in the acute stages of rheumatic fever but also many years later even when there is no clinical evidence of activity of the diseases. An area of the posterior wall of the left ventricle may appear hyperaemic and oedematous. This is known as McCallum's patch, and the endocardium here may be the site of attachment of thrombus.

More subtle changes may be present in the mitral and aortic valves. On the lines of closure where opposing cusps meet there may be minute vegetations, composed of fibrin and platelets (Fig. 1.5). On microscopy the underlying cusps show oedema and vascularisation, sometimes with patchy fibrinoid necrosis and a mild inflammatory infiltrate of lymphocytes and plasma cells. Among these occasional Aschoff cells and Anitschoff cells may be seen.

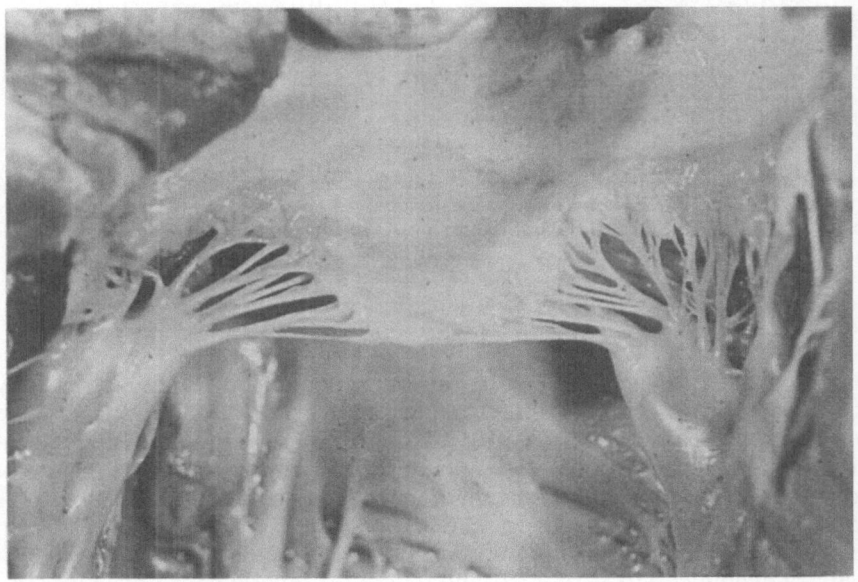

Fig. 1.5. Rheumatic endocarditis. The mitral valve from the same patient as the two previous figures, showing minute vegetations on the lines of closure.

Clinical Features

Introduction

Rheumatic fever can present in all degrees of severity. At its most inconspicuous it may cause little more than fleeting joint pains and no fever, and in roughly half there is no carditis. However, the systemic and the cardiac manifestations of the disease are not necessarily present in similar degree. An apparently symptomless attack may be associated with damaging carditis while at the other extreme an acutely painful febrile illness is not necessarily accompanied by carditis (Feinstein and Spagnuolo 1962). Arthritis and chorea rarely appear together, mainly because chorea arises at a much later stage after the streptococcal infection than does the arthritis. The differing patterns of presentation are well expressed in the Venn diagrams of Fig. 1.6.

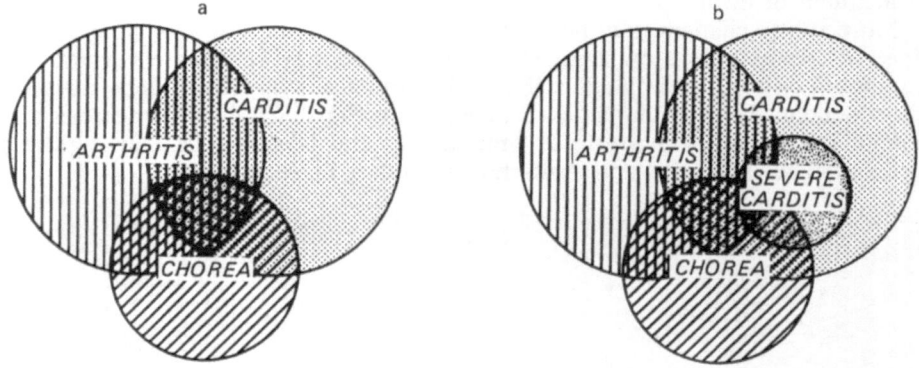

Fig. 1.6. Rheumatic fever: clinical patterns. Venn diagrams illustrating patterns of clinical presentation of rheumatic fever with and without carditis. Even severe carditis (*b*) is not necessarily accompanied by arthritis. (Feinstein 1966; by courtesy of the *Bulletin of Rheumatic Diseases*).

Onset

The mode of onset ranges from gradual to acute and abrupt. Although usually starting 10–14 days after the onset of a streptococcal throat infection, the interval may be three weeks or more. Typically, the symptoms of the throat infection have subsided and the patient, if a child, is recuperating but may not yet have returned to school when rheumatic fever begins. If acute, the symptoms develop within a few hours or overnight.

The fever is of variable degree and duration. In a moderately severe case it will swing at evening up to 39 or 40 °C and persist for several days – even weeks – before subsiding gradually. There may be one or two relapses of fever before it finally settles. It is accompanied by tachycardia, perspiration and prostration. In a milder case the fever and systemic upset are slight and settle in a few days.

The arthritis, if severe, will develop acutely in one or two joints, which may be any of the main limb joints – knee, ankle, wrist or elbow – but the hands, fingers, shoulders or spine may also be affected. Pain is acute and the child cries and cannot move the affected limb. The inflamed joints are swollen, warm and tender with reddening of the overlying skin. An effusion may be detected in the larger joints although examination is limited because of pain.

The arthritis subsides in a few days, even without treatment, but as initially-affected joints improve others may become affected, only to settle in their turn within a few days i.e. the arthritis is transitory and migratory, although in mild cases only a single joint may be affected. In individual bigger joints, such as the knee, symptoms may settle more slowly and an effusion may still be present after two or three weeks as in Case History 1.1. In general, adults tend to be affected less acutely than children, usually without carditis, but this is not invariably the case (Adatto et al. 1965; Al-Rawi and Al-Khateeb 1982; Hart 1985).

Case History 1.1

Mild rheumatic fever
No carditis

Miss S. H., Student, born 1955

11 July 1975	Developed sore throat: recovered in 3 days Given brief course of penicillin
25 July	Ill again with fever, transient generalised macular rash and swollen painful L knee
28 July	Admitted to hospital. Fever, 37.7 °C, P 100 L knee still painful and swollen Normal heart and ECG Throat swab: no haemolytic streptococci ESR 120. ASO titre 700 (normal below 200) Given oral penicillin 250 mg and aspirin 600 mg 6-hourly
4 August	Fever settled. ESR 115. L knee improved
7 August	ASO 500. ESR 96
11 August	Well apart from small residual L knee effusion
24 September	Fully recovered. Normal heart and ECG Penicillin V 250 mg b.d. prophylaxis started
Comment	An uncomplicated attack affecting one joint only. The knee effusion persisted for over 2 weeks but might have cleared more quickly with bigger doses of aspirin. The initial brief course of oral penicillin was insufficient to protect her from rheumatic fever

---

The only lasting sequel of the arthritis, mainly of historical interest, is the Jaccoud type of "arthritis" of the metacarpo-phalangeal joints. Repeated severe attacks of rheumatic fever may result in residual fibrosis around the capsule of these joints causing an ulnar deviation deformity superficially resembling rheumatoid arthritis. However, there is no true chronic arthritis present and other joints are unaffected (Girgis et al. 1978; Grahame et al. 1970).

The Heart

If carditis is present the most obvious clinical evidence is tachycardia, persisting after the acute arthritis and fever have subsided. Four-hourly monitoring of the pulse rate is important and a record of the sleeping pulse rate is valuable, particularly in children, as tachycardia continues during sleep if carditis is present. The heart sounds change in quality, becoming softer or muffled as carditis develops. A mitral pansystolic murmur is commonly heard, probably indicating a temporary phase of mitral regurgitation secondary to left ventricular dilatation. This commonly disappears and is not necessarily a sign of future valve lesion. The short mid-diastolic murmur of Carey Coombs may be heard probably indicating temporary swelling of the mitral valve cusps. This too may disappear as carditis subsides but is a likely indicator that a permanent valve lesion may result. A soft aortic diastolic murmur may be heard if the aortic valve is affected but this too is not necessarily permanent.

Pericarditis is revealed by a friction rub and sometimes precordial pain, in a minority of patients. It does not appear in isolation but as part of a pancarditis. It is usually a "dry pericarditis" though an effusion may form, detectable on X-ray films or, with more precision, on echocardiography. The accompanying ECG changes are usually slight and not diagnostic e.g. confined to T wave flattening as the characteristic full pattern of the ECG changes of pericarditis is not often seen. Rarely an effusion large enough to cause tamponade may form, requiring aspiration (Tan et al. 1983).

Myocarditis, if severe, causes dilatation of the heart, detected clinically by shift of the apical impulse to the sixth intercostal space and the anterior axillary line. Cardiac dilatation is confirmed by X-ray examination, although this will not distinguish between dilatation and pericardial effusion, as echocardiography will. With myocarditis there is a softening of heart sounds and the addition of a soft third heart sound with protodiastolic gallop. The murmurs of mitral and tricuspid regurgitation will probably accompany myocarditis, and possibly a pericardial friction rub.

Severe myocarditis will cause congestive heart failure, with engorgement of neck veins and liver, possibly with oedema of lower limbs and trunk. Pulmonary oedema results from left ventricular failure, with basal rales, a rapid respiratory rate and orthopnoea. Chest X-ray films show oedema in the lung fields as well as enlargement of the cardiac shadow.

The Electrocardiogram

The electrocardiogram is a valuable guide to myocardial involvement. The characteristic finding is of first degree heart block with lengthening of the PR interval. If the patient is a child it is important to take into account the child's age and the heart rate in assessing the normal value for the PR interval (more correctly, the PQ interval, being measured from the start of the P wave to the start of the ventricular complex). The younger the child and the faster the tachycardia, the shorter is the normal value for the PR interval. If nomograms showing normal values are available the PR index is calculated, i.e. the ratio between the actual PR interval and the expected normal under the circumstances, a figure over 1.0 being abnormal (Clarke and Keith 1972). Serial study of the PR index, which is independent of the heart rate, gives useful information as to the state of the myocardium during the course of the illness. Abnormality of the PR index may be the only evidence of myocarditis (Sanyal et al. 1976). With recovery the PR index almost invariably returns to normal.

Occasionally higher grades of conduction defect may be found, such as second degree block (Mobitz type I) with Wenckebach periods (Fig. 1.7) or temporary atrio-ventricular dissociation.

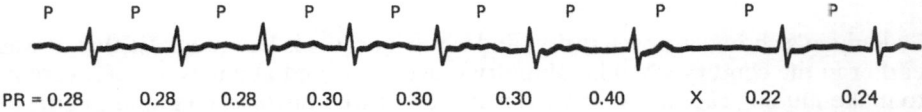

PR = 0.28   0.28   0.28   0.30   0.30   0.30   0.40   X   0.22   0.24

Fig. 1.7. Rheumatic fever. ECG showing second degree heart block in a boy with carditis. Progressive lengthening of the PR interval occurs until a ventricular beat is missed (at *X*) – a "Wenckebach period".

The Skin

Subcutaneous nodules are only seen in the more severe cases and do not appear until 3 or 4 weeks after the onset. Such patients usually have carditis. Nodules may persist for some weeks before spontaneously disappearing, but the appearance of fresh crops signifies that the disease process is still active. A typical nodule is small, firm and mobile beneath the skin, feeling like a small pea; it is not tender. Larger nodules, in greater numbers, are associated with more severe forms of the disease. Nodules usually form over the extensor surfaces of joints such as the knuckles, wrists and elbows, knees and ankles, but may also be found on the flexor aspect of the wrist, close to the flexor tendons, or over the occiput.

The classical rash associated with rheumatic fever is erythema marginatum. In florid cases it covers the trunk and limbs forming well-marked slightly raised irregular rings of erythema with a pale centre. The rash is not fixed, for each ring tends to spread over a matter of days, leaving a central area of clear skin as the ring widens and finally fades. In milder cases the ring is evanescent and seen on the trunk only, or it may come and go over a period of some weeks.

The intensity of the rash does not necessarily match the severity of the disease. It may appear to be the only manifestation of rheumatic fever, in which case it probably indicates that a mild attack has occurred in the recent past without being recognised.

Other rashes of a post-streptococcal nature may be seen, such as erythema nodosum or erythema multiforme. These are indicators of a recent streptococcal infection but are not necessarily a sign of rheumatic fever.

Other Symptoms

Abdominal pain may be one of the presenting symptoms; it is usually fleeting
and transient, but may be severe enough to suggest peritonitis or early
appendicitis. It normally subsides within a day or two. Back or neck pain may
also occur in the acute stage, probably attributable to involvement of spinal
joints. Epistaxis has often been noted during the acute stage of rheumatic fever.

Chorea

Sydenham's chorea is now a rarity, and when it occurs is less dramatic than it was
earlier in the century when involuntary movements and ataxia were so severe as
to make nursing care a problem. It is twice or three times as common in girls as
in boys and is seen at a slightly older age than the average case of rheumatic
fever, i.e. between 10 and 20 years. Its onset is usually insidious and may be
noticed by an astute school teacher if not by the child's family. The child is
emotionally upset, fretful, tearful and unhappy. Ataxia becomes noticeable,
particularly in hand movements: articles are dropped and broken, hand-writing
deteriorates and clumsiness affects fine movements such as dressing, doing up
buttons, putting on gloves. The involuntary movements are characteristic:
sudden twitching and writhing movements of the hands, arms or of the whole
body, or facial grimacing. The movements are non-repetitive and in this are
unlike the movements of a nervous tic or habit spasm. When asked to put out
her tongue the child's response is so sudden that the movement has been called
the "jack-in-the-box tongue". When asked to hold out her outstretched arms,
the forearms turn into a position of pronation and it is difficult or impossible to
keep the hands and arms still.

Rarely there is a degree of muscle weakness affecting one side of the body and
limbs (chorea mollis) when movement and power are much reduced on the
affected side. Muscle tone is flaccid.

The course of chorea is unpredictable but the symptoms usually persist for a
few weeks. There may be evidence of recent streptococcal infection but this is
uncertain as the causative infection precedes the onset of chorea by several
weeks. Arthritis fortunately does not coincide with chorea although it may have
occurred previously. Carditis is present in about half of the patients with chorea,
as with rheumatic fever.

Chorea gravidarum appears at a later age, during pregnancy, sometimes
affecting patients who have had Sydenham's chorea in earlier years. Carditis is
an unlikely complication.

Investigations

Throat Swab

In the early stages of rheumatic fever throat swabs may well be positive for
Group A beta-haemolytic streptococci. Swabs should be repeated during the
course of the illness to ensure that antibiotic therapy has eradicated the
organism.

Blood Count

A neutrophil leucocytosis is found if the illness is acute, with fever and arthritis, but is not necessarily seen in milder cases or in the later stages with carditis alone. A normochromic anaemia is likely to develop in the course of a protracted attack.

Antibodies

Antibodies to streptococci in rising titre are proof of recent streptococcal infection. In more than 70% of cases the titre of antistreptolysin A is raised. Other antibodies likely to be present are antihyaluronidase and antistreptokinase. Raised titres of one or more of these three will be found in virtually all cases.

Acute Phase Reactants

A raised ESR, an increased plasma viscosity or a raised C-reactive protein (CRP) will all be found while active carditis persists. Weekly monitoring of one or more of these is a valuable aid in assessing progress.

Electrocardiogram

This should be recorded weekly during the active phase of the illness. In most cases of rheumatic fever the ECG is normal but a prolonged PR interval or a PR index greater than 1.0 is strong evidence of carditis (see p. 12). It may even be the only evidence of carditis.

Chest X-ray

The X-ray film may show enlargement of the heart shadow, which may be due to pericardial effusion or cardiac dilatation or both. Pulmonary oedema may be seen in the lung fields if carditis causes left ventricular failure. "Rheumatic pneumonia" is probably a form of persistent pulmonary oedema, only seen in gravely ill patients.

Echocardiogram

This is of value in identifying enlargement of individual cardiac chambers and in revealing the presence of a pericardial effusion. With the Doppler technique minor degrees of valvular regurgitation may be detected (p. 53).

Diagnosis

Diagnosis presents few problems in the classical case of acute rheumatic fever but can be difficult if the attack is mild or if there is carditis without any arthritis. As there is no single specific diagnostic test, diagnosis must depend upon the recognition of a group of features.

The Duckett Jones criteria (Stollerman et al. 1965; Table 1.3) are helpful in this respect. The presence of two major criteria is clearly diagnostic of rheumatic fever, but often only one is present and diagnosis then depends on the presence of two supporting minor criteria combined with evidence of preceding streptococcal infection.

Table 1.3. The Duckett Jones criteria for rheumatic fever (as revised by the American Heart Association 1966; Stollerman et al. 1965)

Major Criteria
  Carditis
  Polyarthritis
  Chorea
  Erythema Marginatum
  Subcutaneous nodules
Minor Criteria
  History of previous rheumatic fever or established rheumatic heart disease
  Arthralgia
  Fever
  Acute phase reactants (ESR, WBC, CRP)
  ECG: prolonged PR interval
Plus supporting evidence of preceding streptococcal infection
The Diagnosis of rheumatic fever is highly likely if two major criteria are present, or one major and two minor criteria, providing that there is evidence of recent streptococcal infection

The differential diagnosis includes a wide variety of possibilities, but a brief period of observation and investigation usually clarifies the diagnosis with little difficulty. Some viral infections cause sore throat, fever and limb pains and a few, such as rubella and mumps, can produce a frank polyarthritis. Rheumatoid arthritis may in its initial phases cause migratory joint symptoms and systemic illness, and Still's disease classically presents with high fever and a rash leading subsequently to a polyarthritis. Osteomyelitis and septic arthritis, with localised acute pain affecting a single joint may, at the onset, resemble rheumatic fever. Brucellosis is another cause of fever, malaise and occasionally arthritis. Sickle cell disease may present with acute limb pains mimicking arthritis.

Chorea is difficult to recognise at first as the onset is usually gradual. It needs to be differentiated from habit spasm, where movements or grimaces are repetitive. In chorea the position of the outstretched hands and arms is characteristic, the wrists being slightly flexed and the metacarpophalangeal joints hyperextended with the forearms somewhat pronated. The typical abruptness of movements is seen in the "jack-in-the-box" tongue. The associated ataxia and emotional upset are an essential part of chorea.

Difficulty may arise over heart murmurs. The mitral and/or aortic murmurs of previously established rheumatic heart disease may be present in a patient who is now suffering a new recurrent attack of rheumatic fever. A commonly heard functional murmur in children is a soft low-pitched systolic murmur at the base of the heart i.e. in the aortic and pulmonary valve areas. Its loudness is much influenced by changes in posture and by respiration, being loudest when the patient is sitting upright and leaning forwards, and in expiration. The two elements of the second sound remain normal i.e. the split or interval between them widening on inspiration and narrowing on expiration. The basal systolic murmur usually softens and disappears as the child grows older although it sometimes may persist into adult life.

Another murmur of benign nature is the late systolic murmur heard at and medial to the cardiac apex, due to mitral cusp prolapse. It is usually accompanied by a systolic click. This murmur, too, may disappear or may continue into adult life usually without sequelae or complications. However, there may be associated arrhythmias, left-sided chest pain or ultimately significant mitral regurgitation (see p. 234).

The presence of an innocent murmur does not rule out the possibility of the patient having rheumatic fever and carditis. It is important therefore to examine the heart carefully and repeatedly during the illness, noting any changes in murmurs, sounds and heart size which would indicate the presence of an active carditis. Echocardiography is helpful in assessing the significance of murmurs, and should be repeated at intervals where appropriate.

Treatment

General Care

The patient with rheumatic fever needs bed rest, good nursing care and monitoring of temperature and pulse which should be 4-hourly at first but less often as the acute stage subsides. If there is tachycardia it is important to check the sleeping pulse rate, especially in children. Drugs are needed for the relief of pain and an antibiotic, first as therapy and later as prophylaxis, which should be continued as part of long-term supervision. With recovery graded exercise and rehabilitation are needed appropriate to the degree of cardiac involvement. Where children require long periods of hospitalisation some form of schooling is valuable within the limits imposed by confinement to bed or to the ward.

Bed Rest

Total bed rest is advisable at first and pillows should be allowed, as slight elevation of the head and shoulders is better tolerated than lying flat. If there are no signs of carditis mobilisation can be started as soon as fever and joint pain have subsided. But in the presence of carditis bed rest should continue with monitoring of pulse and temperature and a check at least weekly on the cardiac physical signs, blood count, ESR or CRP, antibody titres as necessary, throat swab and ECG. Usually mobilisation can begin after 6 weeks at most and physical activity is then permitted in accordance with the state of the heart.

Pain Relief

Protective bandaging and light-weight splints may be needed at first for acutely painful joints. Aspirin is still the best analgesic and is said to have a specific effect on pain and fever in rheumatic fever, so that the response to aspirin may be used as a confirmatory factor in diagnosis. The use of aspirin is justifiable in spite of its occasional association with Reye's syndrome of encephalopathy and hepatic failure. In the treatment of rheumatic fever aspirin should only be withheld if a child is known to be exposed to infective hepatitis or viral influenza, both of which are known causes of Reye's syndrome. A loading dose of 140 mg/kg is given for the first day or two, administered 4-hourly (with a maximum of 10 g/day for an adult) continuing at 70 mg/kg thereafter, given 6-hourly (maximum 5 g/day for an adult). This may be continued for 4 to 6 weeks, with reduction of dosage before this if progress is good. There is no evidence that prolonged administration of aspirin in high dosage influences the outcome in terms of heart damage. Aspirin overdose induces hyperpnoea, deafness and tinnitus, in which case the drug should be withdrawn temporarily and then started again at a lower dose. Adverse reactions to aspirin include rash, asthma and gastric bleeding; if any of these occur the drug must be stopped and a different analgesic given, such as paracetamol, ibuprofen or naproxen.

Antibiotics

Penicillin should be given in bactericidal doses as soon as the diagnosis has been made in order to eradicate streptococci from the throat. Benzyl penicillin (penicillin G) is best, given intramuscularly twice daily in doses of 0.5 or 1 mega unit depending on the patient's weight. This should be continued for a minimum of 10 days or until throat swabs become negative for streptococci. This should be followed by oral phenoxymethyl penicillin (penicillin V) at first 250 mg 6-hourly, soon reducing to 125 or 250 mg twice daily as prophylaxis. So far the haemolytic streptococcus has shown no signs of becoming penicillin-resistant. If the patient is allergic to or intolerant of penicillin an alternative bactericidal antibiotic, e.g. erythromycin, should be substituted as therapy, followed by a sulphonamide for prophylaxis.

Corticosteroids

Corticosteroids have not been shown to have any long-term benefit in rheumatic fever. However, the prompt symptomatic relief given by steroid therapy makes this preferable to aspirin for the patient with a severe attack, with much joint pain or with carditis producing heart failure. An initial dose of 1 mg/kg prednisone is appropriate, reducing gradually as improvement follows, with the aim of withdrawal of prednisone after 4 to 6 weeks depending on the course of the illness.

Chorea

There is no specific therapy for chorea. The aim of management should be a quiet tranquil atmosphere in a room or in a quiet corner of the ward. Hypnotics such as diazepam up to 20 mg/day may be needed at first. Aspirin is not indicated. Monitoring of the pulse rate, the heart, throat swabs, blood and ECG should be followed as for rheumatic fever. If streptococci are found in the throat penicillin is given until swabs become negative; otherwise it is sufficient to start the long-term prophylaxis with phenoxymethyl penicillin 125 or 250 mg twice daily. Hospital admission is usually preferable to home treatment at first for the sake of observation and monitoring, but if home conditions are good return home should be possible in 2 to 4 weeks and bed rest thereafter is not necessary unless there is evidence of carditis.

Further Course

Most children can return to school within 3 months of the onset of rheumatic fever or chorea unless there is still an active carditis. Children should be allowed to take part in games, although these should be of non-competitive nature at first. The presence of a heart murmur should not be a bar to physical activity. It is important to avoid an attitude of invalidism on the part of the patient and, even more, on the part of the family and school teachers. Regular follow-up, at 2 or 3-monthly intervals initially, is advisable to assess the state of the heart, to see that penicillin prophylaxis is being continued and to see that invalidism is being avoided.

Prophylaxis

The standard recommendation is that this should continue for 5 years or for as long as the patient is at school or college. Normally phenoxymethyl penicillin (penicillin V) 250 mg twice daily orally is given or, if there is an allergy or intolerance to penicillin, a sulphonamide e.g. sulphadiazine 0.5 g twice daily. WHO also recommends as an alternative a monthly depot injection of benzathine penicillin (Penidural) 1.2 mega units for a child or the same dose 3-weekly for an adult (Editorial (*Lancet*) 1982).

A careful appraisal of the prophylactic effectiveness of penicillin was made over a 6-year period at Irvington House, New York (Albam et al. 1964). It showed a clear superiority for the depot injections over oral penicillin. Patients receiving the depot injection had only about one-third of the attack rate of streptococcal throat infection and one-tenth the attack rate of rheumatic fever compared with patients on the oral regime.

The same study showed that the children most at risk for recurrences of rheumatic fever with carditis were those who had already had one or more attacks with carditis. But the risk of rheumatic fever with carditis was low in those who had previously had an attack of rheumatic fever without carditis. That is, recurrent attacks of rheumatic fever tended to repeat the pattern and severity of previous attacks in the individual patient, thus making it possible to identify high-risk and low-risk patients.

For maximum protection of the high-risk child with an already damaged heart prophylaxis is best given with monthly depot injections, even for 5 years; the benefits justify the inconvenience and the local discomfort of the injection, particularly where cooperation over oral prophylaxis is likely to be unreliable. For the low-risk child oral penicillin is adequate, and a shorter period of prophylaxis, say, of 2 years, may be considered on the understanding that subsequent throat infections should be promptly reported and treated.

References

Adatto IJ, Poske RM, Pouget JM et al. (1965) Rheumatic fever in the adult. JAMA 194: 1043–1048

Agarwal BL (1981) Rheumatic heart disease unabated in developing countries. Lancet II: 910–911

Albam B, Epstein JA, Feinstein AR et al. (1964) Rheumatic fever in children and adolescents. A long term epidemiologic study of subsequent prophylaxis, streptococcal infections and clinical sequelae. Ann Intern Med 60: Suppl 5

Al-Rawi ZS, Al-Khateeb N (1982) Clinical features of first attack of rheumatic fever in adults. Rheumatol Rehabil 21: 195–200

American Heart Association (1966) Revised Duckett Jones Criteria. In: WHO Technical Report Series No 342 "Prevention of Rheumatic Fever". WHO, Geneva

Besterman EF (1970) The changing face of acute rheumatic fever. Br Heart J 32: 579–582

Bland EF (1960) Declining severity of rheumatic fever. A comparative study of the past four decades. N Engl J Med 262: 597–599

Clarke M, Keith JD (1972) Atrioventricular conduction in acute rheumatic fever. Br Heart J 34: 472–479

Congeni B, Rizzo C, Congeni C, Streenvasan VV (1987) Outbreak of acute rheumatic fever in northeast Ohio. J Pediatr 111: 176–179

Coombs FC (1920) The incidence of fatal rheumatic heart disease in Bristol 1876–1913. Lancet II: 226

Editorial (1982) Prevention of rheumatic heart disease. Lancet I: 143–144

Editorial (1985) Decline in rheumatic fever. Lancet II: 647–648

Feinstein AR (1966) The natural histories of acute rheumatic fever. Bull Rheum Dis 17: 423–428

Feinstein AR, Spagnuolo M (1962) The clinical patterns of acute rheumatic fever. A reappraisal. Medicine (Baltimore) 41: 279–305

Gelfand MC, Maclay M, Shin ML, Green I, Frank MM (1981) Binding of IgG sensitised erythrocytes by mitral and aortic cardiac valves: a possible clue to the pathogenesis of human valvular heart disease. Clin Immunol Immunopathol 19: 151–160

Giardina AC (1987) Resurgence of acute rheumatic fever. N Engl J Med 317: 507–508

Girgis FL, Popple AW, Bruckner FE (1978) Jaccoud's arthropathy. Ann Rheum Dis 37: 561–565

Gotsman MV (1984) Rheumatic fever in the Eighties. In Ansell BM, Simkin PA (eds) The heart and rheumatic disease. Butterworths, London, pp 234–267

Grahame R, Mitchell ABS, Scott JT (1970) Chronic post-rheumatic fever arthropathy (Jaccoud's). Ann Rheum Dis 29: 622–625

Gross L, Ehrlich JC (1934) Studies on the myocardial Aschoff body. I. Descriptive classification of lesion. Am J Path 10: 467–488

Hart FD (1985) Acute rheumatic fever in adults: the disease. J Rheumatol 12: 193–194

Kaplan MH (1969) The cross-reaction of Group A streptococci with heart tissue and its relation to induced autoimmunity in rheumatic fever. Bull Rheum Dis 19: 560–567

Kaplan MH (1976) Autoimmunity in rheumatic fever. In: Dumonde DC (ed) Infection and immunology in the rheumatic diseases. Blackwell, Oxford, pp 113–118

Land MA, Bisno AL (1983) Acute rheumatic fever: a vanishing disease in suburbia. JAMA 249: 895–898

Perry CB (1969) The natural history of acute rheumatism. Ann Rheum Dis 28: 471–476

Perry CB, Roberts JAF (1937) A study on the variability in the incidence of rheumatic heart disease within the city of Bristol. Br Med J 2: Suppl 154–158

Sanyal SK, Thapar MK, Sharma DB (1976) Atrioventricular conduction in children with acute rheumatic fever. Am J Dis Child 130: 473–476

South East Asia Rheumatic Fever and Rheumatic Heart Disease Conference (1975) Jap Circ J 39: 151–201

Stollerman GH (1976) Global view of rheumatic fever today. In: Russek HI (ed) Cardiovascular problems, perspectives and progress. University Park Press, Baltimore, p 381

Stollerman GH, Markowitz M, Taranta A, Wannamaker LW, Whittemore R (1965) Jones criteria (revised) for guidance in the diagnosis of rheumatic fever. Circulation 32: 664–668

Strasser T (1978) Rheumatic fever and rheumatic heart disease in the 1970s. WHO Chronicle 32: 18–25

Tan ATH, Mah PK, Chia BL (1983) Cardiac tamponade in acute rheumatic carditis. Ann Rheum Dis 42: 699–701

Taranta A, Markowitz M (1981) Rheumatic fever: a guide to its recognition, prevention and cure with special reference to developing countries. MTP Press Ltd, Boston

Veasy LG, Wiedmeier SE, Orsmond GS et al. (1987) Resurgence of rheumatic fever in the intermountain area of the United States. N Engl J Med 316: 421–427

Wagner BM, Siew S (1970) Studies in rheumatic fever. V. Significance of human Anitschoff cell. Human Pathology 1: 45–71

Zabriskie JB (1976) Rheumatic fever: a streptococcal induced autoimmune disease. In: Dumonde DC (Ed) Infection and immunology in the rheumatic diseases. Blackwell, Oxford, pp 97–111

Chapter 2

Rheumatic Heart Disease I

Introduction

Rheumatic heart disease is the late, chronic stage of heart disease resulting from one or more attacks of rheumatic fever. The most important lesions are those affecting the valves, particularly the mitral and aortic, where various combinations of stenosis and incompetence can occur. In the myocardium there may be some degree of fibrosis following rheumatic myocarditis and, if severe, this seriously impairs ventricular function. Some pericardial adhesion is usually present but this is never sufficiently dense to affect ventricular function and does not progress to form constrictive pericarditis.

Incidence

Rheumatic fever has now virtually disappeared in Western countries. The declining prevalence of resulting rheumatic heart disease in younger women in the post-war years is well illustrated by a report from large antenatal clinics in Newcastle and Edinburgh (Szekely et al. 1973). In 1942–7 rheumatic heart disease was found in 3.5% of patients, but by 1966–9 this figure had fallen to 0.7%. The severity of the disease was also diminishing, with a significant fall in the incidence of major complications such as pulmonary oedema, right heart failure and atrial fibrillation during pregnancy.

Nevertheless, a considerable legacy of rheumatic heart disease remains in older adults, providing an appreciable work load for the cardiac surgeon. For example, in the Wessex Cardiology Centre, Southampton, 3000 open heart operations were performed in the period 1972–81: over half were valve replacements, the majority being for rheumatic heart disease (Monro et al. 1983).

As a cause of death, rheumatic heart disease is of diminishing importance, particularly when contrasted with ischaemic heart disease. In 1986 in England and Wales the total number of deaths from ischaemic heart disease was nearly

160000, a figure that was at last beginning to fall slightly, with a male predominance of 1.28:1. In the same year rheumatic heart disease caused 2619 deaths, a figure that had been falling steadily for decades, having a female predominance of 2.8:1 (OPCS Monitor 1987). There is consequently a steadily rising ratio between the numbers of deaths from the two diseases, rising from 15:1 in 1963 to 25:1 in 1973 and 60:1 in 1986.

In poor countries rheumatic heart disease is more nearly equal in importance to ischaemic heart disease. In India, Mathur (1976) found that 28% of hospital cardiac patients had rheumatic heart disease, 28% coronary disease, 16% hypertensive heart disease and 15% cor pulmonale.

Pathology

General

The heart is usually enlarged due to a combination of dilatation and hypertrophy affecting individual chambers according to the nature and severity of valvular disease. The main lesions involve the left side of the heart.

Left atrial dilatation and hypertrophy result from mitral stenosis, with generalised thickening of the atrial endocardium. Frequently thrombus is present, particularly in the atrial appendix and if there is atrial fibrillation. When the mitral lesion is predominantly one of incompetence left atrial enlargement is less striking, but the left ventricle is also then affected, with both dilatation and hypertrophy.

The *left ventricle* is markedly affected by aortic valve lesions. Predominant aortic valve stenosis results in concentric hypertrophy of the ventricle while aortic incompetence produces both dilatation and hypertrophy. When there is considerable regurgitation through an incompetent aortic valve a jet lesion of thickened endocardium forms on the septal wall of the ventricle over the area on which the regurgitant blood stream impinges.

Right atrial dilatation and hypertrophy are associated with tricuspid valve stenosis. Dilatation of both atrium and ventricle result from tricuspid incompetence, which may be caused by a rheumatic tricuspid valve lesion or by stretching of a normal tricuspid valve as a result of congestive heart failure. Thrombus may form in the dilated right atrium.

Right ventricular hypertrophy most frequently develops as a result of pulmonary hypertension secondary to mitral stenosis. Pulmonary valve lesions are rare and are unlikely to affect the right ventricle except in the uncommon situation of pulmonary valve incompetence secondary to severe pulmonary hypertension, when the right ventricle is both dilated and hypertrophied.

Valve Lesions

The heart valves are affected with different frequencies in approximately the following proportions: mitral 85%, aortic 45%, tricuspid 10%–15% and the pulmonary valve rarely (Wood 1968). Involvement of two or three valves together is common. Aortic and tricuspid lesions are not found in isolation but always in combination with a mitral lesion.

The small endocardial vegetations and oedematous thickening of affected valve cusps that characterise acute rheumatic endocarditis are followed by slowly progressive changes that may take many years to evolve. Adhesions form between the cusps, beginning at the commissures. In some cases the adhesions remain confined to the commissural regions and have little effect on valve function, but in others the process advances producing a stenosed valve with a significantly narrowed orifice.

At the same time the affected valve cusps become thickened and fibrotic, associated with increased vascularity and cellular infiltration seen at the base of the cusps (Fig. 2.1). The resulting rigidity of cusp tissue and fibrous shrinkage give rise to valvular incompetence. In later years secondary calcification may develop in the thickened valve (Fig. 2.2).

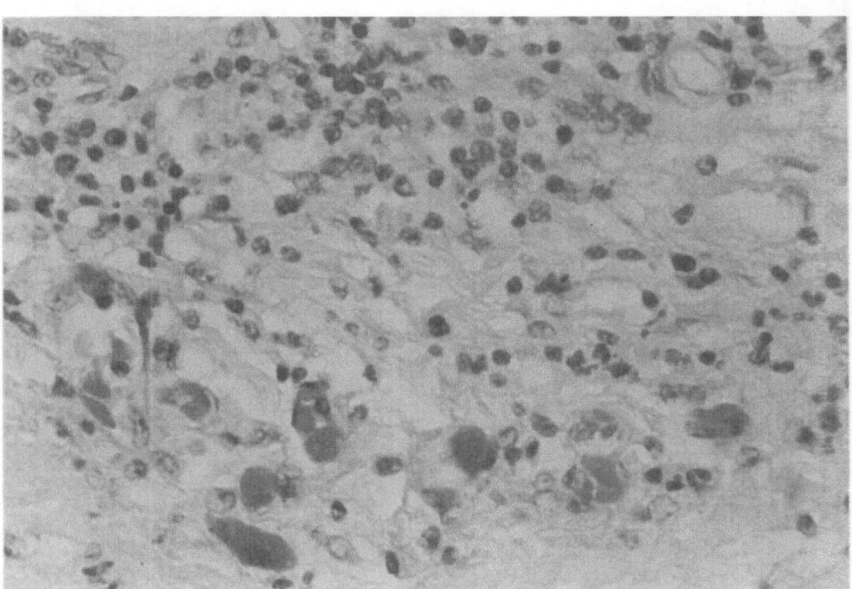

Fig. 2.1. Chronic rheumatic carditis. Photomicrograph (× 180) of the base of the mitral valve showing round cell infiltration and increased vascularity.

In the case of the mitral and tricuspid valves the chordae tendineae become thickened and shortened, tending to fuse together or to fuse with the adjoining ventricular wall. This tethering of the cusps is a further factor leading to mitral or tricuspid incompetence.

In affected valves one or another of these processes usually predominates but commonly the end result is a damaged valve whose function is impaired by a combination of stenosis and incompetence in varying degree (Selzer and Cohn 1972; Siegel and Fishbein 1984).

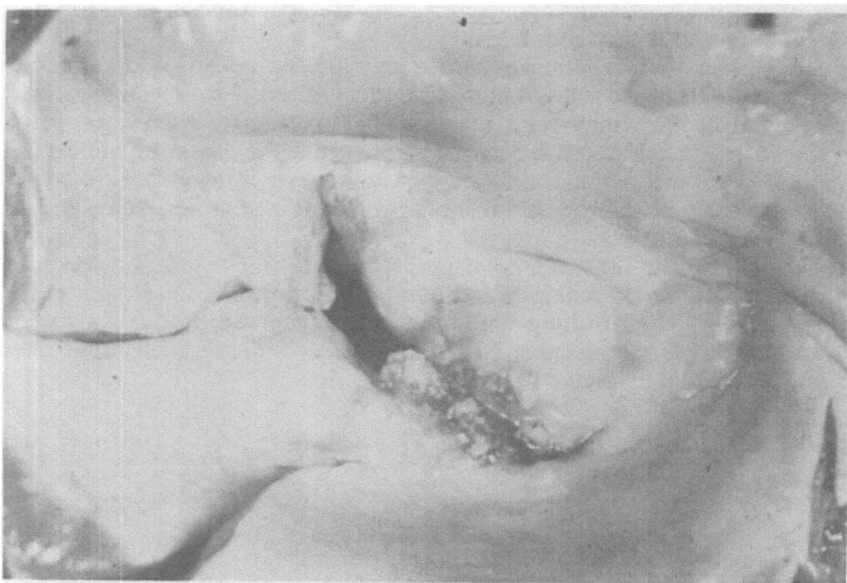

Fig. 2.2. Mitral stenosis. Mitral valve seen from the atrial aspect. The valve orifice has been reduced to a slit-like opening and there are warty calcific vegetations on the opposing aspects of the two cusps, principally on the anterior cusp. The atrium is dilated and its endocardium is thickened, white and fibrous.

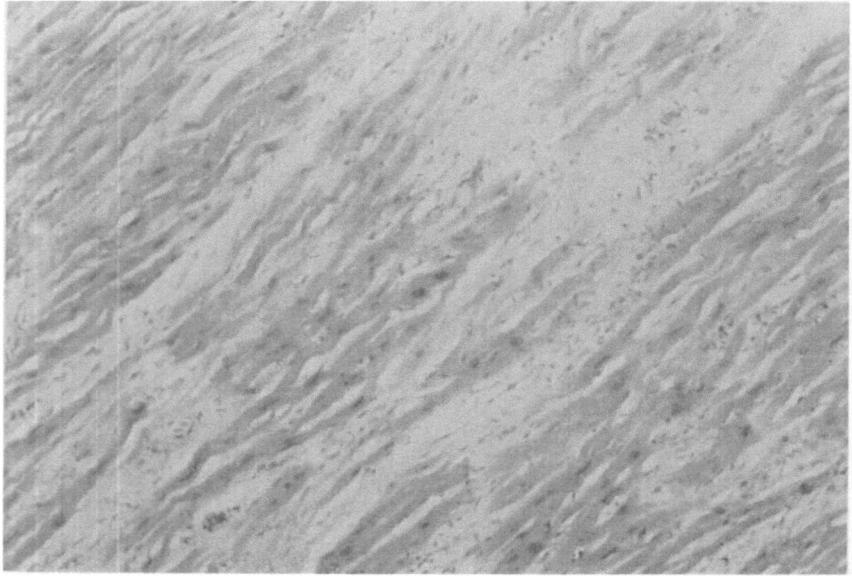

Fig. 2.3. The myocardium ($\times$ 45) in chronic rheumatic heart disease, showing the effects of previous myocarditis. Many of the myocardial cells are fragmented or destroyed and replaced by fibrous tissue.

Myocardium

Following the myocarditis of the acute stage of rheumatic fever there is a gradual resolution of the interstitial cellularity and of the Aschoff bodies resulting in fibrotic scarring. In some areas myocardial cells are destroyed, being replaced by fibrous tissue (Fig. 2.3). However, long after all clinical signs of activity of carditis have subsided, Aschoff bodies may still be identified in tissues removed at surgery or at autopsy in the interstitial layers of the atrial or ventricular myocardium or in the deeper layers of the endocardium, implying that some form of low grade inflammatory activity is still proceeding. The gross hypertrophy and dilatation of the myocardium is secondary to valvular disease rather than to these microscopic changes.

Pericardium

The acute fibrinous pericarditis of the acute stage of rheumatic carditis subsides, with absorption of any effusion and the formation of fibrous adhesions between the two layers of the pericardium. The result is partial or total obliteration of the pericardial sac. However, the adhesions are not dense or progressive, and do not restrict the filling of the cardiac chambers. Constrictive pericarditis has never been known to develop as a result.

The Lungs

Acute pulmonary oedema may flood the alveoli with fluid as a result of left ventricular failure or following an acute rise in pulmonary venous pressure due to mitral stenosis. Chronic vascular congestion is present when there is congestive heart failure, with the appearance of "heart failure cells' i.e. macrophages, in the alveoli. When mitral stenosis has led to pulmonary hypertension the pulmonary arterial and arteriolar walls become thickened, with an increase in the muscular coat, reduplication and fragmentation of the internal elastic lamina and diffuse endothelial thickening. To some extent all three of these changes may be present, representing the effect of back pressure on the lungs possibly complicated by pulmonary hypertension.

Natural History

Approximately half of the patients who have suffered a first attack of rheumatic fever are left with some sign of a heart lesion, most often an apical systolic murmur. After a second or third attack the proportion affected is appreciably higher. In individual patients the situation may appear to change in the first few years after an attack. In some a murmur may disappear suggesting healing of a valve lesion and in others, who at first appeared to have normal hearts, a murmur may later appear (Perry 1969).

In addition, signs of rheumatic heart disease may be found in later life in patients never known to have had rheumatic fever, implying that they had at some time suffered an unrecognised attack of rheumatic carditis, probably without arthritis. In the case of mitral stenosis as many as 30%–40% of patients may be in this category.

After recovery from rheumatic fever the patient with a valve lesion has a symptom-free latent period of some years. The length of this period is very variable, ranging from a minimum of two years up to 30 years or more, depending on the severity of valve and myocardial damage. Occasionally a valve lesion remains static and causes no symptoms throughout the rest of a patient's life and may be revealed only as an incidental clinical finding in later years.

Mitral Stenosis. Wood (1968) found an average latent period of 19 years before patients with mitral stenosis developed symptoms, after which there was progression to a state of severe disability in a further 5–10 years. Olesen (1962) confirmed the poor prognosis under conservative treatment of patients with symptomatic mitral stenosis. At initial review over half of his patients had atrial fibrillation and cardiac enlargement: their survival rate at 10 years was 34% and at 20 years only 14%. The outlook was similar for those with pure mitral stenosis and for those with a mixed lesion of stenosis and incompetence. But now cardiac surgery has entirely altered the natural history of mitral valve disease (Portal 1984; and see p. 59).

Aortic Valve. The natural course of aortic incompetence differs from that of aortic stenosis. An appreciable degree of aortic incompetence may be tolerated without symptoms for many years in a young person with good myocardial function, although grosser incompetence or an impaired myocardium will inevitably lead to symptoms in time. Aortic stenosis produces a more serious situation as major complications may arise within a very few years. Here again, cardiac surgery has greatly and favourably affected the natural history of aortic valve disease.

In poorer parts of the world the rate of progression of rheumatic heart disease is much quicker. In India, for example, a quarter of all patients with disabling mitral stenosis are under 20 years of age and "juvenile mitral stenosis" is all too familiar (Mathur 1976). Combined mitral and aortic lesions of some severity in young patients under 30 years of age in South India are described by Vijayaraghavan et al. (1977). In Egypt Ibrahim (1979) reported significant impairment of left ventricular function in young adults resulting from previous rheumatic myocarditis.

Case History 2.1 illustrates a case of juvenile mitral stenosis in a Sicilian who later developed severe pulmonary hypertension.

Case History 2.1

Juvenile mitral stenosis, pulmonary hypertension
Mitral valvotomy: re-stenosis: repeat valvotomy

Mr. N.S., Clerk, Sicilian, born 1946

1959   Rheumatic fever and carditis, residual mitral lesion

1961	Mitral stenosis, pulmonary oedema, emergency *mitral valvotomy* with relief
1968	Dyspnoeic. Mitral re-stenosis Pulmonary hypertension. ECG: RV hypertrophy (Fig. 2.4) Dilated pulmonary artery, pulmonary valve incompetence (Figs. 2.5, 2.6)
1969	Respiratory infection precipitated atrial fibrillation and pulmonary oedema. Cardiac catheter confirmed pulmonary hypertension (90/35 mmHg) *Second mitral valvotomy* Sinus rhythm later restored by cardioversion
1970–77	Fair progress. Atrial fibrillation recurred Repeated cardioversion failed to restore sinus rhythm
1979	Dyspnoea, pulmonary hypertension, mitral incompetence Mitral valve replacement advised
Comment	Rapidly developing mitral stenosis, requiring surgical relief only 2 years after rheumatic fever. Subsequent pulmonary hypertension, severe enough to cause pulmonary valve incompetence. Pulmonary diastolic murmur disappeared after second valvotomy

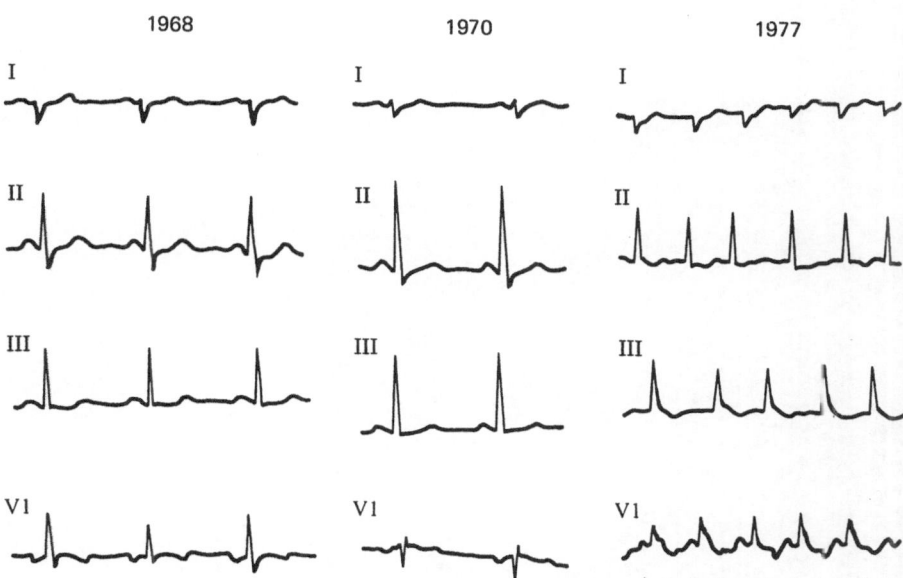

Fig. 2.4. Mitral stenosis. ECGs of the patient described in Case History 2.1. In 1968 there is marked R axis shift and RV hypertrophy, shown by the prominent R wave in lead V1. In 1970 after mitral valvotomy the RV hypertrophy has receded and there is only a small R wave in lead V1. In 1977 RV hypertrophy has returned. In the upper three leads the rhythm appears to be atrial fibrillation, although in the lowest lead, V1, the pattern suggests a rapid atrial arrhythmia, probably atrial flutter with 2:1 AV block.

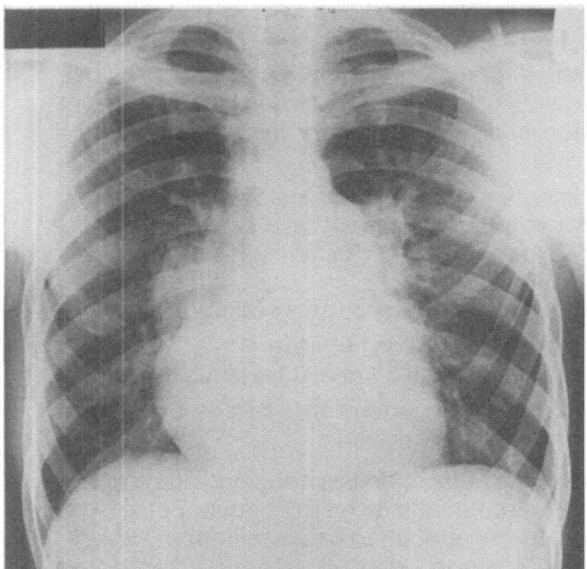

Fig. 2.5. Mitral stenosis and pulmonary hypertension. Chest X-ray film (PA) of the patient described in Case History 2.1. The heart is enlarged with prominence of the right atrium and the main pulmonary artery.

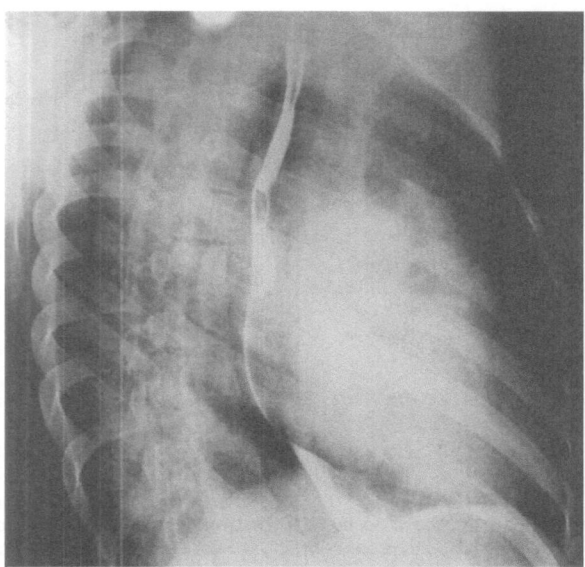

Fig. 2.6. Mitral stenosis. Chest X-ray film (R anterior oblique) of the patient described in Case History 2.1 showing prominence of the left atrium, displacing and narrowing the barium-filled oesophagus.

Mitral Valve Lesions

Mitral Stenosis: Haemodynamics

The normal mitral valve when open has an orifice whose area is of 4 sq cm or more. When stenosis has reduced this to 2 sq cm symptoms develop and further reduction to 1 sq cm or less produces a serious state of affairs, usually calling for surgical relief. At operation a stenosed mitral valve may be found to be reduced to an oval orifice about 1 cm by 0.5 cm (Fig. 2.2).

The first effect of mitral stenosis is to produce a rise in pressure in the left atrium and pulmonary veins. It is this which is largely responsible for the main symptom, dyspnoea on effort, and for occasional haemoptysis. Raised pulmonary venous pressure also may give rise to pulmonary oedema, particularly when exercise or emotion lead to an increase in right ventricular output, adding to the pressure in capillaries and veins. This form of pulmonary oedema causes urgent dyspnoea of rapid onset, sometimes with copious watery sputum which may be tinged with blood. This is more often seen in younger patients, usually women, whose right ventricular function is still good. It is more frequent with sinus rhythm than with atrial fibrillation, which reduces right ventricular output.

Left atrial pressure is measured by advancing the cardiac catheter through the right atrium and ventricle into a pulmonary artery until the tip occludes a branch of the artery. The "wedge pressure" then measured is virtually identical with pulmonary venous and left atrial pressure. In mitral stenosis the left atrial pressure is raised from its normal 5 or 6 mmHg to 15 mmHg or more, and a pressure of 30 mmHg is sufficient to precipitate pulmonary oedema. Exercise further increases the left atrial pressure and a useful assessment of the severity of the obstruction at the mitral valve may be made by monitoring the wedge pressure during a test period of exercise.

In some patients with mitral stenosis, for reasons that are not entirely clear, the pulmonary vascular resistance rises leading to pulmonary hypertension. The pulmonary arterial systolic pressure may rise from its normal value of 15 to 20 mmHg to 60 or 80 mmHg or even more, and rises further still on effort (Fig. 2.7). The increased work load on the right ventricle is met by ventricular hypertrophy and ultimately is a factor in causing right heart failure. However, on the credit side, the increased pulmonary vascular resistance protects the pulmonary capillaries from raised forward pressure making pulmonary oedema less likely. Such patients have a low, relatively fixed cardiac output which cannot effectively rise on exertion. Their facial appearance of malar flush and slight cyanosis of cheeks and lips constitutes the "mitral facies".

Left atrial dilatation and atrial fibrillation increase the risk of thrombus formation in the atrium and the possibility of systemic embolism. Atrial fibrillation may be temporary or episodic before becoming permanently established. If congestive heart failure finally develops it is always in the presence of atrial fibrillation.

Mitral Stenosis: Clinical Effects

The physical signs of pure mitral stenosis are as follows: a tapping "right ventricular" type of apical impulse which is not displaced to the left: a crescendo

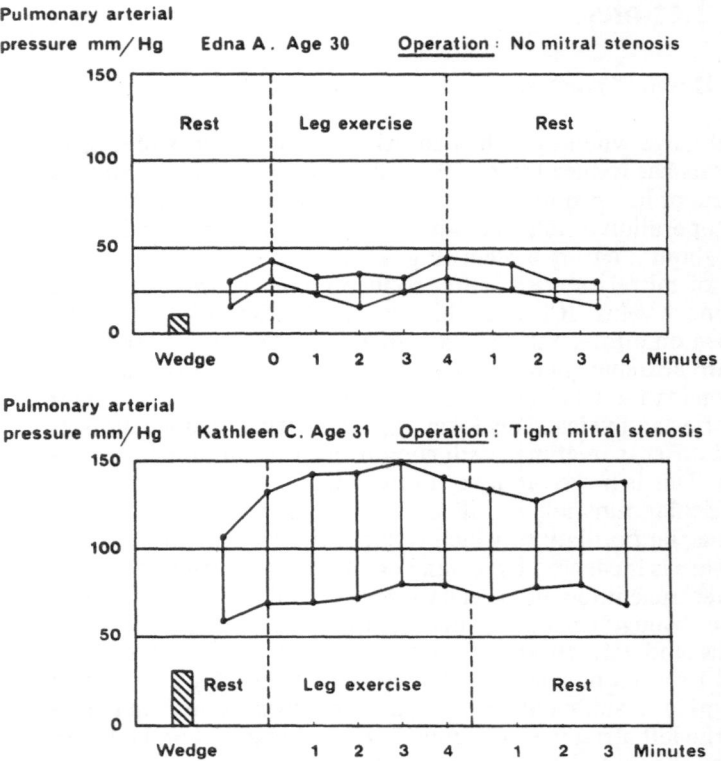

Fig. 2.7. Pulmonary arterial pressure during exercise. *Above*: normal pulmonary arterial pressure in a patient with a normal mitral valve. The pressure is not increased by a 4-minute period of exercise. Note that the left atrial (wedge) pressure is normal. *Below*: pulmonary hypertension in a 31-year-old woman with tight mitral stenosis. The pulmonary arterial pressure is raised still further by the period of exercise. Note that the left atrial pressure is markedly raised (30 mmHg).

presystolic murmur at the apex, leading up to an accentuated first heart sound: no systolic murmur: a loud pulmonary (second) element to the second sound: an opening snap shortly after this, followed by a low pitched rumbling mid-diastolic murmur (Fig. 2.8). If the diastolic murmur is loud it causes a palpable thrill at the apex. Both the presystolic and mid-diastolic murmurs are accentuated by a brief period of exercise and by auscultation with the patient lying on the left side. The presystolic murmur is due to the atrial systole driving blood through the narrowed mitral valve and is therefore lost when the rhythm changes to atrial fibrillation.

Rarely, severe pulmonary hypertension may dilate the pulmonary artery and valve ring and cause pulmonary valve incompetence. The resulting early diastolic murmur sounds very like an aortic diastolic murmur, but differs in being heard best in the pulmonary valve area, to the left of the upper sternum and in following an accentuated pulmonary element in the second heart sound (see Case History 2.1 and Figs. 2.4, 2.5 and 2.6).

Mm/Hg

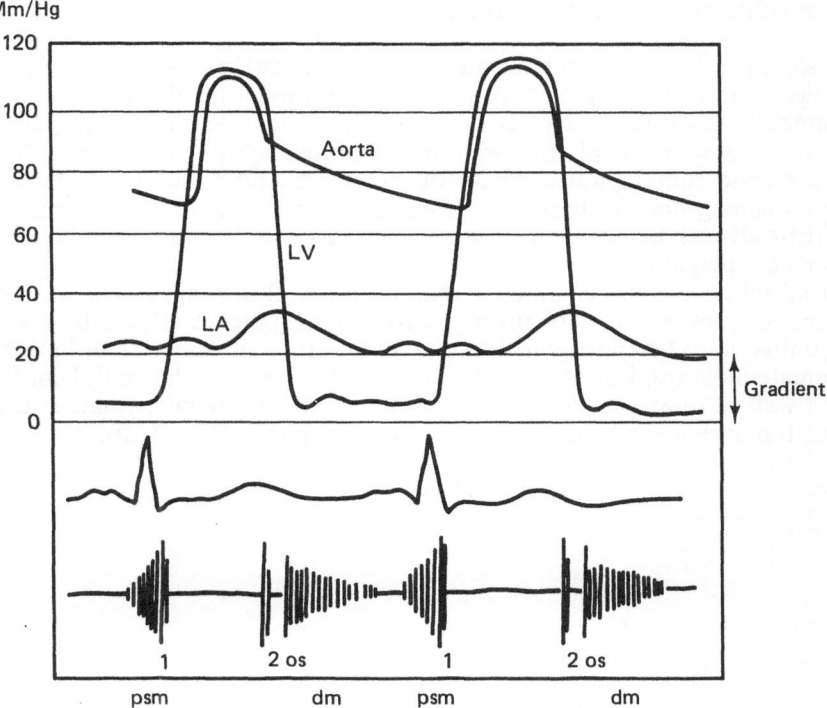

Fig. 2.8. Mitral stenosis. Pressure relationships in left ventricle, aorta and left atrium. Note the pressure gradient in diastole between atrium and ventricle. A crescendo presystolic murmur (*psm*) leads up to the first heart sound. The second sound is followed by the opening snap (*os*) of the mitral valve, leading on to the decrescendo diastolic murmur (*dm*).

Mitral Incompetence: Haemodynamics

With mitral incompetence too the left atrial and pulmonary venous pressures are raised, though not to the same degree as with mitral stenosis. The forceful regurgitant flow of blood from left ventricle into atrium produces greater dilatation of the atrium than with stenosis and on radioscopy expansile pulsation of the atrium may be seen in time with systole. The left ventricle has to eject a bigger stroke volume to achieve adequate forward output into the aorta as well as regurgitation into the atrium and the ventricle enlarges and hypertrophies in order to achieve this. If there is gross mitral regurgitation the peripheral pulse is small and collapsing.

Calcification of the mitral valve is more often seen when it is incompetent than when stenosed. The complication of infective endocarditis is also commoner and is usually found with sinus rhythm rather than with atrial fibrillation. Pulmonary hypertension is not associated with mitral incompetence to the degree that it is with mitral stenosis.

Mitral Incompetence: Clinical Effects

The physical signs of pure mitral incompetence are: a heaving "left ventricular" type of apical impulse, which is displaced to the left and downwards i.e. approaching the anterior axillary line and possibly in the sixth intercostal space: a loud first sound immediately followed by a long loud systolic murmur lasting up to the second sound (holosystolic): the second sound is not accentuated: there is no opening snap or diastolic murmur (Fig. 2.9). The systolic murmur is characteristically well heard at the apex and further laterally in the axillary line: there may be a palpable thrill with it.

Mixed mitral lesions are commoner than pure mitral incompetence, so that the physical signs of both may be present. Mitral incompetence affects the sexes equally, unlike mitral stenosis which occurs more often in women than in men with a female:male ratio of about 4:1. Another difference is the complaint of fatigue as well as dyspnoea associated with mitral incompetence, whereas the patient with mitral stenosis complains mainly of dyspnoea (Fig. 2.10).

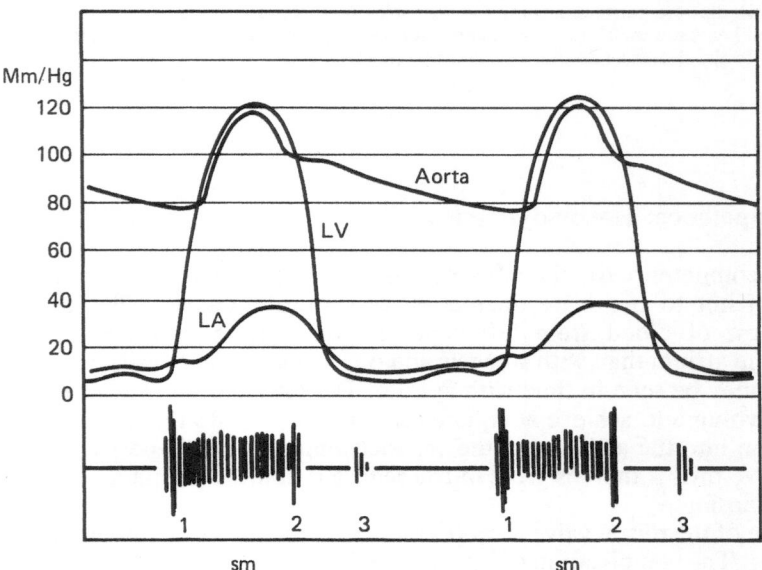

Fig. 2.9. Mitral incompetence. Pressure relationships in left ventricle, aorta and left atrium. Note the significant rise in left atrial pressure during systole and the holosystolic murmur. A third heart sound in diastole is also indicated.

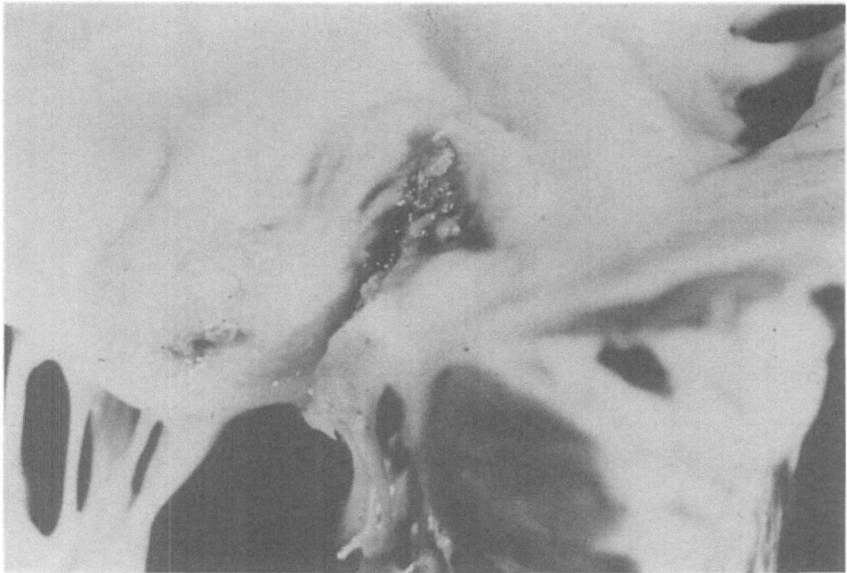

Fig. 2.10. Mitral valve showing mixed stenosis and incompetence. The chordae are thickened and fused and there is thickening of the left atrial endocardium. There is an area of calcification in the valve commissure.

Aortic Valve Lesions

Rheumatic heart disease may produce either incompetence or stenosis or a combination of the two at the aortic valve, but is more likely to cause incompetence in the early years. In later years sclerosis and calcification in the damaged cusps may add an obstructive element resulting finally in a degree of stenosis (Fig. 2.11). In Britain rheumatic heart disease is no longer the predominant cause of aortic valve disease. In patients requiring surgical valve replacement, degenerative disease with calcification, or the late results of congenital malformation are now at least as frequent as rheumatic heart disease as underlying causes (Cosh and Lever 1984; Davies 1980).

Rheumatic aortic valve lesions are found in males more often than in females, unlike mitral stenosis, in which females are more often affected.

Aortic Incompetence: Haemodynamics

The blood regurgitating into the left ventricle through an incompetent aortic valve, added to the normal diastolic inflow from the left atrium, increases the diastolic filling volume of the ventricle and the work required in systole. With a moderately damaged valve a quarter or more of the blood ejected in systole returns immediately to the ventricle; e.g. to achieve an effective stroke output of

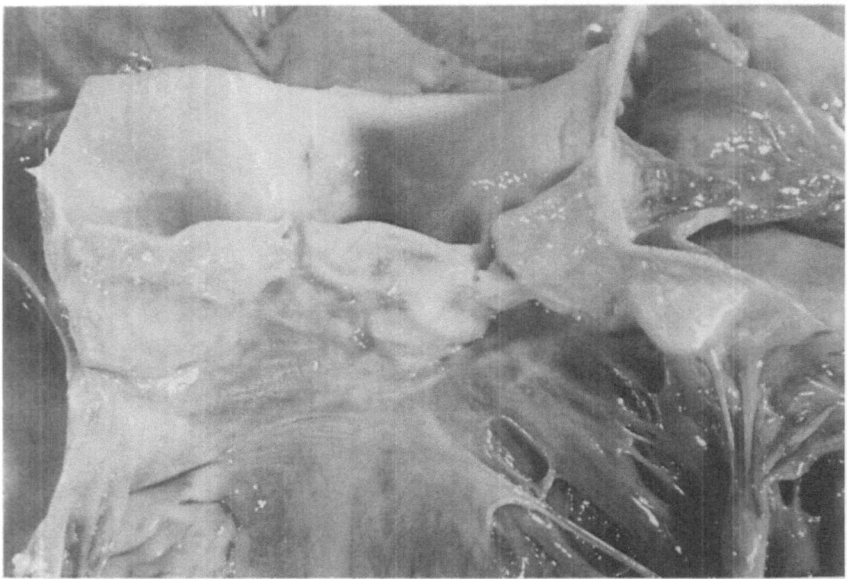

Fig. 2.11. Aortic valve showing fusion between the right coronary and non-coronary cusps.

70 ml the ventricle may have to eject 100 ml, of which 30 ml immediately returns in diastole.

The resulting "volume overload" is met by dilatation and hypertrophy of the ventricle. If the myocardium is healthy this is achieved without difficulty and the additional work load may be performed satisfactorily for many years. However, ventricular function may be impaired by previous rheumatic myocarditis or in later years by the addition of coronary disease or by degenerative changes in the myocardium. The end-diastolic pressure in the ventricle then rises leading to raised pressure in the left atrium and pulmonary veins; pulmonary oedema and finally congestive failure result.

If deterioration in the aortic valve advances rapidly, as with cusp rupture or infective endocarditis, or if ventricular function is adversely affected by arrhythmia, there is insufficient time for the ventricle to adjust to the extra work load and left ventricular failure quickly develops.

Aortic Incompetence: Clinical Effects

Minor aortic incompetence that is well compensated produces no symptoms and the only clinical effect is the early diastolic murmur. Detection requires careful auscultation in quiet surroundings, with the diaphragm of the stethoscope applied to the left of the sternum and the murmur is best heard with the patient sitting upright or leaning forwards and in expiration. The murmur is soft and high pitched, like the whispered word "Ah" immediately following the second heart sound. There may also be an aortic systolic murmur, either from some degree of associated aortic stenosis or, when there is free aortic regurgitation, simply from the turbulence of the vigorous ejection of blood into a somewhat dilated aorta.

Significant aortic incompetence causes an increase in pulse pressure to a half or more of the systolic pressure instead of the normal one-third (Fig. 2.12). The peripheral pulse is collapsing in nature producing the characteristic "waterhammer" effect, which is in part due to compensatory peripheral arterial dilatation.

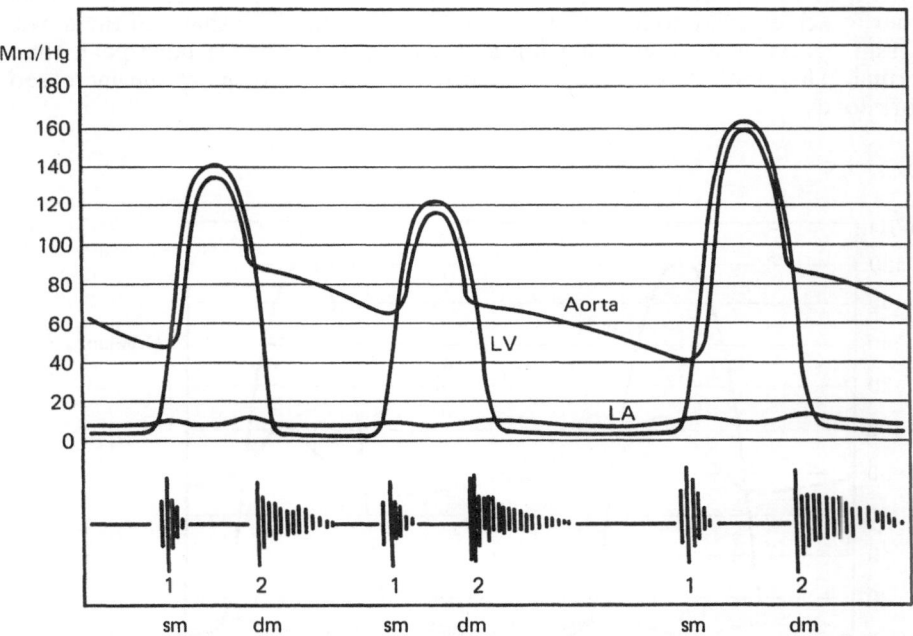

Fig. 2.12. Aortic incompetence. Pressure relationships. The pressure in the aorta falls off markedly in diastole. In atrial fibrillation, as represented here, the fall in diastolic pressure is greater in the longer diastolic period. A brief systolic murmur is shown at the start of ejection into the dilated aorta, but the main murmur is the decrescendo diastolic murmur which begins as soon as the aortic valve closes.

The regurgitant stream of blood may be sufficiently forceful to set up vibration in the anterior cusp of the mitral valve, shown on echocardiography as a "fluttering" of the cusp (Fig. 3.7). Full opening of the mitral valve in diastole may be hindered producing, in effect, a functional mitral stenosis. It is this which gives rise to the Austin Flint murmur, a low-pitched mid-diastolic murmur heard at the apex, mimicking mitral stenosis.

Aortic Stenosis: Haemodynamics

The orifice of the normal aortic valve has a diameter, on average, of 3.2 cm, giving a cross-section area of about 8 sq cm. When fusion of the valve cusps has reduced this area to half or less of the normal, i.e. a diameter nearing 2 cm, a pressure gradient develops across the valve in systole. Serious obstruction, e.g. with a diameter of 1.0 cm or less, produces a pressure gradient up to 60 mmHg or more. However, extremes of stenosis, or stenosis without incompetence are unusual with rheumatic heart disease, which is the only one of the rheumatic diseases giving rise to aortic stenosis.

Figure 2.13 illustrates the pressure patterns found with a gradient of 80 mmHg, in which the ventricle has to reach a peak systolic pressure of 180 in order to achieve a systolic pressure of 100 in the aorta. The shape of the aortic pressure curve is affected, showing a slower upstroke and a later peak than normal. The ventricle develops concentric hypertrophy to meet the increased work load.

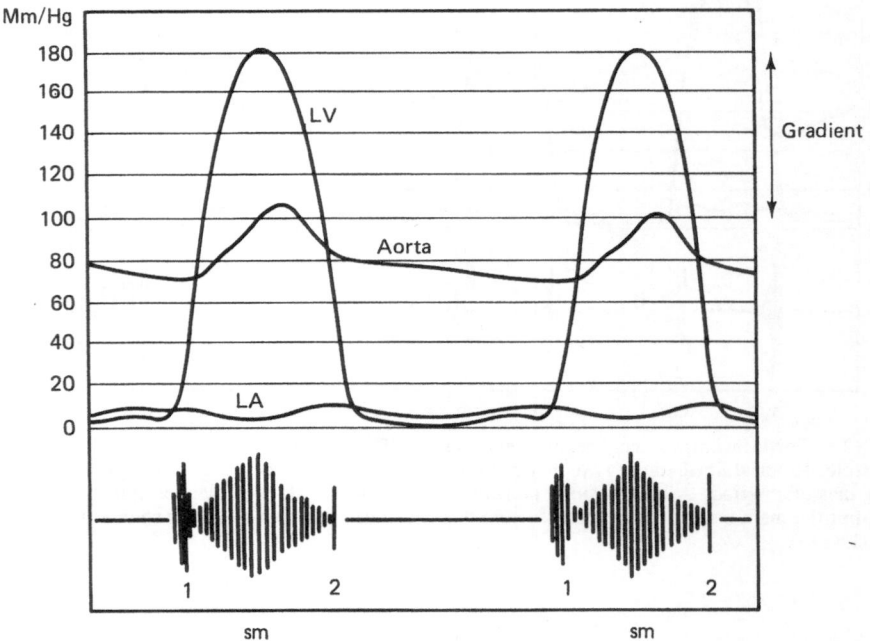

Fig. 2.13. Aortic stenosis. Pressure relationships. A systolic gradient of 80 mmHg is shown, meaning that the ventricle has to produce a peak systolic pressure of 180 mmHg in order to achieve a systolic pressure peak of 100 mmHg in the aorta. A diamond-shaped systolic murmur accompanies ejection through the stenosed aortic valve.

Over the course of years sclerosis increases in the valve cusps and they may calcify. If the calcific deposits are florid they may encroach on the coronary ostia. These factors increase the stress on the ventricle, especially if in addition there is valve incompetence, previous damage by rheumatic myocarditis or coronary atheroma. The result may be angina, syncope due to low output, arrhythmias or left ventricular failure with pulmonary oedema.

Aortic Stenosis: Clinical Effects

With lesser degrees of stenosis cardiac function is unaffected, there are no symptoms, and the only clinical abnormality may be the systolic murmur. This is characteristically a loud rasping murmur which has been likened to the sound of a saw cutting wood; it is widely heard over the precordium though usually loudest at and below the aortic valve area. The murmur is conducted upwards into the neck and if very loud is accompanied by a systolic thrill. On phonocardiography the murmur produces a diamond-shaped pattern of sound (Fig. 2.13). The second sound is soft and the aortic element may be lost so that the second heart sound is caused only by pulmonary valve closure.

With severe stenosis the peripheral pulse is small in volume and slow rising. The pulse pressure is reduced. With left ventricular hypertrophy the apical impulse becomes heaving and powerful and may be displaced outwards and downwards. Gallop rhythm may be heard, with an added third or fourth heart sound.

Angina is a common symptom arising either from obstruction to the coronary ostia, or from coincidental coronary atheroma, or simply from the increased mass of muscle failing to receive an adequate arterial blood supply.

Syncope on exertion is an ominous sign that ventricular output has become severely limited. Usually recovery from syncope is spontaneous and follows within a few minutes of the patient falling, but if unconsciousness is prolonged it may be followed by convulsions. Another serious cause of syncope is ventricular arrhythmia – paroxysmal tachycardia or ventricular fibrillation. This is a potential cause of sudden death.

Ultimately the ventricular muscle fails to meet the demands upon it: the ventricle dilates, end-diastolic pressure rises and leads to raised left atrial and pulmonary venous pressure. There is increasing dyspnoea on effort and there may be attacks of paroxysmal dyspnoea or frank pulmonary oedema. The final picture is one of congestive heart failure, usually with atrial fibrillation.

Tricuspid and Pulmonary Valves

The tricuspid valve is never affected alone in rheumatic heart disease, but always in association with a mitral lesion and sometimes with an aortic valve lesion too. In consequence, the signs of tricuspid disease are masked by the more serious and more obvious effects of the other lesions.

Tricuspid valve lesions may be a combination of stenosis and incompetence together, as with mitral and aortic valve lesions, but in practice the clinical picture is that of whichever process predominates. Functional tricuspid incompetence is commoner than organic tricuspid disease and arises when the valve ring stretches as part of a general dilatation of the right ventricle. This may be the result of pulmonary hypertension or of congestive heart failure and so tends to be a feature of the later stages of rheumatic heart disease.

Tricuspid Stenosis. As with the mitral valve, the tricuspid orifice has to be reduced to less than half of its normal area before significant symptoms develop. Pressure rises in the right atrium and is transmitted back into the great veins. Jugular venous pressure is visibly raised in the neck and there is a prominent "a" wave in the venous pulse as long as sinus rhythm is maintained. Pressure is also increased in the inferior vena cava leading to liver enlargement and tenderness and if severe progressing to cirrhosis and ascites. Oedema develops in the lower limbs and trunk.

On auscultation there is a mid-diastolic murmur resembling the murmur of mitral stenosis, best heard near the lower sternum and varying with respiration. It is louder during inspiration due to the temporary increase in venous return into the thorax and in blood flow through the tricuspid valve.

Tricuspid Incompetence. Whether organic or functional, tricuspid incompetence is characterised by forceful regurgitation from the right ventricle into the atrium in systole. The atrium is enlarged, with expansile pulsation in systole. The raised pressure in the right atrium as well as the accentuated systolic venous pressure pulse are transmitted back into the great veins. A prominent "v" wave is seen in the engorged jugular veins. The liver is enlarged and tender, and with gross tricuspid incompetence an expansile pulsation can be felt in the swollen liver.

The right ventricle dilates and hypertrophies in order to deal with the increased stroke volume. The cardiac apex is displaced to the left with an accentuated palpable lift: the systolic thrust of the hypertrophied right ventricle can also be felt below the left costal margin near the xiphisternum. On auscultation there is a pansystolic murmur maximal at the lower left sternal edge and this murmur too is louder during inspiration.

The Pulmonary Valve. This valve is rarely directly affected by rheumatic heart disease. However, it may become incompetent if severe pulmonary hypertension develops: the main pulmonary artery dilates under the increased pressure and slight stretching of the pulmonary valve ring can result. The murmur of pulmonary regurgitation, the Graham Steell murmur, is a high-pitched soft diastolic murmur, best heard to the left of the sternum, following immediately after the accentuated second sound. Of the two elements of the second sound it is the second, pulmonary, element which is the louder. The diastolic murmur is very similar to that of aortic incompetence but is distinguished from it by its association with evidence of right ventricular hypertrophy and pulmonary hypertension (Case History 2.1).

The Myocardium

With a good myocardium the extra work load imposed by a valve lesion is surprisingly well tolerated, which largely explains the long latent period, of perhaps 20 years, before symptoms develop. However, if one or more attacks of rheumatic fever have damaged the myocardium the subsequent clinical course is different.

Destruction of myocardial cells and their replacement by fibrosis impairs myocardial function and limits the effectiveness of compensatory hypertrophy when this is required. In the presence of a mitral or aortic valve lesion the cardiac output cannot be increased sufficiently to meet the demands of effort. There is dilatation of the heart and end-diastolic pressure rises, most importantly, in the left ventricle. There is reduction in the ejection fraction, that proportion of the ventricular diastolic volume which is ejected in systole.

The resulting increase in left atrial and pulmonary venous pressure leads to dyspnoea on effort and possibly pulmonary oedema. A corresponding increase in pressure in the right side of the heart leads to the manifestations of congestive failure. Arrhythmias, particularly atrial fibrillation, are more likely, further impairing cardiac efficiency. The success of possible cardiac surgery is jeopardised.

References

Cosh JA, Lever JV (1984) The aortic valve. In: Ansell BM, Simkin PA (eds) The heart and rheumatic disease. Butterworths, London, pp 83–119

Davies MJ (1980) Pathology of the cardiac valves. Butterworths, London, pp 1–59

Ibrahim MM (1979) Left ventricular function in rheumatic mitral stenosis. A clinical and echocardiographic study. Br Heart J 42: 514–520

Mathur KS (1976) Rheumatic heart disease: problems and promises (Sarabhai Oration 1976). J Ass Phys India 24: 373–382

Monro JL, Ross JK, Manners JM et al. (1983) Cardiac surgery in Wessex. Br Med J i: 361–365

OPCS Monitor (1987) Office of Population Censuses and Surveys, No 3

Olesen KH (1962) The natural history of 271 patients with mitral stenosis under medical treatment. Br Heart J 24: 349–357

Perry CB (1969) The natural history of acute rheumatism. Ann Rheum Dis 28: 471–476

Portal RW (1984) Editorial: Mitral stenosis: the picture changes. Br Med J i: 167–168

Selzer A, Cohn K (1972) Natural history of mitral stenosis. A review. Circulation 45: 878–890

Siegel RJ, Fishbein MC (1984) The mitral valve. In: Ansell BM, Simkin PA (eds): The heart and rheumatic disease. Butterworths, London, pp 120–150

Szekely P, Turner R, Snaith L (1973) Pregnancy and the changing pattern of rheumatic heart disease. Br Heart J 35: 1293–1303

Vijayaraghavan G, Cherian G, Krishnaswami S et al. (1977) Rheumatic aortic stenosis in young patients presenting with combined aortic and mitral stenosis. Br Heart J 39: 294–298

Wood P (1968) In: Somerville W (ed) Diseases of the heart and circulation. Eyre and Spottiswood, London (Reprinted 1975)

Chapter 3

Rheumatic Heart Disease II

Symptoms

The symptoms associated with individual valve lesions have been described, but can now be summarised in general.

Dyspnoea is the cardinal symptom of rheumatic heart disease. At first it is only noticed after considerable effort, but it is more readily induced as the cardiac reserve diminishes. Urgent dyspnoea can develop rapidly, sometimes progressing to frank pulmonary oedema in younger adults without severe pulmonary hypertension, in sinus rhythm rather than in atrial fibrillation, or from left ventricular failure due to aortic valve disease: here the first development may be paroxysmal dyspnoea, often at night and resolving spontaneously within an hour or two. In either case the tendency is to progress in due course to pulmonary oedema and to congestive heart failure.

Fatigue is also associated with a diminishing cardiac reserve. In mitral valve disease it is associated more with mitral incompetence than with stenosis.

Palpitation as a symptom has varying significance depending on the patient's nature and on the underlying mechanism. It may merely mean an awareness of tachycardia induced by effort. It may also be a feature of aortic incompetence, due to the more marked cardiac action. More significantly, "palpitations" may indicate rhythm disturbances, especially if these are intermittent.

Respiratory infections are more frequent and more persistent in patients with pulmonary vascular congestion, and are associated with mitral valve disease.

Haemoptysis can arise in various circumstances. The most striking is the sudden copious bleed caused by the rupture of a pulmonary vein in the patient with mitral stenosis. A less severe haemoptysis may come from engorged capillaries and may accompany pulmonary oedema. A bronchial vessel may rupture during the course of bronchial or pulmonary infection producing staining of sputum. Haemoptysis is also a feature of pulmonary embolism.

Complications

Arrhythmias

Atrial fibrillation (Fig. 3.1a) develops sooner or later in most patients with rheumatic heart disease of any severity. It is associated more with mitral than

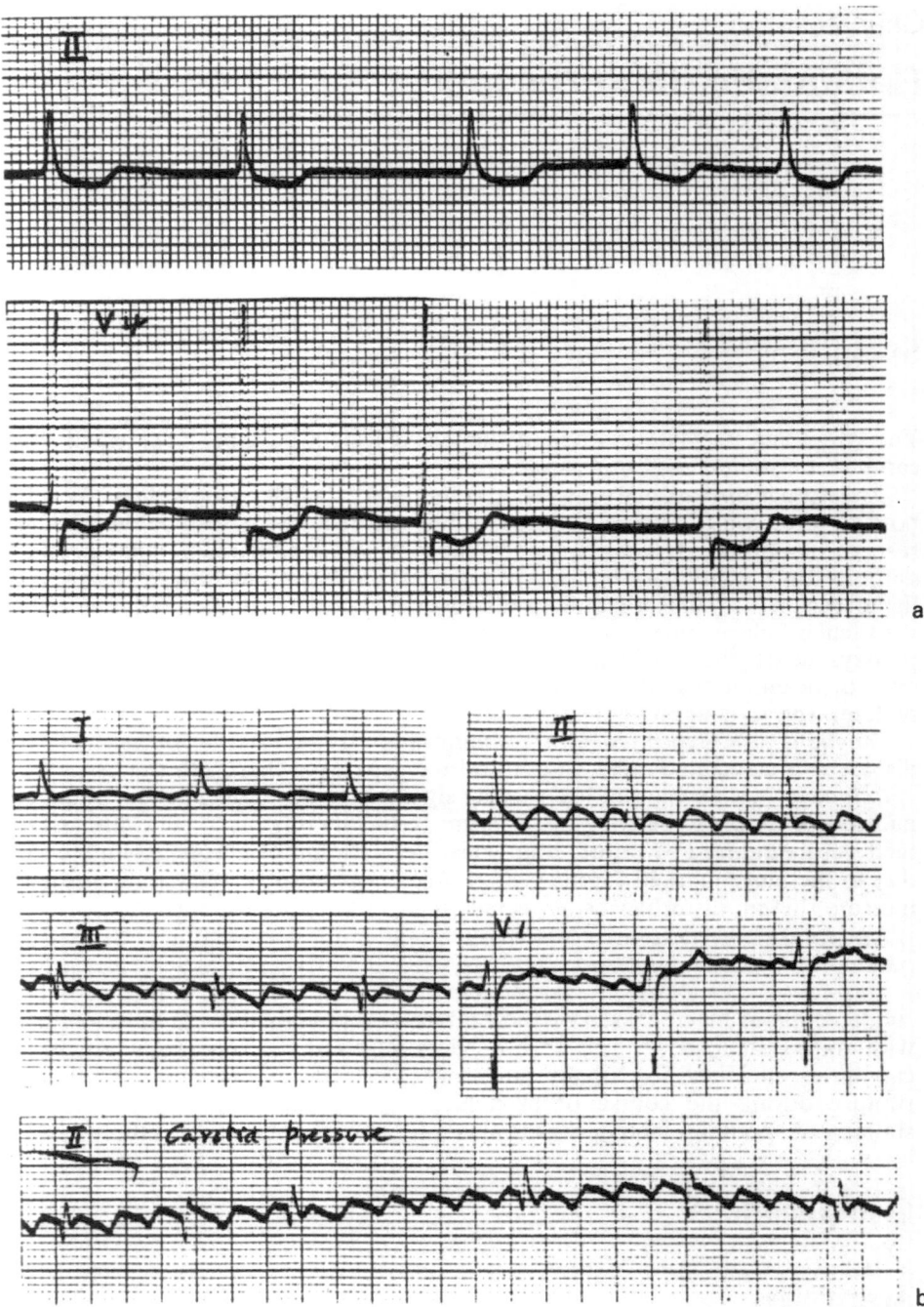

Fig. 3.1a,b. Electrocardiograms. **a** Atrial fibrillation with bradycardia and ST depressions due to digitalis effect. **b** Atrial flutter with 4:1 A:V conduction. In the lowest tracing A:V conduction starts at 3:1 but changes to 6:1 and 4:1 as the result of carotid pressure.

with aortic valve lesions. It may be paroxysmal at first, in episodes of minutes or hours, before becoming permanently established. Frequent changes of rhythm are disturbing to the patient, mainly as an added cause of dyspnoea due to the further impairment of cardiac function during the arrhythmia.

Atrial ectopic beats in isolation have no particular significance, but if they arise with increasing frequency they may indicate that a change from sinus rhythm to atrial fibrillation is imminent.

Atrial flutter (Fig. 3.1b) is much less common than atrial fibrillation but has the same basic cause: mitral valve disease with dilatation and disturbed function of the left atrium. Atrial flutter too may be paroxysmal. If it becomes established for a period it is unlikely to be permanent, but while it is established the patient may be conscious of sudden changes in heart rate as the degree of A:V block changes. 1:1 A:V conduction gives rise to a heart rate of 250 to 300/minute but is fortunately uncommon; it is distressing and may cause faintness or syncope in the older patient due to the sudden fall in cardiac output. The heart rate may drop spontaneously or as a result of treatment to 140 or 70/minute as A:V conduction changes to 2:1 or 4:1. These step-wise changes in heart rate are disturbing to the patient, who will prefer it when atrial flutter ultimately changes to sinus rhythm or, as is more likely, to atrial fibrillation.

Ventricular ectopic beats are common, as they are in normal hearts, and are not necessarily of any significance. However, in the patient receiving digitalis they may be a sign of digitalis toxicity.

Atrial paroxysmal tachycardia, too, may be a sign of digitalis toxicity, and is more likely if there is also potassium deficiency, possibly as a result of diuretic treatment. The atrial rate is slower than with 1:1 atrial flutter, usually between 150 and 200/minute, sometimes with the ventricular rate slower still due to A:V conduction block.

Ventricular paroxysmal tachycardia may arise with aortic valve disease and associated left ventricular hypertrophy and ischaemia. The heart rate is usually between 120 and 180, with the higher rate being found in younger patients. The much reduced cardiac output may cause angina, syncope or left ventricular failure, particularly in older patients. Ventricular paroxysmal tachycardia is a dangerous arrhythmia as it may progress to ventricular fibrillation with fatal results. Prompt treatment is indicated, usually with cardioversion.

Pulmonary Embolism

Pulmonary embolism is a possible hazard in the patient immobilised with congestive failure and venous stasis. The emboli originate in the deep veins of the lower limbs or pelvis. There may be no warning, although a previous history of deep vein thrombosis or of asymmetrical leg oedema, or of being currently on the contraceptive pill, may be a reminder of the risk of venous thrombosis and pulmonary embolism. Isotope scanning of the lung fields is a more informative investigation than an ordinary chest X-ray. The scan reveals the site of pulmonary embolism as an area in which vascular perfusion has ceased although ventilation continues normally. Sites of other unsuspected pulmonary infarcts may be revealed at the same time. Anticoagulant therapy is indicated unless there are strong contraindications.

Systemic Embolism

Systemic embolism is associated with mitral stenosis and is more likely with atrial fibrillation than with sinus rhythm. Emboli originate in the left atrium, particularly in the atrial appendix and are composed of recently formed, loosely attached thrombus. Older thrombus is less dangerous being more firmly attached to the atrial wall.

Over half are cerebral emboli, usually causing a sudden hemiparesis or aphasia, i.e. infarcting the territory of the middle cerebral artery. Fortunately substantial or even complete recovery of function often returns within a matter of days. Small emboli may cause brief attacks of confusion or loss of consciousness without paresis, and may be mistaken for epilepsy of late onset, especially if such attacks recur. Other sites for systemic embolism are renal, with sudden loin pain and haematuria: peripheral, in the lower or the upper limb: saddle embolism at the bifurcation of the aorta: or mesenteric, with central abdominal pain and ileus.

Systemic emboli may well recur, so that a single embolus should be the signal for preventive action by treatment with anticoagulants and consideration of surgical relief of mitral stenosis. The risk of embolisation is much reduced, though not abolished, by effective mitral valve surgery. Valve replacement itself may carry a risk of systemic embolisation from thrombus forming on the prosthesis, so that anticoagulant therapy may have to be continued for an indefinite period after valve replacement with a prosthesis.

Even without surgery and without a history of systemic embolism, some physicians consider that the combination of mitral stenosis and atrial fibrillation is sufficient reason for starting long-term anticoagulant treatment.

Infective Endocarditis

Any rheumatic valve lesion is capable of acting as a focus for infective endocarditis although, with mitral lesions, the risk is greater with mitral incompetence than with stenosis. Also infection is commoner with sinus rhythm than with atrial fibrillation.

Every patient with valvular heart disease should be reminded of the need for antibiotic prophylaxis if undergoing dental or other forms of surgery. The long-term penicillin prophylaxis against recurrences of rheumatic fever is insufficient to protect against infective endocarditis (see Chap. 4).

Diagnostic Procedures

Radiology

Radiology forms an essential part of the clinical examination of the patient with rheumatic heart disease and the file of chest X-ray films covering a number of years gives a useful review of the patient's progress. Fluoroscopic examination of the heart by clinician and radiologist together is valuable when possible.

The Atria. Enlargement of the left atrium is best seen in the right anterior oblique (RAO) view, with displacement backwards of the barium-filled oesophagus (Fig. 2.6). It may also be seen on the postero-anterior (PA) view as a curved prominence on the right heart border, just above and overlapping the border of the right atrium (Fig. 3.12). The enlarged left atrial appendix is seen on the left heart border on the PA view forming a prominence just below the main pulmonary artery. The characteristic "mitral silhouette" is made up of these three components on the PA view: enlargement of the left atrium, of its appendix and of the main pulmonary artery.

Right atrial enlargement causes a generalised curved prominence of the right heart border as seen on the PA view.

Fluoroscopy will reveal expansile pulsation in systole of the left or right atrium if there is significant regurgitation at the mitral or tricuspid valves respectively.

The Ventricles. The right ventricle is seen on the LAO view immediately behind the sternum; when hypertrophied, as with pulmonary hypertension, its outflow tract is prominent in this view right up to the origin of the pulmonary artery. Left ventricular enlargement is seen on the LAO view at the back of the heart. If the enlargement is due to major aortic regurgitation, fluoroscopy will show the exaggerated movement of the left ventricle and the accentuated systolic pulsation of the aorta.

Main Vessels. Prominence of the main pulmonary artery is seen with mitral stenosis if there is pulmonary hypertension. When this is severe there is a visual contrast between the widened main and primary branches and the narrowed and radiologically insignificant secondary and peripheral branches (Fig. 2.5). This has been likened to "pruning" of the pulmonary vascular tree.

The proximal aorta becomes dilated above a long-standing aortic stenosis, without showing much increase in systolic pulsation. When there is free aortic regurgitation, however, the whole of the aortic arch becomes dilated and elongated and shows expansile systolic pulsation.

The Valves. Calcification of the valves should be sought with a penetrating RAO view and also on fluoroscopy. The mitral valve lies a little lower than and posterior to the aortic valve. The motion of the two valves differs: the mitral valve moves in an anticlockwise circle with the heart's action, while the aortic valve moves down and up with systole and diastole respectively.

The Lung Fields. Raised left atrial pressure causes congestion of the pulmonary veins, particularly the upper ones, which become prominent above the main pulmonary arteries. A further rise in venous pressure leads to oedema in the interlobar septa, shown as Kerley's lines. These are best seen in the relatively translucent costophrenic angles (Figs. 3.2, 3.3). Pulmonary oedema causes a diffuse perihilar haze, not always quite symmetrical, and sometimes pleural effusions too. Long-standing high pressure in the left atrium and pulmonary veins may cause miliary mottling from haemosiderosis.

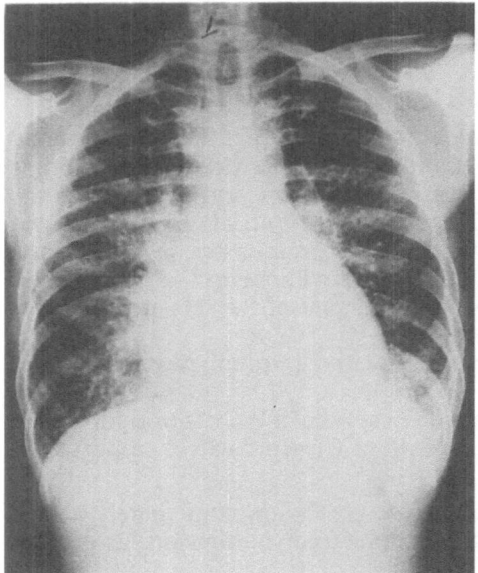

Fig. 3.2. Chest X-ray film (PA) of a patient with cardiomegaly and left ventricular failure causing chronic pulmonary vascular congestion.

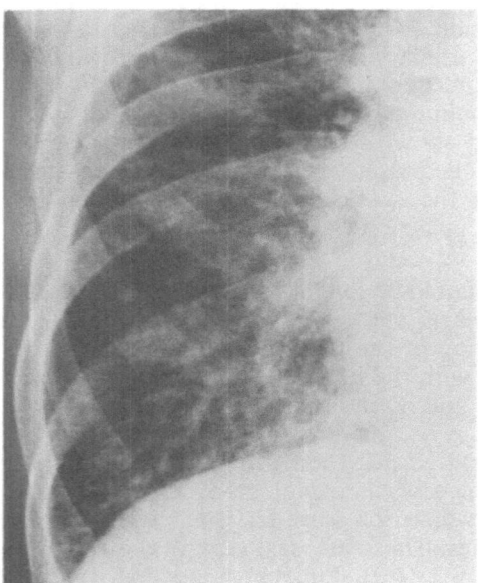

Fig. 3.3. Chest X-ray film. An enlargement of the right lower lung field of the chest film in Fig. 3.2 showing oedema in the interlobar septa, seen as horizontal lines (Kerley's lines) in the costophrenic angle. The interlobar fissure is slightly accentuated with a trace of pleural fluid.

Electrocardiography

The diagnostic abnormalities shown on ECG in rheumatic heart disease mainly relate to hypertrophy of one or more chambers of the heart and to rhythm disturbances which have been reviewed in a previous section, pp. 43-45.

Atrial Hypertrophy. Left atrial hypertrophy in mitral stenosis with sinus rhythm produces a bifid double-humped P wave. This is usually best shown in lead II and in the left chest leads V4 to V6. Right atrial hypertrophy produces a tall P wave with a single peak, best seen in leads II, III and AVF. This is usually associated with right ventricular hypertrophy.

Ventricular Hypertrophy. Left ventricular (LV) hypertrophy is indicated by tall R waves in the left chest leads, V5 and V6 with correspondingly deep S waves in V1 and V2. A common convention is to diagnose LV hypertrophy if the R wave is greater than 25 mm in V5 or V6, or if the sum of the R wave in either of these leads plus the S wave in V1 or V2 is greater than 35 mm. This is not entirely reliable as such ventricular complexes can occasionally be found in normal people. LV hypertrophy is only reliably diagnosed if, in addition, there is T wave inversion in leads aVL and V6 (Fig. 9.10). Right ventricular hypertrophy is indicated by tall R waves in lead V1 and probably V2 combined with T wave inversion in V1 (Fig. 2.4).

Echocardiography

This is a valuable and informative non-invasive procedure available in two forms. In the M mode a single ultrasonic beam is directed through the heart from the fourth or fifth intercostal space at various angles. Returning echoes from structures within the heart are displayed in linear form on a video screen synchronously with the ECG (Figs. 3.4, 3.5, 3.6, 3.7). In the two-dimensional or cross-sectional echocardiogram the ultrasonic beam repeatedly and rapidly sweeps through a sector which views the heart in cross-section. The resulting video display gives a real-time moving image of the heart in cross-section (Figs. 3.8, 3.9) (Hall 1984).

Movement of the mitral valve cusps can be displayed and the rate of valve closure measured. This is reduced in mitral stenosis (Fig. 3.5). The pattern of mitral cusp movement is different in mitral regurgitation (Fig. 3.6) and in mitral cusp prolapse (Fig. 10.6).

Estimates may be made of the diameter of the aorta and pulmonary artery, of the thickness of the ventricular wall and septum, and of the diameter of the left ventricular cavity in systole and diastole. From the latter a figure for the ventricular ejection fraction may be calculated, giving a useful estimate of myocardial function (Table 3.1).

Two-dimensional echocardiography produces a direct display of the left ventricle and mitral valve. Measurement of the valve orifice is possible and thickening of the mitral valve cusps is displayed if present.

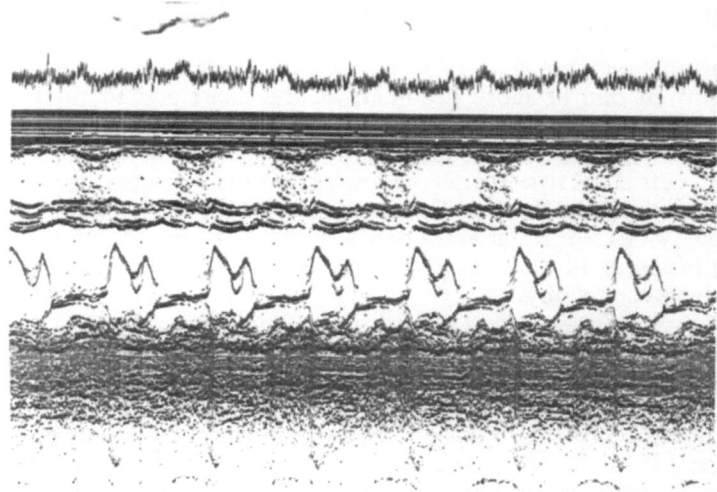

Fig. 3.4. Echocardiogram of normal mitral valve showing the normal two peaks produced by movement of the anterior mitral cusp in the open position in diastole. Figure reproduced by courtesy of Dr. FGM Ross.

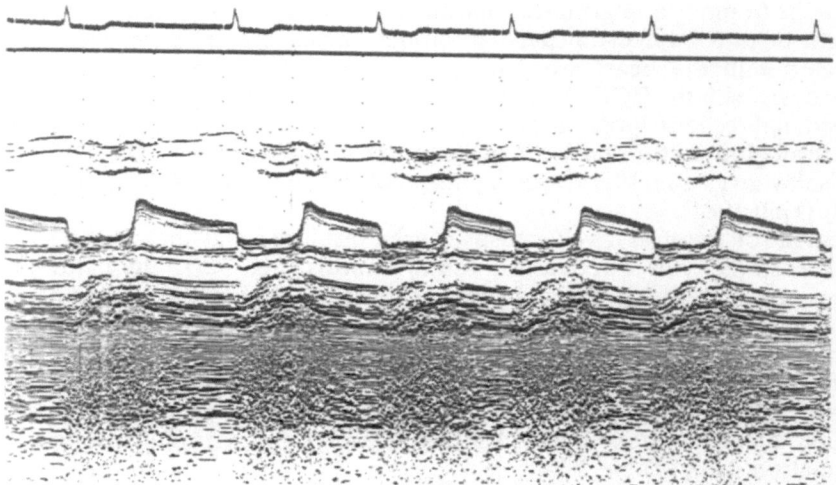

Fig. 3.5. Echocardiogram of mitral stenosis in a patient with atrial fibrillation. The downward slope of valve closure is slowed and the second peak, caused by atrial systole, is lost. Figure reproduced by courtesy of Dr. FGM Ross.

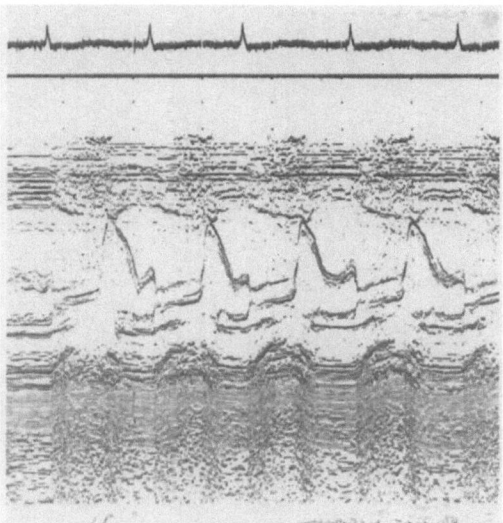

Fig. 3.6. Echocardiogram of mitral regurgitation. The movement of the anterior cusp is exaggerated, both in opening (upward) and closing (downward). Figure reproduced by courtesy of Dr. FGM Ross.

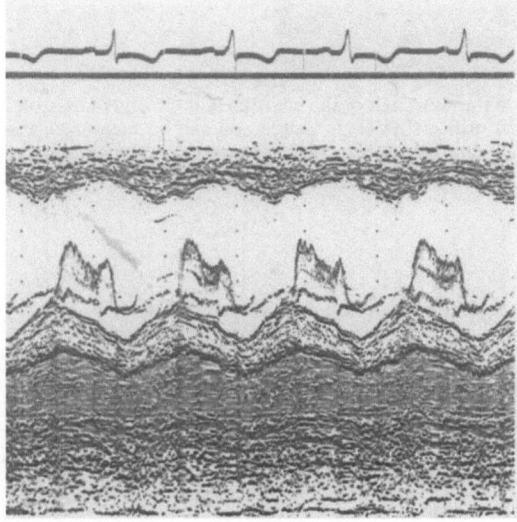

Fig. 3.7. Echocardiogram showing "fluttering" of the anterior cusp of the mitral valve due to free aortic regurgitation. Figure reproduced by courtesy of Dr. FGM Ross.

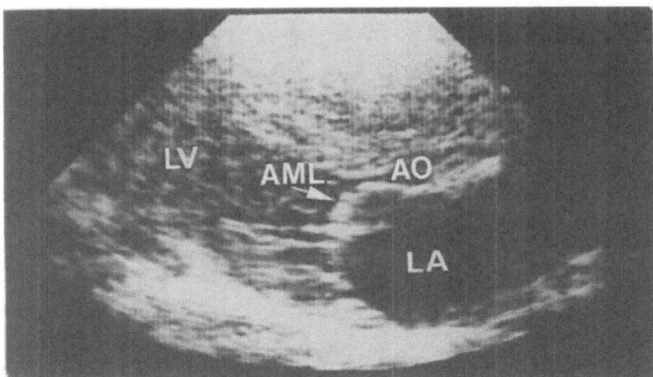

Fig. 3.8. Two-dimensional echocardiogram in the long axis of the heart. The mitral valve is thickened and fixed. Its anterior leaflet (*AML*) is well shown. The left atrium (*LA*) is dilated. The aorta (*AO*) and left ventricle (*LV*) are partially seen.

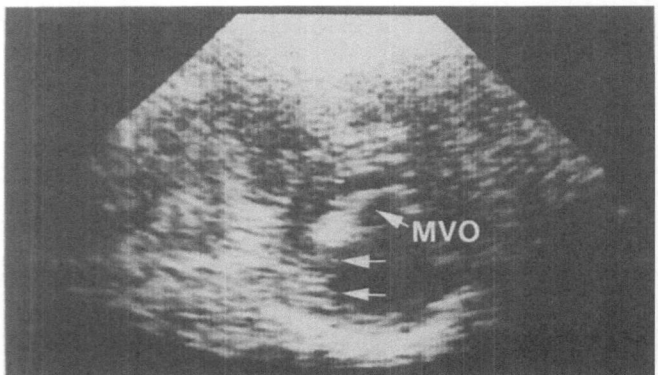

Fig. 3.9. Two-dimensional echocardiogram in the short axis of the heart seen at the end of diastole, from the same patient as Fig. 3.8. The mitral orifice (MVO) is visible and can be measured: the distance between the pair of arrows illustrates 1 cm. Figs. 3.8 and 3.9 are reproduced by courtesy of Dr. RD Thomas.

Table 3.1. Echocardiographic studies in 20 patients with mitral stenosis referred for surgery

	Normal subjects	Patients
L atrial diameter (cm)	3.23	4.3
Stroke volume L ventricle (ml)	72	49
Cardiac output (l/min)	5.02	3.82
Ejection fraction, L ventricle	0.74	0.55
Velocity of circumferential fibre shortening, L ventricle	1.26	0.89

In all the above data the patients' figures were significantly different from normal ($p < 0.001$) (Ibrahim 1979).

Echocardiography also reveals the presence of a pericardial effusion far more effectively than chest X-ray films, giving some indication of the size of the effusion (Fig. 5.16).

As an example of the application of echocardiography to the assessment of myocardial function, Table 3.1 quotes a study by Ibrahim (1979) of 20 patients with mitral stenosis. Echocardiography confirmed enlargement of the left atrium and revealed subnormal average figures for stroke volume, cardiac output, LV ejection fraction and the velocity of myocardial fibre shortening in the LV wall.

Doppler Echocardiography

The development of the Doppler technique has enhanced the applications of echocardiography as a means of non-invasive investigation and diagnosis, as the haemodynamic information that it provides complements the anatomic information given by M mode and cross-sectional echocardiography.

The technique is based on the principle that the frequency of a beam of ultrasonic sound is altered when reflected from a moving jet of blood. The change in frequency is related to the velocity of the blood, being increased when the jet is directed towards the source, and reduced when the jet is away from the source. For accurate measurement the ultrasonic beam must be directed along the axis of the blood flow or jet that is being studied.

The ultrasonic beam may be directed from any point on the chest wall, and it may be a continuous beam or a pulsed one. To achieve precise direction of the beam when assessing intracardiac flow the Doppler technique is used in conjunction with cross-sectional echocardiography.

Valvular regurgitation may be recorded and its severity assessed semi-quantitatively at all four cardiac valves. The method is sufficiently sensitive to detect minor degrees of regurgitation that cannot be detected by any other means, e.g. in rheumatic fever (p. 5). Information of a quantitative nature may be obtained on stenotic valves and the gradient across the stenosis estimated, and the function of a surgically implanted valve can be studied (Hall 1984; Thwaites et al. 1987).

Angiocardiography

Angiocardiography may be required as part of detailed assessment prior to surgery. Any of the cardiac chambers may be studied but visualisation of the left side of the heart is of the greatest importance. The catheter is passed via the femoral or brachial artery to the aortic root or into the left ventricle. Injection of contrast medium is made and a cine X-ray film taken at the appropriate angle or in two planes simultaneously. Injection is made into the left ventricle to show the anatomy and movement of the ventricle, the mitral valve and the degree of mitral regurgitation if this is present. Injection into the base of the aorta shows the aortic valve and possible aortic regurgitation. In candidates for aortic valve replacement who have angina it may be advisable also to undertake coronary arteriography to assess the extent of coronary disease.

Examples are shown of mitral regurgitation (Fig. 3.10) and aortic regurgitation (Fig. 3.11).

Differential Diagnosis

Aortic Incompetence. Rheumatic aortic incompetence is always accompanied by a mitral lesion and usually also by some degree of aortic stenosis. This helps in the differentiation from conditions causing isolated aortic incompetence. These

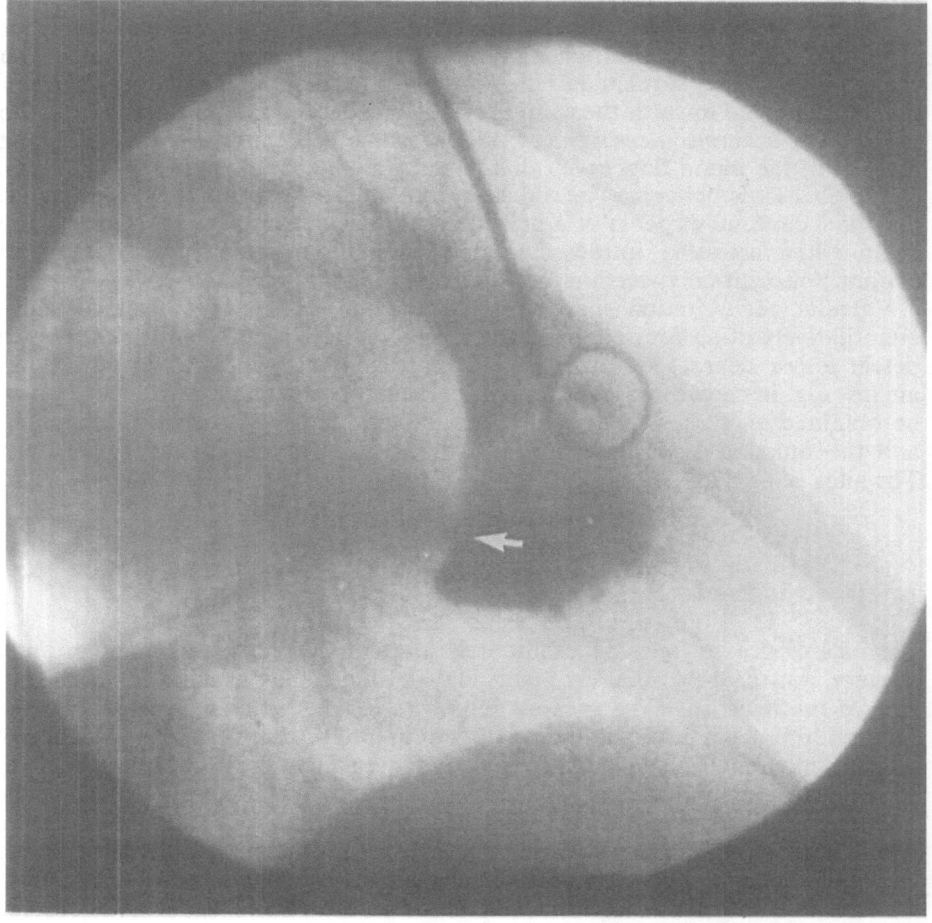

Fig. 3.10a

include aortic atherosclerosis with aneurysm, dissecting aneurysm, Marfan's syndrome and syphilis as well as aortic incompetence due to rheumatoid and spondylitic heart disease, dealt with in later chapters. Isolated aortic incompetence, if severe, may give rise to the Austin Flint mitral diastolic murmur, which suggests the presence of mitral stenosis without other signs of stenosis being present (see p. 37).

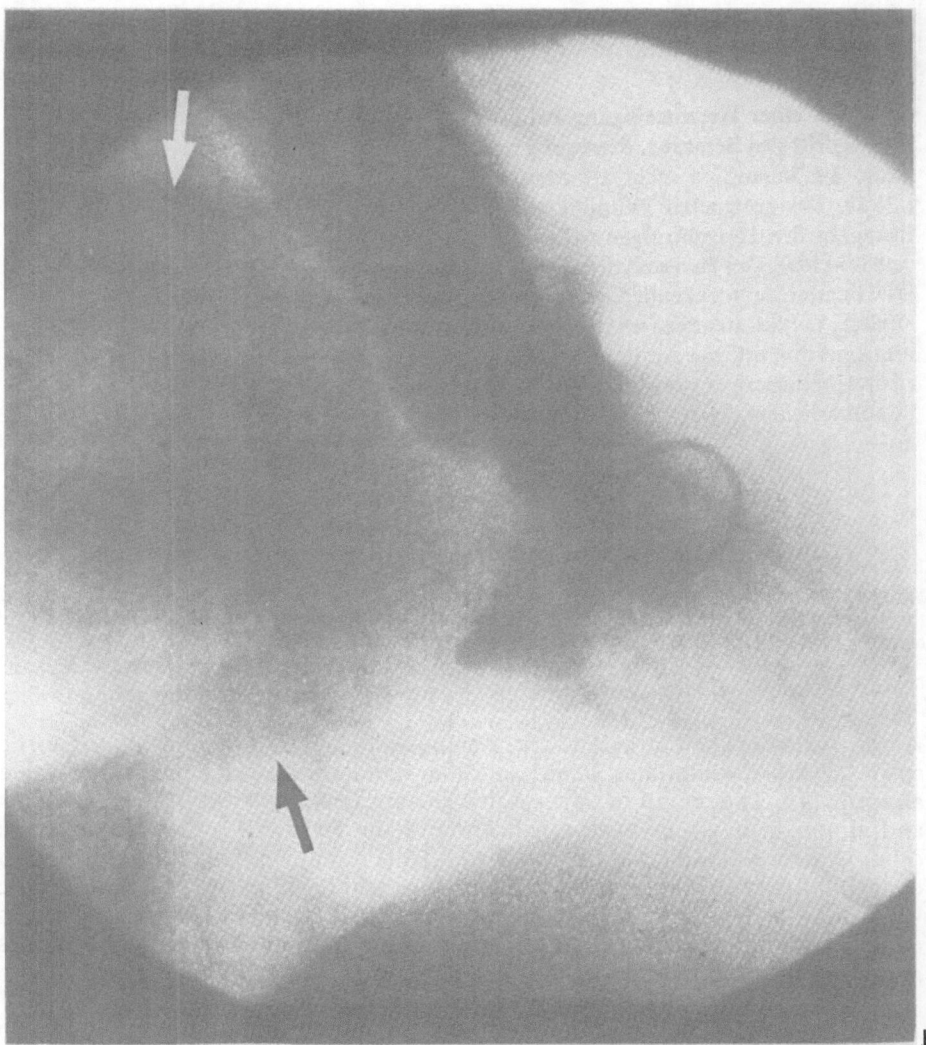

b

Fig. 3.10a,b. Cine angiogram showing mitral regurgitation. In the first frame, **a** *the arrow*, over the left ventricle, indicates the direction of the regurgitant jet into the left atrium. In the second frame, **b**, taken immediately afterwards, the aorta is outlined and the enlarged left atrium is opacified. The *upper and lower arrows* show its margins. Figure reproduced by courtesy of Dr. FGM Ross.

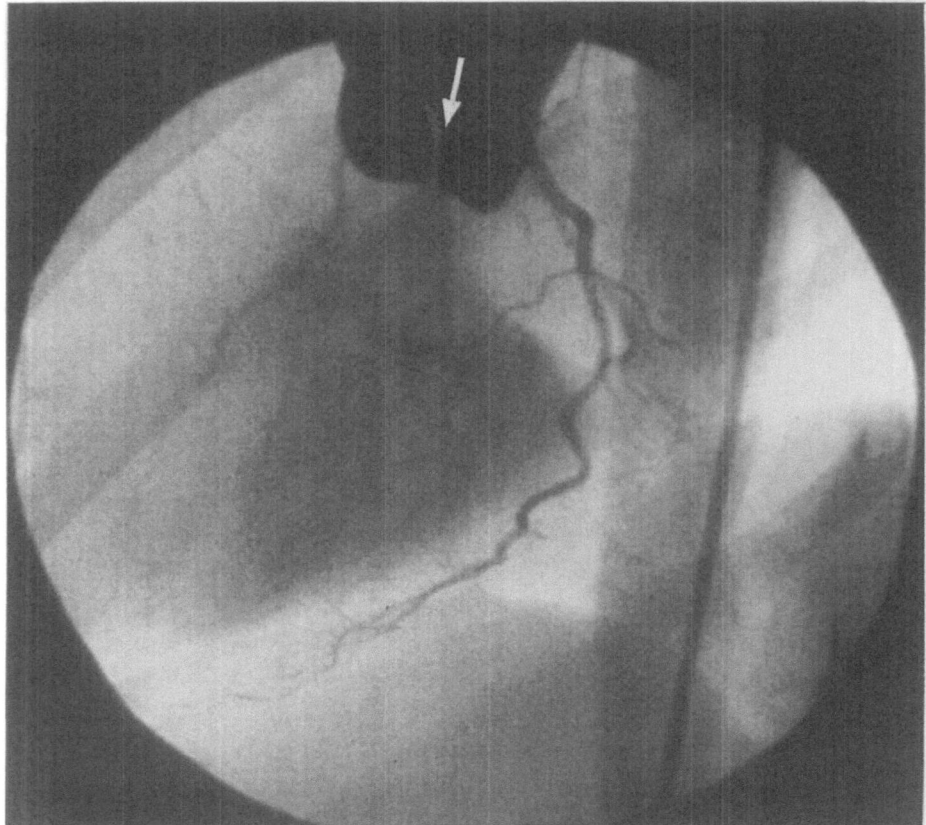

Fig. 3.11. Cine angiogram showing aortic regurgitation. This frame shows the regurgitant jet into the left ventricle in diastole, *arrowed*. The coronary arteries are shown. Figure reproduced by courtesy of Dr. FGM Ross.

Aortic Stenosis. The murmur of aortic stenosis is similar to the murmur of aortic cusp sclerosis, sometimes heard in older adults who have no other valve abnormality. The sound of aortic valve closure is unimpaired in these patients and although they may have calcification of the valve cusps they do not have other evidence of stenosis. In younger patients it may be difficult to distinguish congenital aortic stenosis from a rheumatic lesion. Similarly a bicuspid aortic valve may in later life calcify and produce frank stenosis. In these patients evidence for mitral involvement is lacking. In any case, if valve surgery becomes necessary the aetiological cause of aortic stenosis is of little importance.

Mitral Stenosis. Left atrial myxoma is an uncommon but important benign tumour arising from the wall of the atrium. When sufficiently large it may cause intermittent obstruction at the mitral valve mimicking mitral stenosis or causing syncope. Sometimes this temporary obstruction is related to posture, being associated with sitting upright or leaning forward. There may be thrombus formation in the left atrium and systemic embolism, as in mitral stenosis; also an increased serum globulin, a raised ESR and systemic symptoms which include limb pains and arthralgia (see Chap. 10, p. 238). Atrial myxomas are well shown on echocardiography and once diagnosed require prompt removal.

Mitral Incompetence. A common differential diagnosis here is mitral valve prolapse. This may be present from childhood or may develop later in life in a person who has previously had a normal heart. Characteristically it gives rise to a systolic click and a late systolic murmur, both heard at or near the cardiac apex. A prolapsing mitral valve cusp is usually symptomless but may be associated with left-sided chest pain and ectopic beats but usually with little or no regurgitation. It is well shown on echocardiography (see Chap. 10, p. 234).

Acute mitral incompetence may arise from rupture of chordae tendineae in infective endocarditis or from papillary muscle damage due to cardiac infarction. It causes urgent dyspnoea and may precipitate left ventricular failure.

Prognosis

Rheumatic heart disease progresses at different rates in different patients over the course of years (see Chap. 2, section on Natural History pp. 27–28). However, it is possible to make a prognosis for the individual patient based on a number of factors, favourable and otherwise.

Mitral Valve Disease. Here favourable factors are: history of a single attack of rheumatic fever with mild or unrecognised carditis: good exercise tolerance without dyspnoea: no cardiomegaly: sinus rhythm: little or no evidence of mitral regurgitation: no aortic valve lesion. In such a patient the symptom-free latent period following rheumatic fever is likely to be over the average of 15 to 20 years.

Unfavourable factors are: two or more attacks of rheumatic fever with carditis: reduced exercise tolerance: significant mitral regurgitation: presence of aortic or tricuspid lesion; cardiomegaly: atrial fibrillation. Such a patient has already entered the phase of symptoms and further deterioration is highly likely within the next few years.

Aortic Valve Disease. Favourable factors are: incompetence without stenosis: age under 30 years: good myocardial function. A symptom-free period of 15 to 20 years is likely.

Unfavourable factors are: combined stenosis and incompetence: cardiac enlargement: ECG evidence of left ventricular hypertrophy. Once dyspnoea develops deterioration soon follows and angina and syncope are ominous symptoms. In general aortic valve lesions are poorly tolerated in older adults (Frank et al. 1973; Goldschlager et al. 1973).

Clinical deterioration is often step-wise, with partial recovery after each step, provoked by events such as the development of atrial fibrillation, pulmonary infection, pulmonary or systemic embolism, or an episode of left ventricular failure.

Medical Management

The patient with rheumatic heart disease needs counselling over long-term issues relating to work, physical exercise and child-bearing in addition to medical care and drug treatment should this become necessary. During the course of follow-up an assessment may have to be made of the possible need for cardiac surgery and its timing.

Employment. The younger patient, even if symptom-free, needs advice on suitable employment and should not be committed to work which within a few years may be found too exhausting and have to be abandoned. If a change of employment becomes necessary the help of the medical social worker and possibly the disablement resettlement officer may be needed. Exercise should be allowed virtually without restriction if the patient is symptom-free, with the exclusion only of the more vigorous and competitive sports.

Pregnancy. For the younger woman guidance is needed in the planning and timing of her family. Childbirth is better undertaken sooner rather than later. If she is liable to only slight dyspnoea (defined as dyspnoea induced only by more than usual activity) pregnancy is unlikely to give rise to any difficulty. With moderate dyspnoea (induced by ordinary daily activity) some exacerbation is possible during pregnancy, possibly at the third or fourth month. This can usually be dealt with medically. Serious deterioration and pulmonary oedema may compel consideration of valvotomy, and if necessary this can be undertaken successfully about mid-term with little risk to the foetus. Sterilisation should then be considered.

Dyspnoea. Moderate dyspnoea will be helped by a regular diuretic, e.g. of the thiazide group, usually given with potassium as a compound tablet, or as diuretic combining the potassium-losing quality of a thiazide with the potassium-conserving quality of amiloride.

Dyspnoea associated with atrial fibrillation is an indication for digitalisation. It is usually introduced orally e.g. with digoxin 0.25 mg t.d.s. for the first 2 days, reducing to b.d. for 3 or 4 days and finally 0.25 mg once daily, depending on the response of the pulse rate. In older patients a lower maintenance dose is usually advisable e.g. as digoxin 0.0625 mg up to 3 times daily. If the need is urgent digitalisation may begin with an intravenous dose of 0.75 or 1.0 mg digoxin, subsequent doses being given orally.

Pulmonary Oedema. Pulmonary oedema calls for immediate relief with an intravenous diuretic such as frusemide 20 mg repeated in an hour or two if necessary, or followed by oral frusemide 40 mg. The patient is nursed sitting upright with the support of a bed table, oxygen is given and morphine 10 or 15 mg intravenously if necessary. An alternative intravenous diuretic is aminophylline 0.25 g.

Haemoptysis. Haemoptysis usually settles spontaneously within a few hours. The patient needs reassurance, rest in a semi-recumbent position and may be sedated with diazepam 5 or 10 mg orally or, if necessary, morphine 10 or 15 mg intramuscularly.

Embolism. Pulmonary or systemic embolism require prompt anticoagulant treament. Heparin 10 000 or 15 000 units is given intravenously 6-hourly for 2–4 days, and on the last day of heparin, warfarin is introduced in a dose of 30 to 50 mg. None is given on the following day and thereafter a maintenance dose is given as determined by the prothrombin time.

Congestive Heart Failure. This requires good nursing care, rest in bed or chair and limited gentle mobilisation, with medication basically by digitalis and diuretics. A fluid balance should be kept and plasma electrolytes and renal function monitored. Morphine at night is a great help when necessary for an exhausted and dyspnoeic patient. Venous thromboses and pulmonary emboli are a risk and long-term anticoagulants may be needed.

In patients who have been on digoxin for a long time signs of toxicity must be looked for and estimation of plasma digoxin levels may be of help. Toxicity and arrhythmias due to digoxin are commoner in the presence of potassium deficiency. Where necessary digoxin should be stopped for a few days and then introduced again at a lower dosage. Potassium supplements should be given as necessary.

Angiotensin converting enzyme (ACE) inhibitor (captopril, enalapril) is of help in congestive failure when needed as an adjunct to digitalis and diuretics. By reducing peripheral vascular resistance the ACE inhibitor improves left ventricular output, reducing venous congestion and improving renal function.

Patients with rheumatic heart disease have remarkable powers of recovery from congestive failure and often succeed in regaining an unexpected degree of physical activity.

Surgical Management

The outlook for patients with valvular heart disease has been immeasurably improved by cardiac surgery. Cardiac function is improved, effort tolerance increased and life expectancy extended.

The decision to operate must in every case be based on a careful assessment of the individual patient, the degree of his or her present disability and the current prognosis under medical management compared with the risks of surgery. In most centres the operative mortality for mitral surgery is under 2% and for aortic surgery under 5%.

In general, operation should be undertaken before deterioration is too advanced. Preferably the patient should have good myocardial function and freedom from other conditions such as coronary disease, chronic lung disease and impairment of renal or hepatic function. Age itself is not necessarily a bar to surgery and there is no need to exclude patients who are, say, 70 years of age if other conditions are in their favour (Canepa-Anson and Emanuel 1979).

There are occasions when surgery becomes the only hope for survival irrespective of risk. This is the case with sudden deterioration due to a ruptured aortic or mitral cusp or with uncontrollable infective endocarditis with a resistant organism. In Case History 3.1 the patient had to have repeat surgery to both aortic and mitral valves after major damage to the valves by infective endocarditis, although in this case the infection had been overcome.

Case History 3.1

Rheumatic mitral and aortic lesions
Surgery, infective endocarditis
Repeat surgery

Mr. I. O., Compositor, born 1939

1948	First attack of rheumatic fever
1949–50	Second attack
1951	Mitral systolic & diastolic murmurs Aortic systolic murmur
1955	Symptom-free: started work
1958	Aortic diastolic murmur now heard
1964	Atrial fibrillation; digitalised
1974	Dyspnoea and fatigue; angina
1976	*Aortic homograft & mitral valvuloplasty*

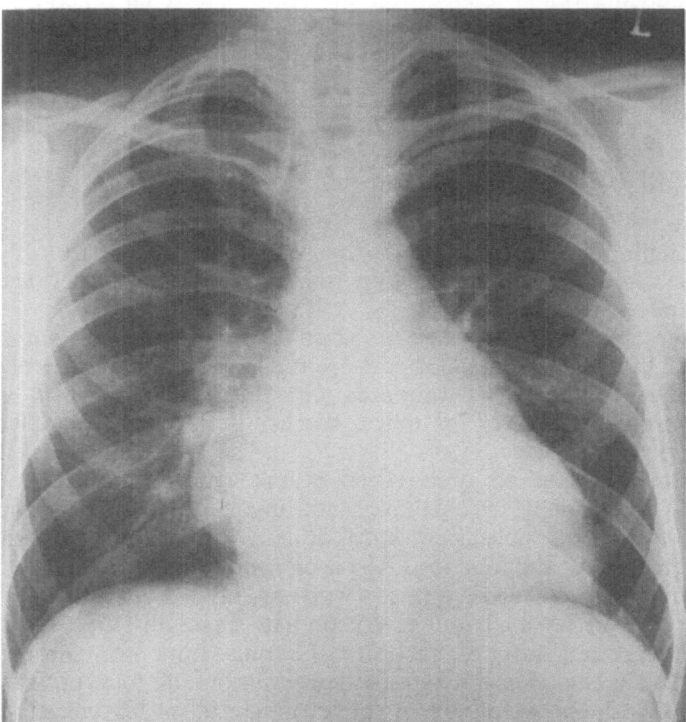

Fig. 3.12.   Chest X-ray film of the patient described in Case History 3.1 after re-operation on the aortic and mitral valves. There is generalised cardiac enlargement with prominence of the left atrium and left ventricle.

1978 Jan   *Infective endocarditis*, streptococcal
            Cured with penicillin + gentamycin
            Major aortic regurgitation; LV failure

1978 June   *Aortic homograft renewed*
            Mitral valve replaced

1979   Recovered, well and working (Fig. 3.12)

Comment   No penicillin prophylaxis after first attack of rheumatic fever:
            it might have prevented the second attack.
            Symptom-free latent period 14 years.
            First aortic homograft largely destroyed by infective
            endocarditis

Mitral Valve Surgery. Closed mitral valvotomy has now been virtually superseded, though it may still have a place in centres or countries where resources are limited (Portal 1984). The closed technique offers satisfactory results with predominant mitral stenosis and pliable cusps free from calcification, but it carries an appreciable risk of re-stenosis as in Case History 2.1.

Open heart surgery under bypass is now the method of choice, offering the surgeon inspection of the mitral valve from its atrial aspect. Commissural adhesions may be divided under direct vision and calcific deposits removed; there is a lower risk of subsequent re-stenosis (Kay et al. 1983). If restoration of valve function cannot be achieved in this way, valve replacement is necessary, usually with a mechanical prosthesis. Case History 3.2 illustrates a successful outcome with a Bjork Shiley tilting disc.

Case History 3.2
Rheumatic mitral and aortic lesions
Mitral valve replacement

Mrs. B. W., Housewife, born 1939

1953   Rheumatic fever, 4 months in hospital, residual systolic
            murmur

1958 ⎫
1961 ⎭   Bore two children without difficulty

1965   Murmurs of mitral stenosis and incompetence and aortic
            incompetence. Slight dyspnoea
            Cardiomegaly, L atrial enlargement. Digoxin

1972   Atrial fibrillation: increased dyspnoea
            Started long-term anticoagulants

1975   Further deterioration
            Cardiac catheter: no pulmonary hypertension; pulmonary
            wedge pressure normal at rest, rising on exercise

LV angiogram: mitral regurgitation
Mitral valve replaced, Bjork Shiley prosthesis

1980   Well, little dyspnoea. Heart still enlarged
            Continues warfarin and digoxin
                (Figs. 3.13 and 3.14)

Comment   19 years latent interval between rheumatic fever and signifi-
            cant symptoms and a further 3 years to surgery. Aortic
            incompetence still present, well tolerated

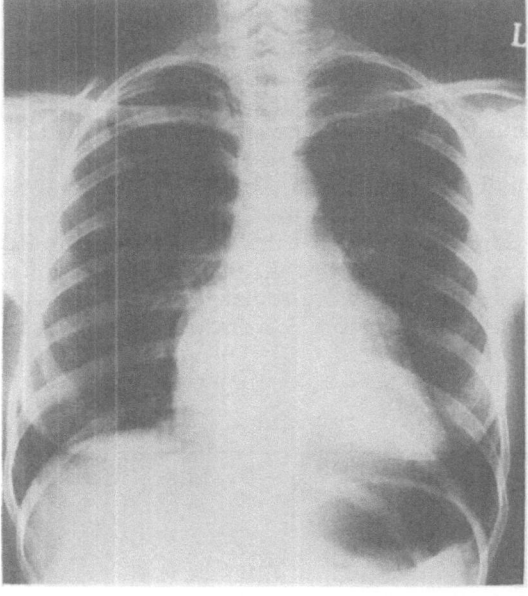

Fig. 3.13. Chest X-ray film of the patient described in Case History 3.2 after mitral valve replacement. There is still left atrial enlargement and prominence of the pulmonary artery.

Aortic Valve Surgery. Here the operative risks are rather higher than with mitral surgery. Valvuloplasty is rarely practicable and for either stenosis or incompetence the usual decision is for valve replacement. Initial post-operative results have been good with homografts and xenografts, which offer a widely opening valve orifice. However, the late failure rate has been such that for long-term reliability a mechanical prosthesis is favoured (Bailey 1984). The Starr valve has the longest record of success in both the mitral and aortic sites although it gives only a limited orifice when open; the Bjork Shiley and St Jude valves are improvements in this respect.

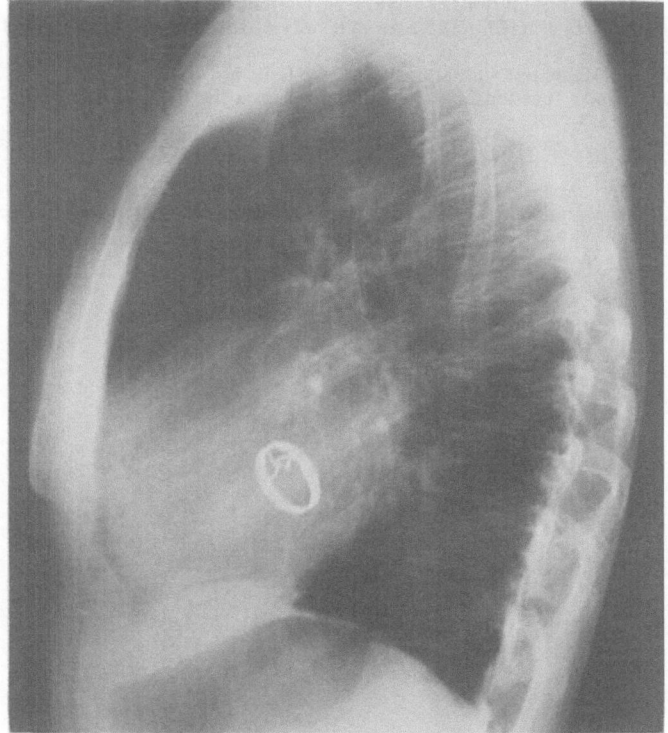

Fig. 3.14. Chest X-ray film, left lateral, of the patient described in Case History 3.2 showing the Bjork Shiley prosthesis.

Multiple Valve Surgery. Simultaneous operation on the mitral and aortic valves is sometimes necessary, or on the mitral and tricuspid valves, or on all three. The operative risks are inevitably higher than with single valve surgery, with an operative mortality of the order of 15%.

After Care. There is a risk of thrombo-embolic complications after insertion of a mechanical valve prosthesis and the risk is rather greater with aortic than with mitral valve surgery. This means that long-term anticoagulant treatment is advisable. Atrial fibrillation increases this risk, meaning that there is an added advantage if sinus rhythm can be restored post-operatively by cardioversion.

References

Bailey JS (1984) Surgical approach to valvular heart disease. Medicine International, Series 2 (18): 777–780

Canepa-Anson R, Emanuel R (1979) Elective aortic and mitral valve surgery in patients over 70 years of age. Br Heart J 41: 493–497

Frank S, Johnson A, Ross J (1973) Natural history of valvular aortic stenosis. Br Heart J 35: 41–46
Goldschlager N, Pfeiffer J, Cohn K et al. (1973) The natural history of aortic regurgitation. Am J Med 54: 577–588
Hall R (1984) Echocardiography. Medicine International, Series 2 (16): 678–687
Ibrahim MM (1979) Left ventricular function in rheumatic mitral stenosis. Clinical echocardiographic study. Br Heart J 41: 514–520
Kay PH, Belcher P, Dawkins K, Lennox SC (1983) Open mitral valvotomy: fourteen years experience. Br Heart J 50: 4–7
Portal RW (1984) Editorial: Mitral stenosis: the picture changes. Br Med J 1: 167–168
Thwaites BC, Shapiro LM, Donaldson RM (1987) The clinical assessment of Doppler cardiac ultrasound in valvular heart disease. J R Coll Physicians Lond 21: 192–195

Chapter 4

Infective Endocarditis

Introduction

Although infective endocarditis is not usually regarded as a rheumatic disease, it has certain features which are very relevant to rheumatology and which justify its inclusion here.

In the first place, the valve lesions predisposing to infective endocarditis include rheumatic heart disease and the specific valve lesions of rheumatoid, spondylitic and other rheumatic diseases or a prolapsing mitral valve cusp. In the second place, infective endocarditis can cause a variety of musculoskeletal symptoms, which include back, limb and joint pains and sometimes a frank arthritis. Thirdly, the development of rheumatoid factor and other antibodies during the course of the disease and the production of lesions due to circulating immune complexes are of interest to the rheumatologist.

The change in the name from "bacterial" to "infective" endocarditis is a reminder that the causative organism is not necessarily a bacterium, but could be a rickettsia (the coxiella of Q fever), chlamydia, or a fungus (e.g. candida or aspergillus).

Aetiology

In the classical descriptions of half a century ago and more, infective endocarditis was seen as a condition mainly affecting younger adults, whose underlying cardiac lesion was usually due to rheumatic heart disease. The majority of infections were caused by the *Streptococcus viridans* group, originating in the mouth and commonly giving rise to bacteraemia after dental treatment. The vegetations on the affected valves, liberating infected material and organisms into the blood were seen as accounting for most of the peripheral features of the disease by the process of embolisation. The concept of peripheral lesions such as those in the kidney, arising from deposition of immune complexes was unknown.

Today fewer than half of patients with infective endocarditis have rheumatic heart disease as the underlying lesion, and a third or more had apparently normal hearts previously (Bayliss et al. 1983b). The patient is now likely to be an older adult, of average age 50 years or more (Hayward 1973). While streptococci of the viridans group are still the commonest agents, organisms from the bowel or genitourinary tract are now being found more often, gaining entry to the bloodstream through investigative procedures as well as from surgery (Bayliss et al. 1984). Some patients are victims of drug addiction, whose casual technique of intravenous injection introduces a variety of organisms which may lead to infection on a previously normal tricuspid valve.

Other patients who are particularly vulnerable are those with a heart valve prosthesis, which may be infected with a streptococcus in the immediate post-operative period, or other organisms if arising later. As patients undergoing cardiac surgery are given antibiotic prophylaxis, any organisms causing infective endocarditis are likely to be resistant to antibiotic and therefore difficult to treat. If the infection cannot be controlled by medical treatment, or if the infection has caused major damage, urgent surgical valve replacement may become necessary in spite of the risks involved (Case History 3.1).

Men are affected twice as often as women, and the male preponderance is seen particularly in the older age groups.

The mortality rate, which was 100% prior to the introduction of antibiotics, then fell to about 30%. There, in general, it has remained, constituting both a challenge and a reproach to the clinician, pointing to the need for early diagnosis as well as constant awareness of the need for prophylaxis (Goodwin 1985). However, one review quotes a mortality rate of 20% (Lowes et al. 1980). The influence of the virulence of the organism on the outcome is clear. In one large series the mortality with staphylococcal infection was found to be 30%, with organisms originating from the bowel 14%, and with other streptococci only 6% (Bayliss et al. 1983b).

Pathology

The frequency with which individual valves are affected, based on autopsy findings, is approximately as follows: mitral 75%, aortic 55%, tricuspid 15% and pulmonary 1%. Two valves may be affected together, most often the mitral and aortic.

The lesions begin with the attachment of platelets at a point of irregularity in the endocardium, either at the site of a valve lesion, congenital or acquired, or due to degenerative changes. The platelet deposits are colonised by micro-organisms from the blood stream, and the growth of organisms is able to proceed as the lesion is beyond the reach of an organised cell-mediated inflammatory response. The addition of fibrin to the deposit and further bacterial growth lead to the formation of the characteristic vegetations of infective endocarditis.

Lesions form most often at sites exposed to high pressure jet streams, which accounts for the more frequent involvement of the mitral and aortic valves, and the greater frequency of infection at an incompetent rather than a stenotic mitral valve.

In general, organisms of low virulence attack mainly abnormal valves and give rise to large vegetations (Fig. 4.1). More virulent organisms may attack previously normal valves, particularly in older or debilitated patients, leading to rapid destruction of the valve cusp and sometimes invasion of the myocardium.

Histologically the vegetations are composed of fibrin and platelets and clumps of organisms are seen growing deep in the lesion where access by circulating antibiotics is limited (Fig. 4.2).

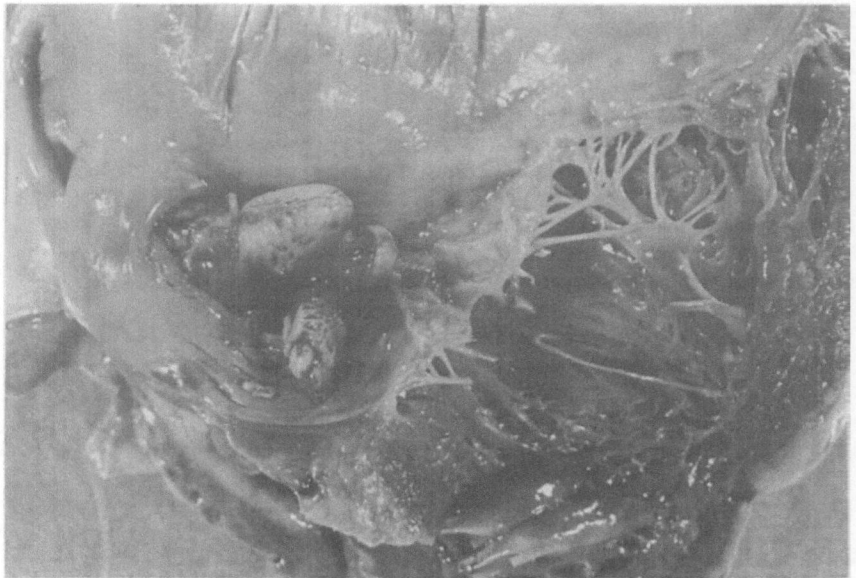

Fig. 4.1. Infective endocarditis. Left side of heart opened to show vegetations involving the anterior cusp of the mitral valve. From a woman aged 68 years with mitral stenosis.

Emboli of infected material are shed into the systemic circulation from vegetations on the mitral and aortic valves, and into the pulmonary circulation from the tricuspid valve. However, many peripheral lesions, particularly of the renal glomeruli, and those due to vasculitis are not embolic in origin but are caused by the deposition of immune complexes.

Immunology

The long continued release of bacterial antigens into the blood stream stimulates the production of antibodies and in the presence of an excess of antigen,

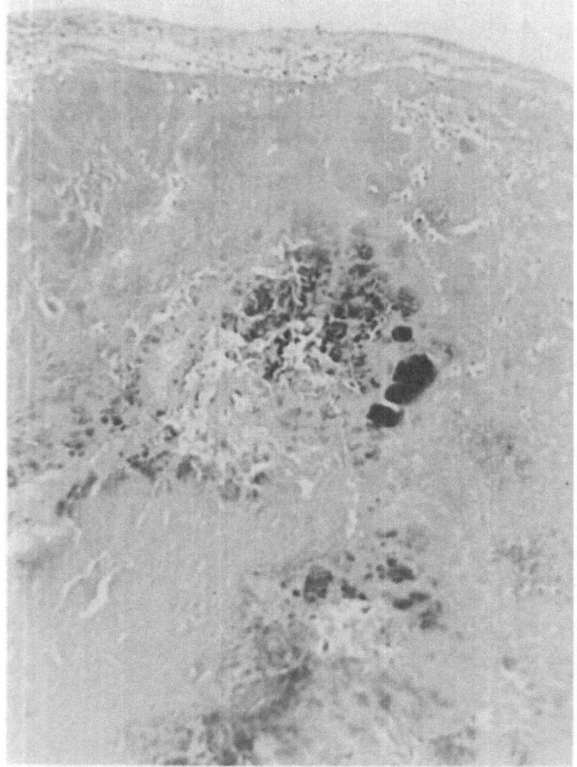

Fig. 4.2. Infective endocarditis. Microscopy of vegetation showing colonies of organisms staining dark in a background of fibrin and platelets (× 150).

complexes of antigen-antibody form in the circulation. After a time, these complexes in their turn evoke the production of antiglobulins which include both IgG and IgM rheumatoid factor. This response is a nonspecific feature of a number of long continuing bacterial infections, and was recognised as occurring with infective endocarditis by Williams and Kunkel (1962).

Deposition of these relatively large immune complexes in the endothelial wall of small vessels is responsible for a transient local vasculitis which is the basis for many of the peripheral lesions which characterise infective endocarditis, e.g. Osler's nodes, splinter haemorrhages, conjunctival petechiae and Roth's spots in the retina (Kauffmann et al. 1981).

In the kidney, circulating immune complexes are filtered out in the glomeruli where, on renal biopsy, they may be demonstrated by electron microscopy as electron dense deposits on the glomerular basement membrane (Gutman et al. 1972). Similarly, in the joint synovia the deposition of these complexes is the probable explanation for the occasional development of synovitis or arthritis during the course of the disease. Consumption of complement with a fall in the plasma complement level is noted with renal lesions in particular.

When infective endocarditis is effectively treated the release of bacterial antigens is brought to an end and in due course the circulating immune complexes and rheumatoid factor disappear (Bayer et al. 1976).

Clinical Features

Classification

The traditional classification of infective endocarditis as either acute or subacute is artificial as there is no real division into two such classes. The severity of the illness in the individual patient is a matter of degree which is determined mostly by the virulence of the infecting organism.

At one extreme, in its most acute form infective endocarditis may be due to a *Staphylococcus aureus* or a haemolytic streptococcus, has an abrupt onset with high fever and rigors, and within a few days the patient has become gravely ill. At the other extreme the illness is due to an organism of relatively low virulence e.g. a streptococcus of the viridans group, and has an insidious onset: its initial symptoms are indefinite and non-specific, or else misleading, being determined by the site of peripheral embolism. Most cases lie between these two extremes, and there may be "rheumatological" manifestations irrespective of the acuteness of the disease.

Clinical Effects

The clinical effects of the disease fall into three main groups: signs of infection, effect on the heart, and peripheral effects.

Signs of Infection

These are more striking in the more acute forms of the disease, but in due course appear in all. There is fever which is high, with rigors in the more acute forms, low or intermittent in others, tachycardia, sweating, weight loss and anaemia. Splenomegaly and finger clubbing may develop in due course. Leucocytosis is unusual. The sedimentation rate and plasma viscosity are raised.

Case History 4.1 describes a case of acute staphylococcal infection developing as a terminal event in a patient with chronic rheumatoid arthritis which was complicated by septic arthritis and septicaemia. The affected valve, the mitral, was previously normal.

Case History 4.1

Chronic rheumatoid arthritis
Staphylococcal arthritis and septicaemia
Terminal infective endocarditis

Mrs D.S., Housewife, born 1905

1952	Onset of rheumatoid arthritis
1962	Arthritis progressive: started prednisone

July 1965	Deteriorating: refused hospital treatment
5 Dec 1965	Admitted to hospital: discharging sinus from front of L shoulder. Culture of pus grew *Staph. aureus*, penicillin sensitive
6 Dec	Started ampicillin, initial improvement Found to be diabetic, started chlorpropamide
13 Dec	Deteriorating: hypotension and tachycardia Changed to cloxacillin + streptomycin Blood culture grew penicillin sensitive staph.
15 Dec	Some improvement
19 Dec	New apical systolic murmur noted
20 Dec	Died suddenly
Autopsy	L shoulder joint disorganised, pus present Heart: single large vegetation on aortic cusp of mitral valve, which was otherwise normal Many systemic infected emboli
Comment	Systemic steroid treatment and diabetes increased the risk of septic arthritis. Septicaemia not controlled with antibiotic. Terminal infective endocarditis developed on a previously normal mitral valve

Effect on the Heart

This may be catastrophic in the acute case, with a virulent organism rapidly destroying the aortic or mitral valve and precipitating left ventricular failure, pulmonary oedema or congestive failure. Similar but less dramatic deterioration may occur over a matter of weeks rather than days in less acute cases. Control of infection with an appropriate antibiotic may not be in time to check this destructive progress and the only hope for survival may be surgical valve replacement, which may have to take precedence over control of infection.

In Case History 3.1 streptococcal endocarditis partly destroyed an aortic valve homograft, inserted 2 years previously. The infection was controlled, but the damage that it had caused was sufficiently severe to require a further aortic valve replacement as a matter of urgency.

Other damaging effects are rupture of chordae producing mitral regurgitation, rupture of a sinus of Valsalva perforating the right atrium, coronary embolism with infarction, various degrees of heart block, and arrhythmias. Nevertheless healing follows effective treatment, although cardiac function is inevitably impaired. There may be calcification at the affected valve as a late sequel to healing.

Case History 4.2 (Figs. 4.3 and 4.4) describes a spondylitic patient who developed mitral regurgitation due to ruptured chordae, with successful valve replacement after control of the infection.

Case History 4.2

Ankylosing spondylitis
Infective endocarditis on mitral valve
Mitral valve replacement

Mr. H.P., Engineer, born 1918

1941	Onset of lumbar back pain and stiffness
1946	Ankylosing spondylitis diagnosed Iritis. Bilateral hip lesions. Radiotherapy
1976	Prostatectomy: benign prostatic enlargement
1977	Urinary tract infection: *Strep. faecalis* Heart apparently normal
Oct 77	*Infective endocarditis*, mitral regurgitation Blood culture: *Strep. faecalis* Cured with penicillin + gentamicin
1978	Cardiomegaly (Figs. 4.3, 4.4) Echocardiogram: ruptured chordae mitral valve *L hip arthroplasty*
1979	*Mitral valve replacement*
1980	Good progress
Comment	The infecting organism probably originated in the urinary tract. No previous mitral valve lesion suspected, but a silent mitral lesion could have been associated with ankylos ng spondylitis

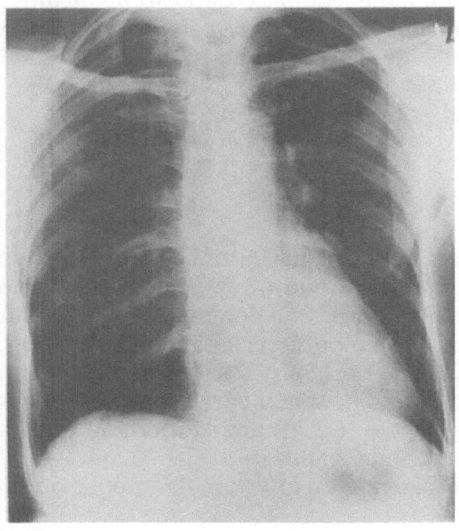

Fig. 4.3. Chest X-ray film of the patient in Case History 4.2 showing cardiomegaly; the appearance is exaggerated by the slight cardiac displacement to the left due to the depressed sternum.

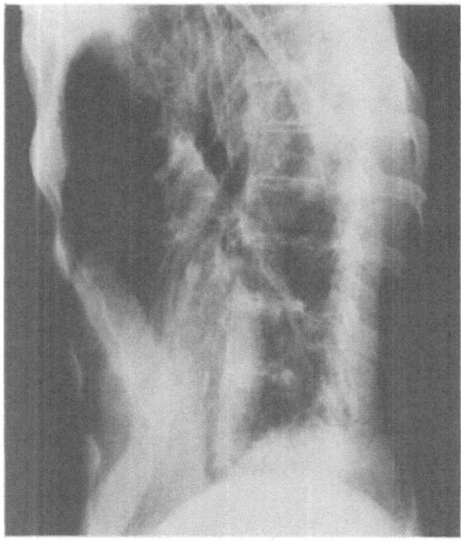

Fig. 4.4. Chest X-ray film. Lateral view of the patient in Case History 4.2 showing the depressed sternum and the spinal changes of ankylosing spondylitis.

Peripheral Effects

Systemic embolisation with infected material may cause infarction in the brain, kidney, abdomen or limbs. Pulmonary infarction and abscess may result from emboli from a tricuspid valve lesion.

Lesions caused by deposition of immune complexes have been mentioned in the previous section. The most important of these is glomerulonephritis, probably present in at least half of patients with infective endocarditis. It is usually symptomless but causes microscopic haematuria and proteinuria; if severe it may impair renal function. Smaller lesions, important diagnostically, and now recognised as being due to immune complex deposition include: petechiae in the mucous membrane of the mouth and palate, or in the conjunctivae, splinter haemorrhages beneath the finger nails, tender Osler's nodes in the fingers and Janeway's nodes in the palms, and small retinal haemorrhages, often with a white central point (Roth's spots).

Musculoskeletal Symptoms

Musculoskeletal symptoms are a feature of about a quarter of cases of infective endocarditis. Limb and joint aches are common, and often ill-defined. Some may be attributable to the general effects of a febrile and debilitating illness, but others are embolic. Back pain, localised in the lumbosacral area is also common, sometimes with sciatica, and may suggest either disc prolapse or embolism and infection in the region of the intervertebral disc or spinal nerve root. Examples of severe back pain are given by Deshayes et al. (1974) and Holler and Pecora (1970). One of the cases quoted by Meyers and Commerford (1977) and two of the four described by de Seze et al. (1965) had proven infection of embolic origin in the vicinity of an intervertebral disc.

Arthritis affecting one or more joints was noted in 24 patients described by Meyers and Commerford (1977), usually affecting the knees and ankles, and sometimes shoulders and elbows. A case of severe disabling polyarthritis, mainly involving knees and ankles is described by Bayer et al. (1975) in a young woman with enterococcal endocarditis. In all cases the arthritis subsided completely once the infection was treated. Examination of joint fluid has only occasionally been possible as the joint effusions are small. In one patient of Meyers and Commerford (1977) the joint fluid had a white cell count of $20\,000/mm^3$ with a reduced level of complement and was sterile on culture. There is good evidence that such cases of arthritis are associated with immune complex formation, either in the blood or in synovial fluid or both. Bayer et al. (1976) found evidence for immune complex formation in 28 of 29 patients with infective endocarditis, associated mainly with long duration of infection and with reduction of plasma complement levels.

Rheumatoid factor and antinuclear factor are frequently present in patients with infection of long duration, and were described in half of the patients studied by Williams and Kunkel (1962). Titres of these factors fell to zero with effective treatment.

Diagnosis

The diagnosis of infective endocarditis should be considered in any patient known to have a heart valve lesion or prosthesis if he or she develops a febrile illness following surgery, major or minor, or genitourinary or gastrointestinal investigation. To this should now be added, as suspect, the older adult without evidence of a valve lesion. If, during observation, a heart murmur changes or develops de novo, this adds to the probability of the diagnosis.

Full clinical examination is essential, including a search for petechiae, retinal lesions and microscopic haematuria. A series of at least three blood cultures must be made. In urgent cases three or more cultures may be taken in the course of a day and treatment started without waiting for the results. In patients with persistently negative cultures the possibility must be considered of infection with coxiella or chlamydia, or a fungus. Fungal infection is of low grade and has an insidious nature, and may be superimposed on a valve prosthesis or may follow antibiotic treatment which has eradicated infective endocarditis caused by a commoner organism.

Echocardiography can be valuable in diagnosis as vegetations may become visible when studied in the two dimensional mode. However, a negative result on echocardiography does not exclude infective endocarditis.

Differential Diagnosis

Valvular heart disease with repeated non-infected emboli may suggest infective endocarditis, and patients who have developed a ball thrombus in the left atrium may have many small systemic emboli. However, there is no fever and blood cultures are negative. Left atrial myxoma also may be associated with small emboli and can give rise to systemic symptoms with a raised sedimentation rate and abnormal plasma globulin.

Seropositive rheumatoid arthritis in the presence of an aortic or mitral valve lesion has features in common with infective endocarditis, but the chronic nature and the pattern of joint involvement differs from the arthritis which may arise with infective endocarditis. Systemic lupus, too may be difficult to distinguish from infective endocarditis as it may present with a valve lesion and a wide range of possible symptoms including fever.

Acute low back pain developing in patients with a heart valve lesion requires close observation to exclude infective endocarditis.

Treatment

As soon as the diagnosis is suspected every effort should be made to obtain confirmation quickly by blood culture and to start treatment. The dangers of delay are such that it is common practice to set up three blood cultures and then start treatment without waiting for the results. This means that the choice of antibiotic must initially be based on clinical judgement, and later revised as necessary in the light of the results of the cultures and of information on the sensitivity of the organism grown (Oakley 1985).

Treatment should be given for a minimum of 4 weeks, and probably for 6 weeks, and two synergistic bactericidal antibiotics should be given. A suitable combination likely to cover most infections in penicillin and gentamicin. They are given by intravenous bolus for the first 2 weeks in doses such as: penicillin 2 mega units four hourly + gentamicin 80 mg 12 hourly. If the infecting organism proves to be sensitive to this regime, oral amoxycillin 1 g 8 hourly can then be substituted for the remaining two to four weeks (British Society for Antimicrobial Chemotherapy (BSAC) 1985).

However, the choice of antibiotic and the dosage depend on the organism and its sensitivity as determined by the minimum bactericidal concentration (MBC) of penicillin, or the minimum inhibitory concentration (MIC), which is rather easier to estimate. Close cooperation between physician and pathologist is necessary to determine the optimum dosage of antibiotic and the duration of treatment.

Older patients and those with impaired renal function are in danger of ototoxicity with gentamicin and there is some evidence that netilmicin may be preferable to gentamicin for them (Kahlmeter and Dahlager 1984).

For staphylococcal infections flucloxacillin should be given instead of benzyl penicillin: a suitable dose would be 2 g 4 hourly by IV bolus, again combined with gentamicin. If the response is satisfactory, after 2 weeks, oral flucloxacillin alone may be substituted.

For the patient allergic to penicillin, or failing to respond to flucloxacillin, vancomycin may be substituted.

The BSAC advise that monitoring of gentamicin peak and trough blood levels should be made twice weekly. If the choice of treatment has been correct temperature and ESR should settle in a week. Failure to respond may indicate the presence of an unusual organism. If infection cannot be controlled or if cardiac deterioration is rapid surgical valve replacement may have to be considered.

Prophylaxis

Antibiotic prophylaxis is indicated for any patient with a known valve lesion, valve prosthesis, congenital heart lesion or past history of infective endocarditis if undergoing any surgical or investigational procedure which might lead to a transitory bacteraemia. The latter include any dental procedure which might induce gingival bleeding, cardiac catheterisation, ureteric catheterisation or cystoscopy, bronchoscopy, colonoscopy, and endoscopy or sigmoidoscopy with biopsy. In patients at special risk e.g. with a valve prosthesis, prophylaxis should be even more widely used, not because the risk of bacteraemia is any greater, but because the treatment of infective endocarditis, should it occur, is so much more difficult.

It is now thought advisable to give antibiotic prophylaxis also to the older individual, over 60 years of age, who apparently has a normal heart.

The choice of antibiotic is determined by the bacterial flora potentially able to enter the blood stream. Basically the agents used are forms of penicillin, given orally or parenterally, with the addition of an aminoglycoside to cover gastrointestinal or genitourinary surgery, or in the presence of a valve prosthesis.

The antibiotic should not be given too far in advance of the operation or procedure: an hour's interval is best. Too long an interval merely allows the bacterial flora time to adapt to the presence of the antibiotic so that surviving organisms are resistant, and remain as a hazard (Durack, 1975).

As for dental prophylaxis, good dental hygiene at all times is probably more important than merely relying on antibiotic prophylaxis at the time of extraction or scaling (Bayliss et al. 1983a).

The recommendations of the British Society for Antimicrobial Chemotherapy were published in 1982, and are given in simplified form in Table 4.1. The recommendations of the American Heart Association's advisory committee (1984) were similar, and were reviewed in detail by Chadwick and Shulman (1986).

Table 4.1. Antibiotic prophylaxis of infective endocarditis (British Society for Antimicrobial Chemotherapy 1982)

1 *Dental treatment with local or no anaesthetic*
  Amoxycillin 3 g orally 1 hour pre-op
  +Amoxycillin 0.5 g orally 6 hours later

  If allergic to penicillin, or penicillin recently given:
  Erythromycin 1.5 g orally 1 hour pre-op
  +Erythromycin 0.5 g orally 6 hours later

2 *Dentistry or surgery with general anaesthesia* (not gastrointestinal or genitourinary)
  (*a*) *Normal risk*:
  Amoxycillin 1 g IM 1 hour pre-op
  +Amoxycillin 0.5 g orally 6 hours later

  If allergic to penicillin use Vancomycin 1 g IV slowly 1 hour pre-op

(b) *Increased risk (prosthetic heart valve)*:
Amoxycillin 1 g + Gentamicin 120 mg IM 1 hour pre-op
+Amoxycillin 0.5 g orally 6 hours later

If allergic to penicillin use Vancomycin 1 g IV slowly
+ Gentamicin 120 mg IV 1 hour pre-op

3 *Gastrointestinal or genitourinary surgery*
As for 2b

4 *Obstetrics, increased risk*
As for 2b

References

American Heart Association (1984) Committee Report on the Prevention of Bacterial Endocarditis. Circulation 70: 1123A–1127A

Bayer AS, Brenner RJ, Galpin JE, Goze LB (1975) Severe disabling polyarthritis associated with bacterial endocarditis. West J Med 123: 404–407

Bayer AS, Teofilopoulos AN, Eisenberg R, Dixon FJ, Guze LB (1976) Circulating immune complexes in infective endocarditis. N Engl J Med 295: 1500–1505

Bayliss R, Clarke C, Oakley C, Somerville W, Whitfield AGW (1983a) The teeth and infective endocarditis. Br Heart J 50: 506–512

Bayliss R, Clarke C, Oakley CM, Somerville W, Whitfield AGW, Young SEJ (1983b) The microbiology and pathogenesis of infective endocarditis. Br Heart J 50: 513–519

Bayliss R, Clarke C, Oakley CM, Somerville W, Whitfield AGW, Young SEJ (1984) The bowel, the genitourinary tract and infective endocarditis. Br Heart J 51: 339–345

British Society for Antimicrobial Chemotherapy (1982) Report of working party on the prophylaxis of infective endocarditis. Lancet II: 1323–1326

British Society for Antimicrobial Chemotherapy (1985) Report of working party on the antibiotic treatment of infective endocarditis. Lancet II: 815–817

Chadwick EG, Shulman ST (1986) Prevention of infective endocarditis. Mod Con Cardiovasc Dis 55: 11–15

De Seze S, Ryckewaert A, Kahn MF (1965) L'endocardite d'Osler en rheumatologie. Rev Rhum Mal Osteoartic 32: 739–744

Deshayes P, Durand JP, Houdent G, Humbert G, Breton G (1974) A propos des manifestations rhumatologiques des endocardites bacteriennes. Rev Rhum Mal Osteoartic 41: 135–141

Durack DJ (1975) Current practice in the prevention of bacterial endocarditis. Br Heart J 37: 478–481

Goodwin JF (1985) The challenge and the reproach of infective endocarditis. Br Heart J 54: 115–118

Gutman RA, Striker GE, Gilliland BC, Cutler RE (1972) The immune complex glomerulonephritis of bacterial endocarditis. Medicine (Baltimore) 51: 1–27

Hayward GW (1973) Infective endocarditis: a changing disease. Br Med J 1: 706–709, 764–766

Holler JW, Pecora JS (1970) Backache in bacterial endocarditis. NY State J Med 70: 1903–1906

Kahlmeter G, Dahlager J (1984) Aminoglycoside toxicity: a review of clinical studies published between 1975 and 1982. J Antimicrob Chemother 13 (Suppl A): 9–22

Kauffmann RH, Thompson J, Valentijn RM, Daha MR, Van Es LA (1981) The clinical implications and the pathogenetic significance of circulating immune complexes in infective endocarditis. Am J Med 71: 17–25

Lowes JA, Williams G, Tabqchali S et al. (1980) Ten years of infective endocarditis at St Bartholomew's Hospital. Lancet I: 133–136

Meyers OL, Commerford FJ (1977) Musculoskeletal manifestations of bacterial endocarditis. Ann Rheum Dis 36: 517–519

Oakley CM (1985) Infective endocarditis. Medicine International, Series 2; 21: 872–878

Williams RC, Kunkel HG (1962) Rheumatoid factor, complement and conglutinin aberrations in subacute bacterial endocarditis. J Clin Invest 41: 666–667

Chapter 5

Rheumatoid Arthritis and Rheumatoid Heart Disease I: Pericarditis

Introduction

Rheumatoid arthritis is a disease whose effects are by no means confined to the joints or even to the musculoskeletal system. In about a quarter of patients the disease involves tissues other than the joints and their related structures, the tendons, tendon sheaths and bursae. The systemic effects of rheumatoid arthritis combined with the existence of extra-articular lesions led to the introduction of the term "rheumatoid disease" by Ellman and Ball (1948) when they first described the pulmonary lesions that may develop. Other organs that may be affected include the skin, eyes, peripheral nerves, pleura, pericardium and the heart itself.

Rheumatoid arthritis as defined by the conventional eleven diagnostic criteria (Ropes et al. 1958) is not a homogeneous disease. It is only among the diagnostically "classical" and "definite" groups of patients who are positive for rheumatoid factor that homogeneity is found. It may be argued that the 25% of rheumatoid patients who are seronegative have a different, milder disease, or diseases, than the 75% who are seropositive (Calin and Marks 1981). Certainly the cardiac and vascular manifestations of rheumatoid arthritis are almost exclusively found among patients with seropositive disease, and it is with those manifestations that we are primarily concerned here.

Immunology

The fundamental cause of rheumatoid arthritis is still unclear, but much is known about the immunological and cellular responses that characterise the disease. An external agent, possibly a virus, acting in an individual who is genetically predisposed, sets up an inflammatory reaction in joint synovia. In a minority of patients there are environmental precipitating factors, traumatic, infective or psychological (Jacoby et al. 1973) but these are not essential. The serious consequence of the initiating inflammation is the generation of new antigenic material that gives rise to a continuing autoimmune inflammatory process with damaging consequences.

The genetic predisposition to rheumatoid arthritis is linked with the presence of cell surface antigens of the HLA-D series, encoded by the major histocompatibility complex (MHC) which is part of chromosome 6. The principal association is with HLA-DR4, originally noted by Stastny (1978), who found this cell marker present in 70% of patients with rheumatoid arthritis compared with 28% of controls. This association has been widely confirmed, but with some ethnic variations. Other antigens in the series such as HLA–A2 are also positively associated, while some (HLA–DR2 and DR7) are negatively associated with rheumatoid arthritis (Jaraquemada et al. 1986). These antigens appear to influence the severity of the disease and probably certain clinical features such as age of onset, the pattern of affected joints and the development of extra-articular lesions and vasculitis (McDermott et al. 1986; Walker and Griffiths 1986).

Inflammation. In rheumatoid arthritis inflammation is a highly complex process. It begins with the infiltration of the synovium with T lymphocytes in a response akin to a hypersensitivity reaction (Decker et al. 1984). Secretion of lymphokines attracts more T cells, as well as B lymphocytes, macrophages and mast cells. B cells, encouraged by helper T cells, are activated to produce plasma cells and antibody. Inflammatory mediators, primarily prostaglandins and interleukin, are responsible for many of the features of inflammation such as increased vascularity and vascular permeability and local oedema.

Immune Complexes. In the continuing synovial inflammation globulin antibodies themselves become antigenic, and antibodies are formed to these. These are the rheumatoid factors, which are found in IgG and IgM classes of globulin. Although rheumatoid factors, particularly of the IgM class, may be found in the sera of some patients with other diseases and some normals, tests for the presence of rheumatoid factors and measurement of their levels are a valid guide to the diagnosis of rheumatoid arthritis and the assessment of its progress (Carson 1982).

The binding of antigen and antibody produces immune complexes of varying sizes depending on the number and size of the participating globulin molecules. After production in the synovium they may enter the synovial fluid and attach to the surface of articular cartilage or they may be phagocytosed by polymorphonuclear leucocytes or by the lining cells of the synovial membrane. Disruption of the phagocytosing cells releases into the synovial fluid damaging agents such as proteolytic enzymes and free oxygen radicals. The immune complexes also bind complement, activating the release of the components of complement which further contribute to cell membrane damage. A major result of this activity is an assault on the integrity of cartilage surface in the joint, producing the erosions of cartilage and finally of underlying bone which are characteristic features (Krane and Simon 1986).

Immune complexes may also enter the blood stream and their dissemination to distant organs and tissues is responsible for the vasculitis and extra-articular lesions found in seropositive rheumatoid arthritis.

Pathology

The Synovium

Normally, the synovial membrane is covered by a single layer of lining cells which have an important phagocytic role in removing cell debris from the joint. They also secrete the synovial fluid, containing hyaluronic acid which maintains joint lubrication. In rheumatoid arthritis the lining cells multiply, producing a layer which is several cells deep. Beneath them the whole synovium is thickened. Within it are aggregations of great numbers of lymphocytes, plasma cells and macrophages (Fig. 5.1). In very active cases, germinal centres containing antibody-producing centroblasts and centrocytes may be seen, but more often these centres produce cells which mature into plasma cells later. Mast cells and dendritic cells are also present. Many new blood vessels develop in the deeper layers of the synovium, which is swollen with oedema and deposition of fibrin. Fibroblasts also appear, laying down collagen as the inflammatory process enters its chronic phase, or heals.

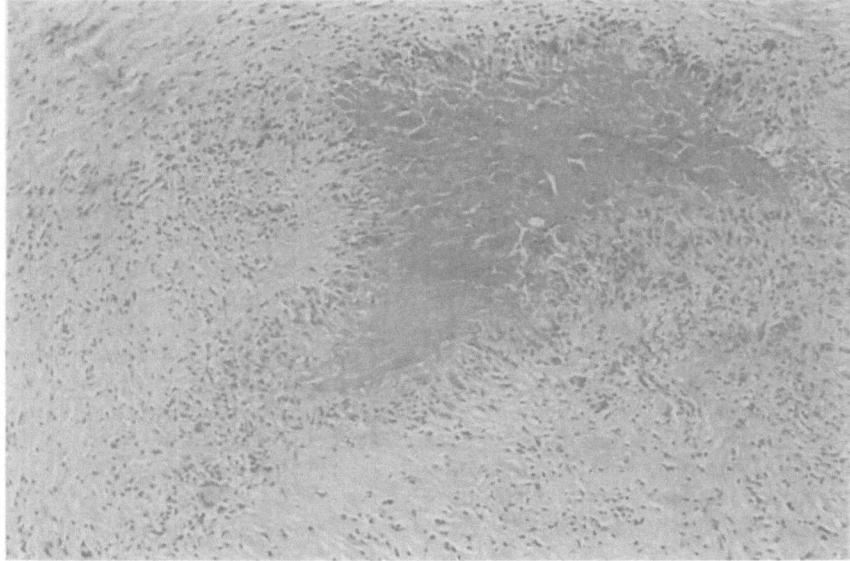

Fig. 5.1. Rheumatoid synovium histology (× 300). This high power view of inflamed synovium shows dense plasma cell infiltration and increased vascularity with dilated capillaries.

Thickening of the synovium is most marked in the angle of the joint, where synovial membrane joins articular cartilage and underlying bone. It is here that a pannus of chronically inflamed tissue proliferates, spreading out over the surface of cartilage and leading to erosions of cartilage and of bone. When the synovitis has become chronic the thickened synovium may form numbers of villi projecting into the joint space, which is distended with fluid (Fig. 5.2).

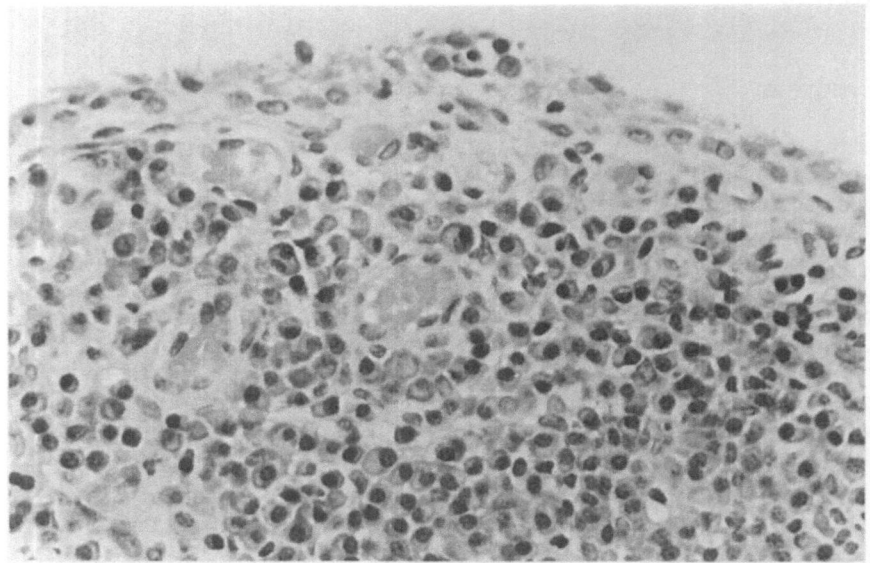

Fig. 5.2. Rheumatoid synovium histology (× 40) This low power view of the same specimen as the preceding figure shows villous proliferation of the synovial tissue with oedema, increased vascularity and a lymphoid aggregate.

The synovial fluid is much increased in volume and is under increased pressure which is exacerbated by muscular contraction and joint movement. The fluid is hazy and opaque and is pale yellow in colour. Its protein level, mainly globulin, is increased to 3 or 4 g per 100 ml and rheumatoid factor is usually present. The cell count is much increased, depending on the acuteness of the inflammation e.g. 10 000 to 20 000 per mm^3. Roughly 75% of the cells are neutrophils; some ("ragocytes") may contain phagocytosed immune complexes containing rheumatoid factor which may be demonstrated by immunofluorescent staining.

To some extent the pathological changes and processes that take place in the synovium are echoed in the pericardium if pericarditis develops as one of the extra-articular lesions in rheumatoid disease.

Nodules

Subcutaneous nodules form at sites such as the elbow or in tendons and tendon sheaths which are subjected to pressure or to shearing stress. They are only seen in seropositive patients. The typical nodule has an acellular centre of necrotic fibrin, surrounded by a palisade of epithelioid cells which are derived from macrophages. Around these are fibroblasts, collagen and scanty infiltration of lymphocytes (Figs. 5.3, 5.4). Nodules may become cystic or may ulcerate. They are of special significance in extra-articular rheumatoid lesions involving the lungs and heart (p. 106).

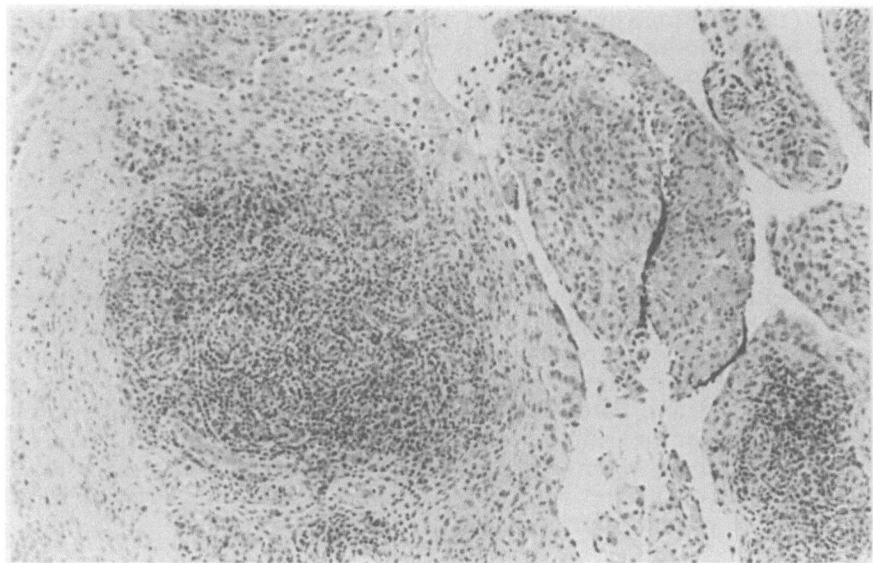

Fig. 5.3. Rheumatoid nodule from elbow; histology (× 20). The central area of necrosis here has a stellate shape. It is surrounded by a palisade of epithelioid cells.

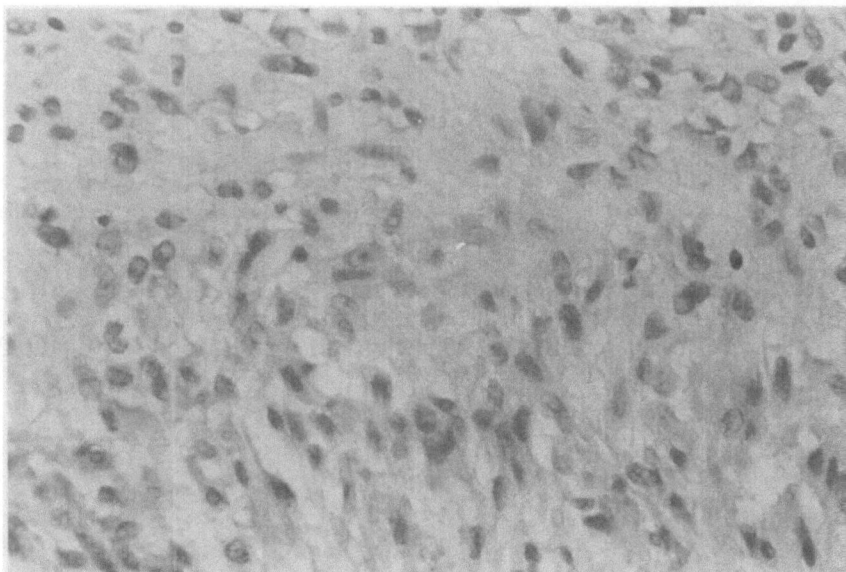

Fig. 5.4. Rheumatoid nodule. Histology (× 180) showing palisading, below, and fibroblasts and lymphocytes, above.

Although there is some evidence that nodules form at the site of a vasculitic lesion this appears to be inconstant. It is more likely that immunoglobulin and complement are deposited at a point of mechanical stress and that a cellular reaction to this accounts for the development of the nodule (Rasker and Kuipers 1983).

Vasculitis

Vasculitis is a feature of seropositive rheumatoid arthritis associated with the release of immune complexes into the circulation following their production in actively inflamed synovial tissue.

The deposition of the complexes in the endothelium of small vessels sets up a local inflammatory reaction of varying severity, determined partly by the size of the vessel involved and partly by the size of the complex. In small vessels vasculitis accounts for the nailfold lesions seen in the fingers (Fig. 5.5). In larger vessels there is a more vigorous inflammatory reaction or even a necrotising arteritis resembling polyarteritis nodosa. Figure 5.6 illustrates arteritis in an arteriole within a peripheral nerve trunk.

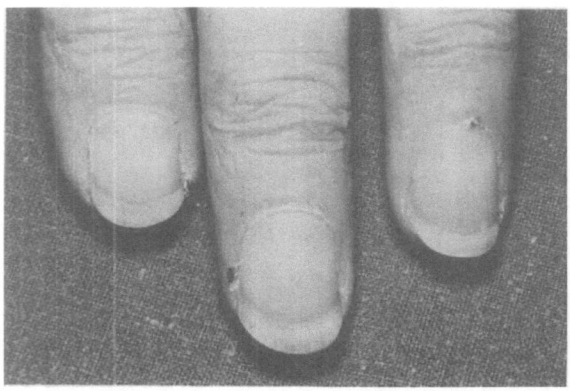

Fig. 5.5. Nailfold lesions. These are tiny infarcts caused by rheumatoid vasculitis. The lesion at the base of the fingernail (right) has almost healed.

Many of the extra-articular lesions of rheumatoid arthritis including some involving the heart are attributable to local vasculitis or to the formation of granulomata which are in effect modifications of the classical rheumatoid nodule.

Clinical Features

Arthritis

Rheumatoid arthritis is found world-wide, in all races and climates, though it appears to be rather more frequent and more severe in temperate zones. It

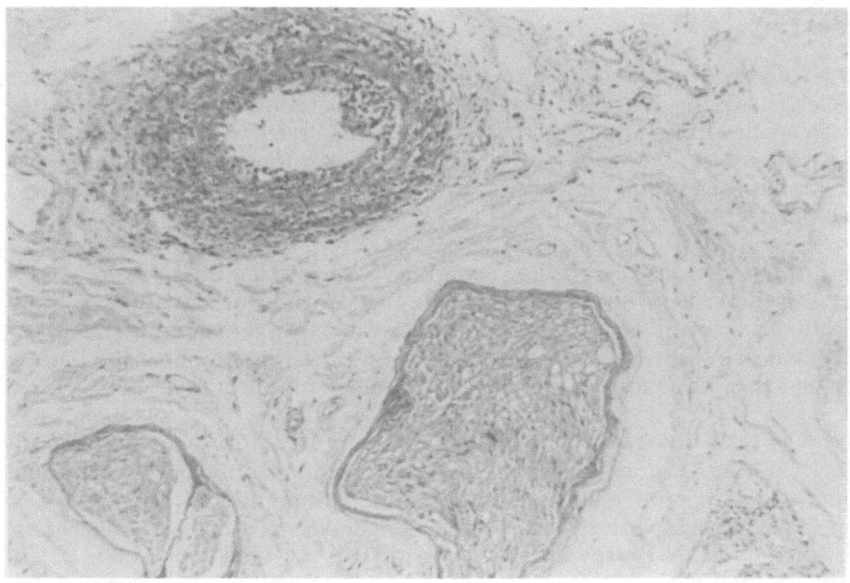

Fig. 5.6. Popliteal nerve. Transverse section (× 20) showing vasculitis in the small artery accompanying the nerve. (By courtesy of Dr. C Knowles.)

affects women two or three times as often as men; it may begin at any age, most often in mid-adult life. In Britain its prevalence is about 3% overall, meaning that there are some 1.5 million patients in the country. The prevalence in men is 2.1% and in women 5.2%, but in individuals over 65 years of age these figures rise to 6% and 16% respectively.

Its onset is most often in the small joints of the hands or feet. It may be unilateral at first, or may begin in a single larger joint such as the knee or shoulder, and symptoms may be intermittent. But as the disease progresses the pattern becomes established of a generalised and symmetrical polyarthritis which is mainly peripheral, although the hips and the cervical spine are also often affected.

The symptoms are joint pain and swelling and restriction of movement, with stiffness which is worst in the early morning or after a period of immobility. Laxity of ligaments, muscle wasting and erosion of cartilage and bone lead to joint instability and deformity. Osteoporosis brings with it a risk of fracture. Systemic effects include lassitude, anaemia and weight loss.

The course of the disease is very variable. Many patients have remissions, but the disease is liable to relapse, particularly in response to trauma or to stress. Ultimately some 25% remain well and active, 40% have moderately impaired function, 25% are quite badly disabled and 10% become confined to a wheelchair. Prognosis is worse in the 75% who are seropositive to rheumatoid factor as they have a higher incidence of extra-articular lesions, some of which are life-threatening (Rasker and Cosh 1981). To some extent the long-term prognosis may be predicted from an assessment of the patient's condition one year after the onset of arthritis (Reilly et al. 1989).

Extra-articular Lesions

Nodules. Nodules occur in a quarter of all patients with rheumatoid arthritis, almost exclusively in those who are seropositive. Common sites are pressure points such as the elbow or sacrum, and they may also form in tendons or tendon sheaths, and cause tendon rupture e.g. of the extensor tendons of the thumb or fingers. Nodules or granulomas of similar pathology may develop in the lungs, pleura or heart.

Cysts and Bursae. Popliteal cysts are common, derived from the knee joint as a result of raised synovial pressure; they may seal off from the joint or may rupture into the calf. Cystic extensions may form from the shoulder or other joints. Bursae, too, may form at sites of pressure or friction e.g. near the elbow, shoulder or knee; infection or rupture are possible complications.

The Eye. Up to a quarter of rheumatoid patients have dry eyes and mouth (Sjogren's syndrome, keratoconjunctivitis sicca) due to atrophy of the lachrymal and salivary glands, the result of autoimmune inflammation. Episcleritis is common and harmless, producing a transient painless red eye, but scleritis is more serious. Scleritis causes inflammation of the full thickness of the sclera anteriorly, probably arising from nodule formation within the tissue of the sclera. The lesion may perforate into the vitreous with loss of sight. Fortunately it is uncommon, affecting under 1% of patients with rheumatoid arthritis.

Neuropathy. Entrapment of the median nerve in the carpal tunnel is a frequent early complication of rheumatoid arthritis due to oedema in the region of the wrist joint. When the disease is advanced, subluxation in the cervical spine may cause pressure on cervical nerve roots or on the cord itself with a danger of paraplegia or quadriplegia. Peripheral neuropathy may arise in two forms. The commoner and less serious form is a symmetrical sensory neuropathy of stocking or (less often) glove distribution. The other, less frequent, form is a mononeuritis of a single peripheral mixed nerve such as the sciatic or popliteal, causing both sensory and motor loss e.g. foot drop. The cause is arteritis in the vessel accompanying the nerve (Fig. 5.6).

Vasculitis. In its simplest form vasculitis causes tiny infarcts in or near the finger tip, such as the classical nailfold lesion (Fig. 5.5). The main digital arteries may also be partially or totally obstructed due to a diffuse thickening of their intima, giving rise to Raynaud's phenomenon or to permanently cold fingers. These arterial lesions are well shown on arteriography. Frank necrosis is uncommon as a result of digital arteritis, but an example is shown in Fig. 5.7. Corresponding lesions in skin vessels of the leg or foot may cause intractable ulceration. Arteritis in bigger vessels is accompanied by a local inflammatory reaction similar to that of polyarteritis nodosa. Rarely such an arteritis may affect a coronary artery (p. 127). Vasculitic lesions are usually multiple and are a sign of a seriously ill patient. Scott et al. (1981) reviewed 50 patients with rheumatoid vasculitis, 15 of whom died as a result of their disease.

The Kidney. Amyloid disease occurs in some 5% of patients with chronic rheumatoid arthritis. The first sign of renal involvement is proteinuria; if the

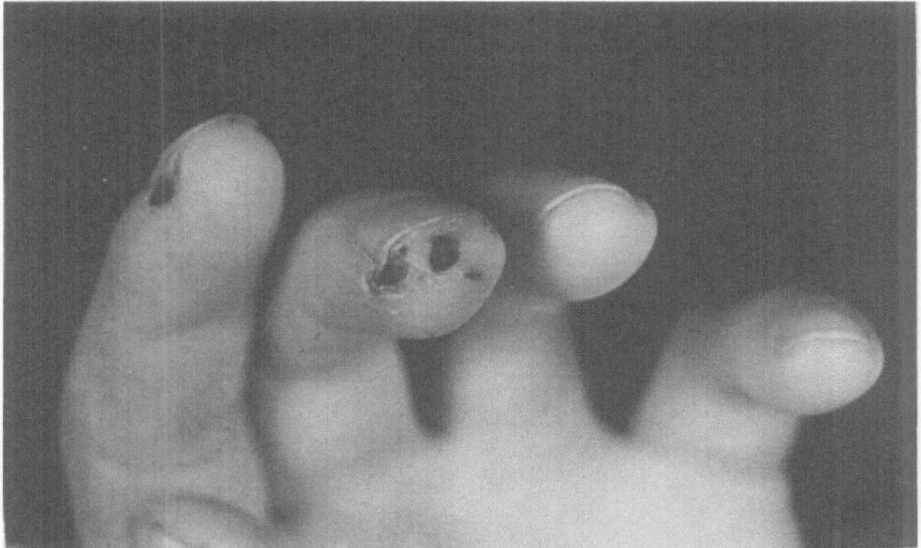

Fig. 5.7. Necrotic lesions at the finger tips due to rheumatoid vasculitis affecting terminal branches of the digital arteries.

renal lesion progresses nephrotic syndrome develops and renal failure is likely to follow. Early diagnosis of amyloid disease can be made on rectal mucosal biopsy. Renal damage may also result from drug therapy, particularly with gold or penicillamine, manifesting with proteinuria. This usually ceases after withdrawal of the drug. Liability to nephrotoxicity is associated with possession of the histocompatibility antigen HLA–DR3.

The Lungs. Rheumatoid nodules may form in the lung tissue, usually towards the apex. The finding of a nodule on chest X-ray films raises diagnostic problems for which the only certain answer is biopsy. Larger nodules may cavitate and if near the pleural surface may rupture and cause pneumothorax. Miners with seropositive rheumatoid arthritis who develop pneumoconiosis tend to develop massive pulmonary nodules and fibrosis, Caplan's syndrome. The most serious pulmonary complication is diffuse interstitial fibrosis. Minor forms of this are not uncommon, but the process can become severe and extensive, producing a form of honeycomb lung with life-threatening impairment of respiratory function.

Pleurisy

Pleurisy, with or without effusion, may occur at any stage of rheumatoid arthritis, presenting subacutely with chest pain and fever. It may accompany the onset of rheumatoid arthritis, and the pleurisy may actually precede the arthritis. Such a presentation is mainly seen in middle-aged men, and the reason for this selectivity is not known. Pleurisy resolves naturally as a rule within a few weeks, although a pleural friction rub may persist painlessly sometimes for months.

Pleural biopsy shows a mononuclear cellular inflammatory reaction with much fibrin. In places an alignment of epithelioid cells is seen, resembling the palisading of such cells in a rheumatoid nodule (Fig. 5.8). The inflamed pleural space has consequently been likened to a large opened-out rheumatoid nodule.

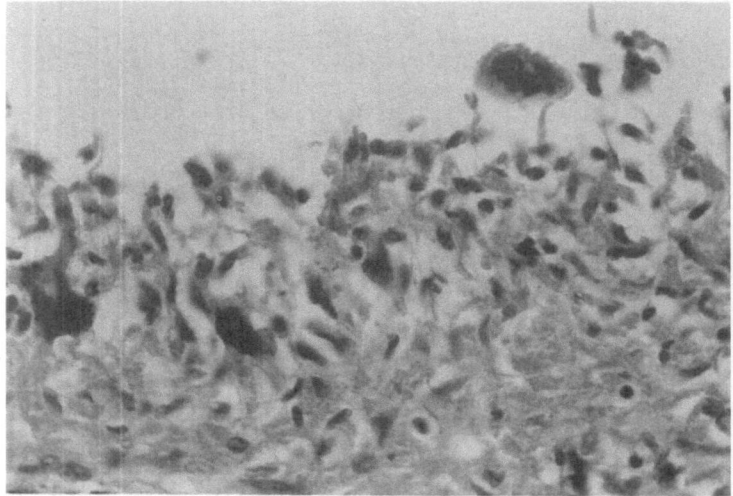

Fig. 5.8. Rheumatoid pleurisy. Section of parietal pleura (× 150) showing the florid cellular response. Note the hint of palisading.

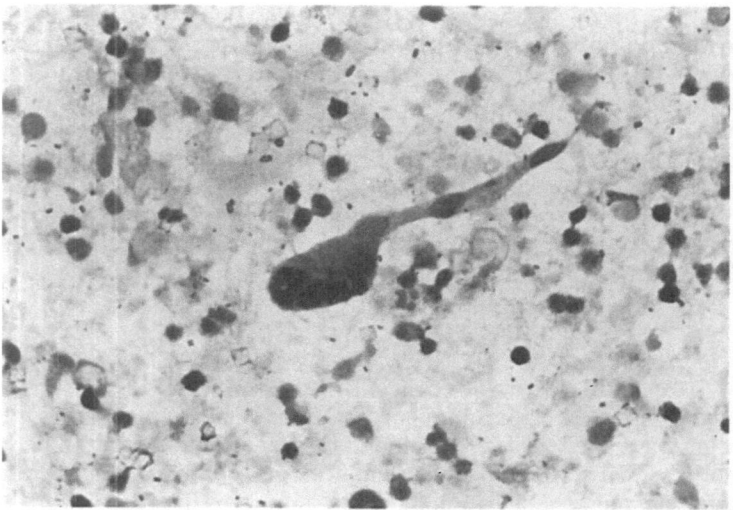

Fig. 5.9. Rheumatoid pleural effusion. Microscopy of centrifuged deposit showing epithelioid "comet cell" (× 150).

The pleural fluid is typically hazy and opaque due to the presence of many cells and cell debris. Among the cells are some, thought to be altered macrophages, with a pink staining cytoplasm which extends into a long narrow tail (Fig. 5.9). These have been called "comet cells' or likened to tadpoles. They are characteristic of rheumatoid pleural or pericardial effusions (Boddington et al. 1971). On centrifuging the fluid an amorphous deposit is obtained in which IgG and rheumatoid factor may be identified. The pleural fluid typically has a low glucose content, well below the plasma level, the difference being attributed to a specific defect in glucose transport across the pleural membrane (Dodson and Hollingsworth 1966)

As a sequel to the effusion there may be much pleural thickening, and it is this which explains the occasional long persistence of a pleural friction rub. If the pleural thickening is so excessive as to hamper the expansion of the lung after the effusion has absorbed, surgical decortication of the lung may be necessary.

Rheumatoid Heart Disease

Summary

Rheumatoid lesions of the heart and pericardium have the same basic pathology as the extra-articular lesions just described, viz. pleurisy, nodules and vasculitis. Different forms of extra-articular lesion, both in the heart and elsewhere, usually occur together.

Pericarditis is the commonest form of cardiac involvement (Table 5.1) and may be accompanied by pleurisy. Although often unrecognised clinically, evidence for current or past pericarditis is found at autopsy in 30% of patients with rheumatoid arthritis.

Table 5.1. Cardiac lesions in rheumatoid arthritis

Pericarditis	Common finding on echocardiography and at autopsy (30%) Often undetected clinically May cause tamponade or constriction
Valve lesions	Uncommon (?1%) Aortic or mitral regurgitation Granuloma in cusp or valve ring or non-specific thickening of cusp May need surgery
Heart block	Rare Granuloma involving conduction system May need pacing
Myocarditis	Pathological finding No apparent clinical significance
Coronary arteritis	Rare

Less often there are granulomas identical in structure with rheumatoid nodules within the heart. They are probably present in 3% at autopsy although they may not have produced any detectable clinical effect. They may develop on the epicardium or in the ventricular myocardium or septum, sometimes in or near the conducting tissue and causing heart block. They may form in the valve ring or in the base of a valve cusp in the mitral or aortic valves causing valvular incompetence. Associated with the granulomas there is usually some infiltration of adjacent myocardium by lymphocytes and plasma cells. This may be extensive enough to be called a myocarditis, but this is a pathological rather than a clinical diagnosis.

Rarely, arteritis in a coronary artery may produce partial or total obstruction of the lumen, resulting in myocardial infarction.

History

Jean-Martin Charcot (1825–1893), renowned for his contributions to neurology, was the first person to recognise pericarditis as a complication of rheumatoid arthritis ("rhumatisme articulaire chronique"). At La Salpetriere he and Cornil made autopsy studies on nine patients with chronic rheumatoid arthritis and found evidence of past pericarditis in four of the nine. He also described the development of acute pericarditis in a woman aged 71 years with rheumatoid arthritis, and in a 10-year-old child during a relapse of juvenile rheumatoid arthritis (Charcot 1881).

Although Charcot himself appears to have distinguished between rheumatic fever and rheumatoid arthritis, it was widely thought at that time that they were merely different phases of the same disease. The occurrence of the Jaccoud type of arthropathy after recurrent attacks of rheumatic fever made this seem possible (see p. 11). Confusion between the two diseases continued well into the twentieth century.

Baggenstoss and Rosenberg (1941) first described the finding at autopsy of granulomatous lesions in the aortic and mitral valves in patients with rheumatoid arthritis. At first they too considered that these were the result of rheumatic fever. But later (1944) they realised that these granulomas were part of the pathology of rheumatoid arthritis.

Bywaters (1950) clarified the issue by showing that rheumatoid heart valve lesions and those that followed rheumatic fever had quite different pathologies. However, as both rheumatoid arthritis and rheumatic fever were (then) common diseases, it was also possible for a patient with rheumatoid arthritis to have, by coincidence, a valve lesion that was the result of rheumatic fever.

Sokoloff (1953) drew attention to the finding of pericarditis in 40% of autopsies on patients with rheumatoid arthritis – more than four times the frequency of its finding in controls. In a later review (1964) he defined specific granulomatous lesions in the heart as a form of rheumatoid heart disease, and differentiated this from rheumatic heart disease and from the aortic valve lesion of ankylosing spondylitis.

Pericarditis

Incidence

Evidence of current or past pericarditis is a frequent autopsy finding in rheumatoid arthritis. Old pericardial adhesions are seen of varying density, sometimes producing complete obliteration of the pericardial sac. Occasionally unsuspected acute pericarditis is discovered. Sokoloff's figure of 40% for the frequency of pericarditis at autopsy has been mentioned above. In other series frequencies ranging from 11% to 50% are given; when eight such series are taken together, totalling 400 autopsies, the frequency of pericarditis averages 30% (Kirk and Cosh 1969).

Yet pericarditis as a clinical finding is unusual in rheumatoid arthritis, and a prevalence of only 2% among 254 hospitalised patients was given by Cathcart and Spodick (1962). The highest figure quoted is 10% among 100 hospitalised patients given careful clinical examination but without echocardiography (Kirk and Cosh 1969; Michet and Hunder 1984).

Jurik and Graudal (1986) during the follow-up of 300 hospital patients with rheumatoid arthritis, without using echocardiography, estimated the annual incidence of pericarditis as 0.34% in women and 0.44% in men. This would mean that among 100 women patients, followed up for 30 years only 10 cases of pericarditis would be found, and among 100 men, only 13 cases.

Echocardiography is the most sensitive method of detecting a pericardial effusion, although it is less able to pick up pericardial thickening or adhesions. A number of reports indicate a prevalence of about 30% in hospital patients found by echocardiography, and a higher figure among patients with nodular rheumatoid arthritis (Bacon and Gibson 1974; MacDonald et al. 1977; Nomeir et al. 1979; Schorn et al. 1976).

Pathology

In its active phase rheumatoid pericarditis repeats in the pericardium the same pattern of inflammatory response as is found in the joint synovium. Both the visceral and parietal surfaces of the pericardium are thickened and oedematous, with the infiltration of lymphocytes and plasma cells which are densely packed in some areas and sparse in others. There is increased vascularity in the deeper layers of parietal pericardium. The pericardial surfaces are covered with a serofibrinous exudate and there is a variable amount of fluid effusion (Figs. 5.10, 5.11, 5.12). After the active inflammatory phase has subsided fibrous adhesions remain, obliterating much of the pericardial cavity. Occasionally there is a thick fibrinous residue with loculi of inspissated fluid, and in rare instances there are adhesions sufficiently dense to constrict the heart's action. In some cases isolated granulomas are found on the epicardial surface, having the histological structure of a rheumatoid nodule (Fig. 5.13); these are not necessarily accompanied by a generalised pericarditis.

The pericardial fluid may be up to 500 or 1000 ml in volume, although 100 to 200 ml is more usual. A volume of fluid above 200 ml appears to be sufficient to produce tamponade. The fluid is pale yellow and is clear or opalescent depending on the amount of fibrin, cells and debris present; it is frankly turbid if there is much fibrin, and it is sometimes blood-stained. The white cells present are mainly polymorphs, in counts up to 5000/mm^3. Some reports describe polymorphs containing inclusion bodies in which IgG and rheumatoid factor have been identified (Ball et al. 1975). "Comet cells" may also be found in the fluid as in pleural effusions (Fig. 5.9).

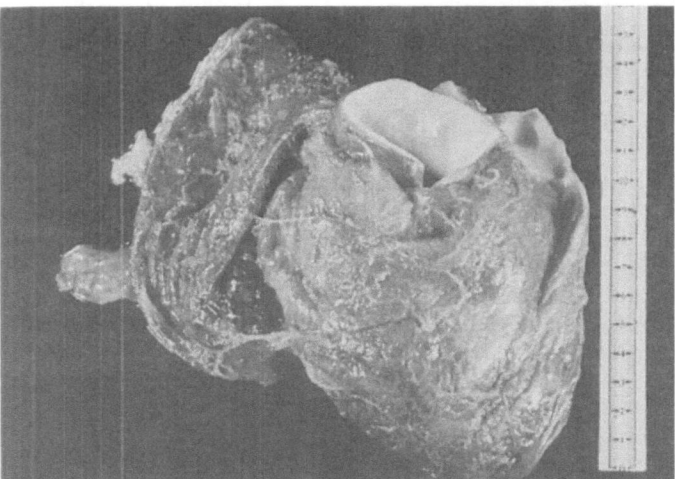

Fig. 5.10. Rheumatoid pericarditis. An active fibrinous pericarditis is seen on both layers of the pericardium; a terminal event in a woman patient with chronic rheumatoid arthritis. She also had aortic incompetence due to a granulomatous valve lesions. (See Fig. 6.4).

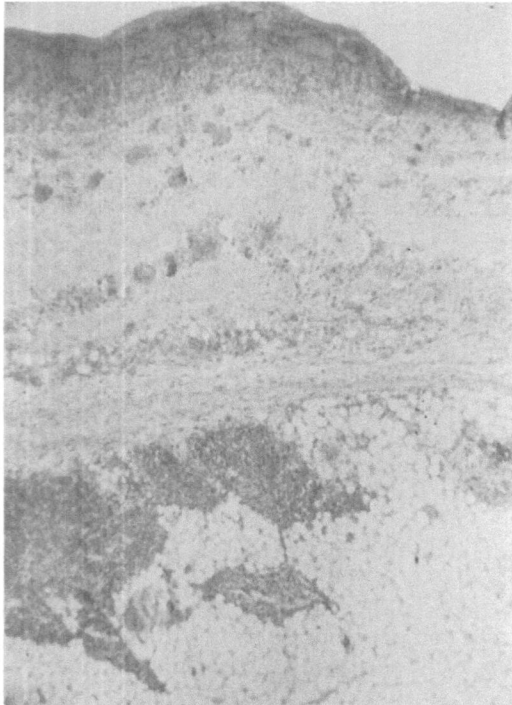

Fig. 5.11. Rheumatoid pericarditis. Histology (× 10) of the pericardium from the same patient as the previous figure. The pericardium is thickened, with oedema, increased vascularity and focal lymphocyte infiltration in the deeper layers.

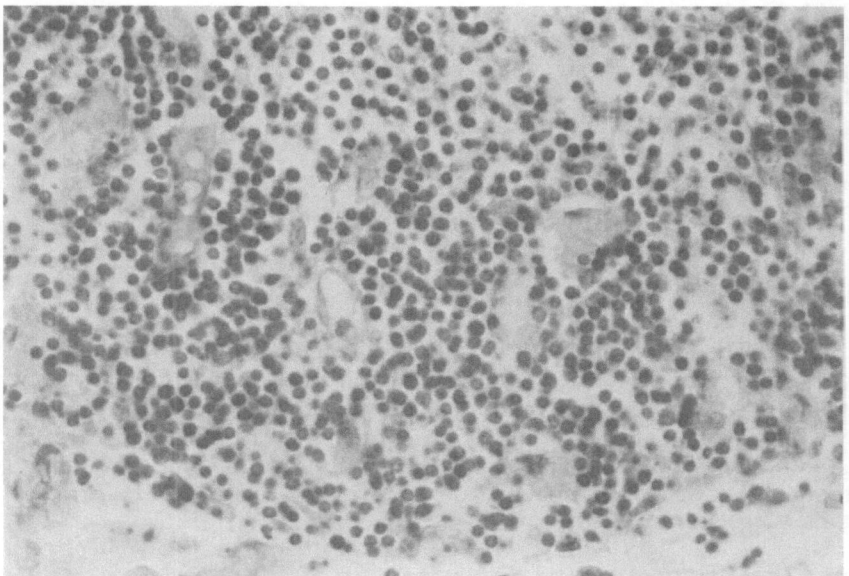

Fig. 5.12. Rheumatoid pericarditis. Histology (× 180) of pericardium from the same patient showing lymphoid aggregation and dilated capillaries.

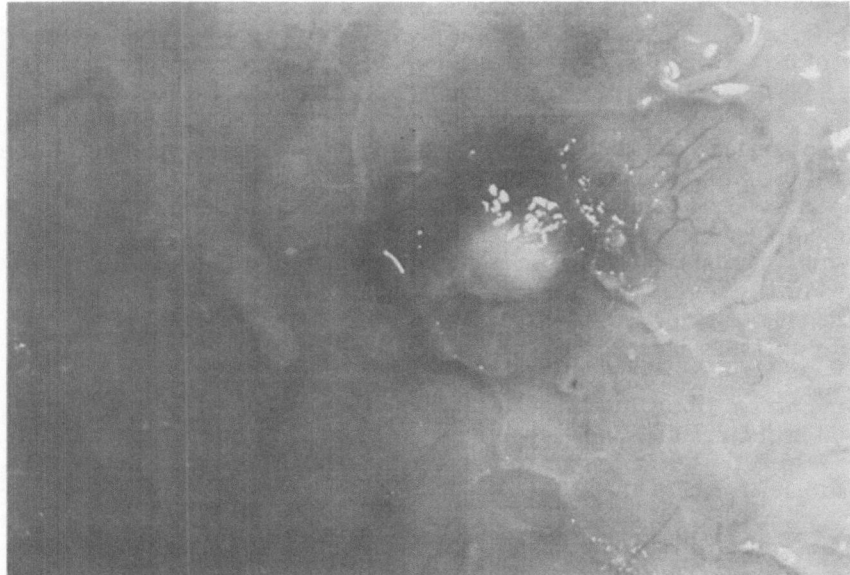

Fig. 5.13. Rheumatoid granuloma 5 mm in diameter, on the surface of the heart.

The fluid contains protein up to 2 or 3 g/100 ml. IgG and rheumatoid factor are found, and immune complexes with a reduced complement level in the fluid, implying that the complexes are being generated locally (Franco et al. 1972; Richards et al. 1976).

The glucose level in the fluid is reduced, even to zero. As with rheumatoid pleural effusions, the low level of glucose is attributed to reduction in glucose transport across the cell membrane of the pericardial lining cells (Dodson and Hollingworth 1966).

Clinical Features

Sex Incidence. The sex incidence of rheumatoid pericarditis shows a female preponderance of 2 or 3 to 1, as for rheumatoid arthritis in general. However, among younger adults the sexes are more equally affected owing to the fact that young and middle-aged men may have pericarditis in the early stages of arthritis. Among the rare cases progressing to constrictive pericarditis there is a definite male preponderance, but this appears to be one of the features of constrictive pericarditis irrespective of its cause.

Duration. The duration of the rheumatoid arthritis at the time of the development of pericarditis is very variable and there is no general pattern. Some patients have pericarditis within months of the onset of arthritis, or even as a presenting feature, while others may have had arthritis for up to 30 or 40 years. The average interval between onset of arthritis and the development of pericarditis in different reports ranges from 3.5 to 10 years (Kirk and Cosh 1969).

Disease Activity. Pericarditis is only found in the presence of active rheumatoid arthritis. Even if the disease seems clinically quiescent, examination will show signs of inflammatory activity such as raised ESR, plasma viscosity or CRP. There is no clear parallel between the severity of the arthritis and the presence of pericarditis, but, in general, pericarditis is more likely to develop in patients with widespread evidence of active arthritis. Virtually all affected patients have classical or definite rheumatoid arthritis and 90% are seropositive. Other extra-articular lesions are usually present as well. About half have nodules, compared with a quarter in rheumatoid arthritis generally. Pleurisy may accompany the pericarditis. There may be signs of vasculitis and the lesions that go with it, such as polyneuritis, scleritis and intracardiac rheumatoid lesions causing aortic or mitral incompetence or heart block (Franco et al. 1972; Kirk and Cosh 1969; Sinclair and Cruickshank 1956).

Juvenile Chronic Polyarthritis. Pericarditis occurs in the polyarthritis of childhood with much the same frequency as in the adult but the situation differs in some respects. This and other forms of cardiac involvement in children are described later (p. 127).

Symptoms. Pericarditis occurs painlessly at least as often as it causes pain. When there is pain it may be a dull retrosternal oppressive ache, or a stabbing central pain, worsened on inspiration and influenced by posture, being worse on lying and relieved when upright. Sometimes the pain of pericarditis is overshadowed by the sharp unilateral pain of accompanying pleurisy. Other symptoms are dyspnoea and cough, and there may be oedema if the pericardial effusion is causing tamponade.

Physical signs. The most significant and pathognomonic sign is a pericardial friction rub; this is not always present, in which case pericarditis can be recognised on other evidence. The intensity of the friction rub ranges from a loud "to and fro" creaking bruit present throughout the cardiac cycle and widely heard over the precordium, to a soft friction sound, heard in a limited area only, and sometimes confined in timing to a part of the cardiac cycle. It may be confused with a soft systolic murmur but is recognisable by its frictional quality. The rub may persist in some patients over a period of weeks or months, and is not necessarily associated with pain; in others it is evanescent being only heard for a day or two or perhaps intermittently. In the absence of a rub pericarditis may be diagnosed from the evidence of X-ray films, electrocardiogram or echocardiogram. Fever is not uncommon while the pericarditis is active, and may reach 39° or more.

Pericardial Effusion. Usually the amount of effusion formed is too small, e.g. under 200 ml, to be detected except by echocardiography. An effusion of moderate size, 200 to 500 ml, is likely to produce radiological changes, and may be enough to cause a rise in central venous pressure. Engorged jugular veins are then seen when the patient lies in a semi-recumbent position, and the height of the venous column of blood may be 10 to 15 cm above the sternal angle (Case History 5.1). With a large effusion, of 500 to 1000 ml, there is an increase in the area of cardiac dullness to percussion, and the friction sound disappears or softens while the heart sound becomes fainter. A big effusion may compress the left lower lobe of lung sufficiently to cause Ewart's sign, namely, dullness to percussion below the left scapula, with bronchial breath sounds in that area.

Case History 5.1

**Rheumatoid pericardial effusion and tamponade
Aspiration of effusion**

Mr. A.H., Transport officer, born 1913

1964	Onset of seropositive arthritis
1966	Disabling lesions in knees
1966/67	Bilateral knee synovectomies and arthroplasties Returned to work
1977	Reactivation arthritis knees and shoulders
1978	General deterioration
22 Nov	Pericardial friction rub Echocardiogram confirms effusion Jugular venous pessure up. Hepatomegaly

6 Dec	Pericardial effusion bigger
	L pleural effusion (Fig. 5.14)
	Pericardial aspiration: 120 ml removed
	Relief of tamponade
	Fluid contained IgG and RF; complement level low
1979	Further deterioration. Hip lesions
	Ischial nodules and ulcer
	Died with bronchopneumonia
Comment	Pericardial effusion and tamponade developing at a late stage, 14 years after onset of RA. Aspiration relieved tamponade. Active progressive seropositive disease

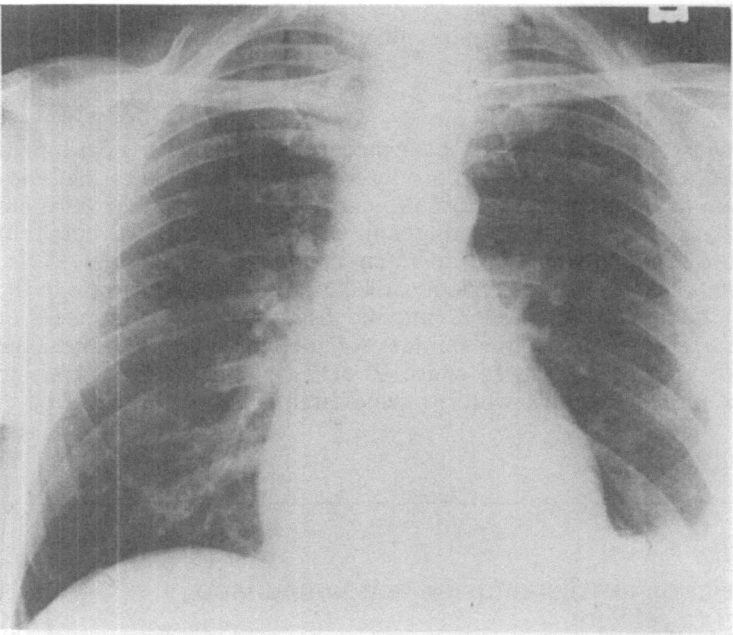

Fig. 5.14.   Rheumatoid pericarditis. Chest X-ray film of the patient described in Case History 5.1. The heart shadow is enlarged owing to the presence of a pericardial effusion; there is also a left pleural effusion.

Cardiac Tamponade. Cardiac tamponade is the disturbance to the heart's action caused by the pressure of fluid surrounding it in the pericardium. It is uncommon in rheumatoid pericarditis, and was seen in only 3 out of 33 patients in one series (Kirk and Cosh 1969). Clinically, tamponade produces changes similar to congestive heart failure: increased jugular venous pressure, engorged and tender liver, dependent oedema and possibly ascites.

Pulsus paradoxus may be seen with tamponade: a brief fall in blood pressure on inspiration. It is due to inspiration causing an increase in the volume of vena caval blood returning to the thorax. This momentarily increases the filling of the right atrium and ventricle and their output. Simultaneously there is a fall in the venous return to the left atrium and ventricle with a reduction in their output, accounting for the brief fall in pulse volume and pressure, lasting only for a few beats. There is still debate as to the reason for the brief reduction in left ventricular function (Fowler 1978). A likely explanation is that the temporary increase in volume of the right atrium and ventricle, within the limited space of the tensely filled pericardium, prevents the left atrium and ventricle from filling normally. There is immediate relief of tamponade on aspiration of the effusion: removal of 120 ml was sufficient in the example given in Case History 5.1.

The production of tamponade is determined as much by the speed of accumulation of an effusion as by its size. An effusion of 200 to 300 ml forming within a day or two may be more disturbing to cardiac function than a much bigger effusion collecting gradually over the course of a month.

Course. The course of pericarditis is usually one of natural resolution over a matter of a week or two. This may happen silently in some cases without the pericarditis ever having been recognised. In a few cases the signs persist for weeks or months before resolving, with the friction rub continually present, usually without pain, as well as the ECG and echocardiographic changes. Ultimately these nearly always return to normal.

Diagnosis of Pericarditis

Pericarditis should be suspected in a patient with active seropositive rheumatoid arthritis who develops chest pain, breathlessness or pleural effusion. A pericardial friction rub should be sought by careful auscultation, repeated daily if necessary, as a friction sound may be faint or transient, but is diagnostic if heard. In the absence of audible friction, the diagnosis may be made on the findings of X-ray, ECG and echocardiography.

If a patient with rheumatoid arthritis presents with signs of congestive heart failure for no obvious reason, tamponade or constrictive pericarditis should be considered. The diagnostic investigations may include paracentesis if investigations suggest a pericardial effusion.

There may be difficulty in recognising pericarditis in the presence of a large pleural effusion or bilateral effusions. If the pleural fluid has a low glucose content rheumatoid disease is the probable cause and pericarditis may well co-exist. Evidence for a pericardial effusion should then be sought by echocardiography.

Chest X-ray. Chest X-ray films show the presence of a pericardial effusion as an overall increase in size of the cardiac shadow, which has a globular shape (Fig. 5.14). With small effusions the only change may be a straightening out of the normal slight concavity of the left border of the heart. Serial films are valuable.

Electrocardiography. The classical ECG change in pericarditis is elevation of the ST segment, with upward-facing concavity, during the acute stage. Subsequently, usually within a matter of days, the ST segment returns to base-line level and the T waves become inverted. This change is due to the effect of the inflammation on the epicardium and as the damage subsides and heals the T waves return to normal. There are no Q waves. But in rheumatoid pericarditis it is unusual to see the full classical changes and in mild cases the ECG may remain normal throughout the episode of pericarditis. This was so in 12 of the 33 cases of rheumatoid pericarditis described by Kirk and Cosh (1969). When there are ECG changes they are of a limited nature, such as temporary flattening or inversion of T waves in all leads (Fig. 5.15). Transient rhythm changes may occur, usually atrial or ventricular ectopic beats or even episodes of atrial fibrillation.

Echocardiography. This is the most sensitive method of demonstrating the presence of a pericardial effusion, which can be shown either by M mode or by

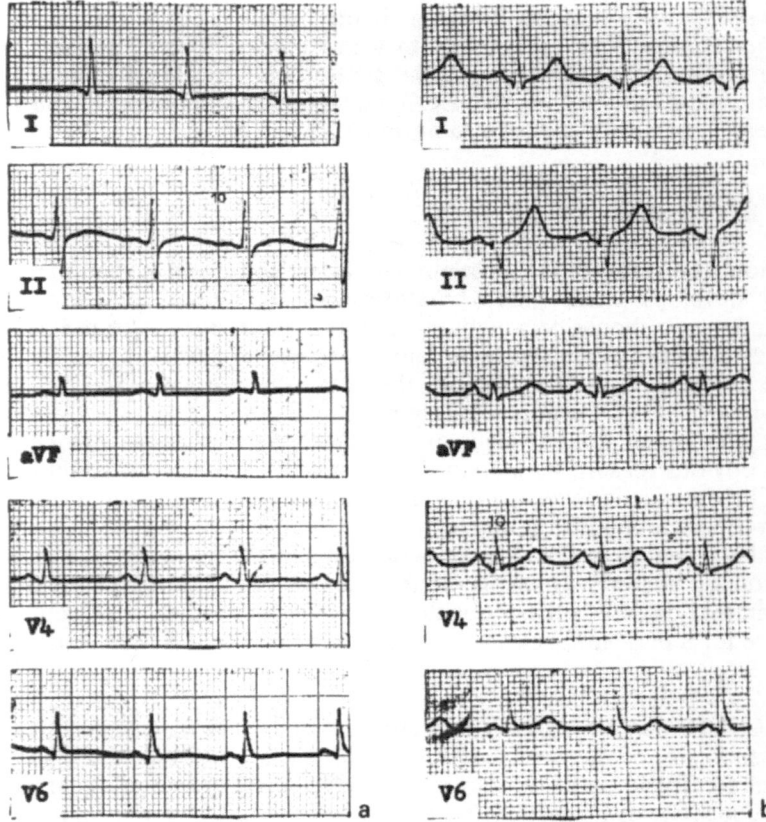

Fig. 5.15a,b. Rheumatoid pericarditis, electrocardiogram. **a** While the pericarditis is active there is general flattening of T waves. **b** Three months later, when the pericarditis has healed, the T waves have returned to normal. (Reproduced with permission from the Quarterly Journal of Medicine).

cross sectional display. A space of up to 2 cm may be shown separating the posterior wall of the left ventricle from the posterior mediastinum, this space corresponding to the fluid in the pericardium. Fluid may also be shown anteriorly as in Fig. 5.16. Sometimes the fluid may be shown to be loculated, mainly posteriorly, and to be surrounded by a thickened pericardium. Other echocardiographic findings in rheumatoid heart disease, relating to the valves, are discussed in the next chapter.

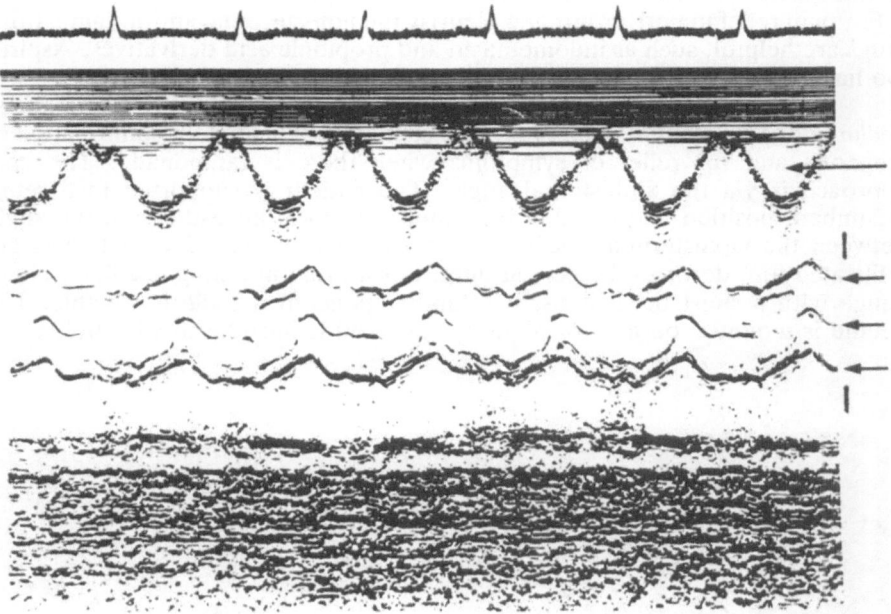

Fig. 5.16. Echocardiogram showing pericardial fluid anteriorly (*upper arrow*) in a patient with rheumatoid pericarditis. The *lower three arrows* show the walls of the aorta and (*centre*) the aortic cusps opening and closing. (By courtesy of Dr. FGM Ross.)

Laboratory Investigations. The blood changes are those of active seropositive rheumatoid arthritis and there are no specific changes associated with pericarditis. Leucocytosis is not a feature. Tests for circulating antibodies are likely to be positive, with reduction in complement level.

Treatment of Pericarditis

The treatment of rheumatoid pericarditis is basically the treatment of rheumatoid disease itself, with aspiration of an effusion if necessary, combined with intra-pericardial steroid injection. Rarely surgical relief may be needed for chronic tamponade or for pericardial constriction.

Whenever there are serious extra-articular lesions such as pericarditis or vasculitis it is important that therapy should include long-term anti-inflammatory drugs such as gold, penicillamine or immunosuppressants. Systemic corticosteroid treatment may be considered advisable for an acutely ill patient but should be regarded as a remedy that should be reduced and withdrawn when possible, or at least continued at a low maintenance dose of not more than 5 mg prednisone or its equivalent daily. In combination with steroid treatment one of the long-term anti-inflammatory agents is introduced. It is doubtful whether systemic steroids have any effect in hastening the resolution of pericarditis or an effusion, but an intra-pericardial steroid injection does appear effective, just as an intra-articular steroid injection is in an inflamed joint.

For pain relief in pericarditis and pleurisy the non-steroidal anti-inflammatory drugs are helpful, such as indomethacin and propionic acid derivatives. Aspirin too has a place.

Technique of Pericardial Aspiration. Paracentesis is indicated for confirmation of diagnosis and for relief of symptoms when there is tamponade. The best approach is via the xiphisternal angle. The patient is supported in a semi-recumbent position and the skin infiltrated with local anaesthetic in the angle between the xiphisternum and the left costal margin. The deeper tissues are infiltrated too, down to the pericardium. For aspiration a long needle of No. 1 gauge with a short bevel is used; a lumbar puncture needle is suitable. The needle is mounted on a 20 or 50 ml syringe and is introduced with full sterile

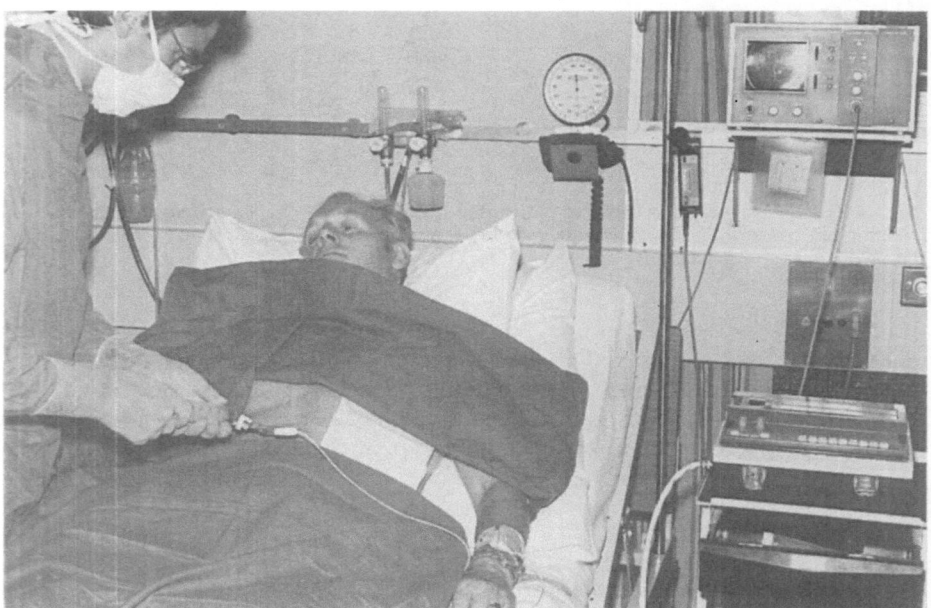

Fig. 5.17. Aspiration of pericardium seen here in the setting of the coronary care unit. The xiphisternal approach is being used and the aspirating needle is connected to the ECG monitor. Aspiration may equally well be carried out in the ward. (By courtesy of Dr. RD Thomas.)

precautions, with the patient relaxed and breathing quietly. The needle is directed inwards and slightly upwards and laterally, as though aiming at the inferior angle of the left scapula (Fig. 5.17). At a depth of about 5 cm the needle tip is felt to penetrate the diaphragm. It is then advanced gently while keeping up suction on the syringe. Fluid should now be obtained. If there is much to be withdrawn a 3-way tap is helpful between syringe and needle, and unnecessary needle movements should be reduced to a minimum during the procedure.

The risk of penetrating the myocardium is slight. But if there is movement at the tip of the needle suggesting that the surface of the heart has been touched, the needle is withdrawn slightly and advanced again in a slightly lower direction. As a precaution paracentesis may be done under ECG control by attaching the chest lead electrode to the base of the aspirating needle, while the limb electrodes are attached in the normal way. Should the needle tip penetrate the myocardium a change in the pattern of the recording from the chest lead is seen, with a current of injury, i.e. ST elevation and T wave changes.

An alternative approach to the pericardium is via the cardiac apex. The appropriate entry point is chosen with the help of a current chest film or with fluoroscopy. The entry point is in the 5th or 6th intercostal space, just within the limit of the cardiac shadow but just lateral to the apex beat, if this is palpable. On entry the needle is directed inwards, upwards and medially, as though aiming at the point of the right shoulder.

If tamponade is present, as much fluid as possible should be withdrawn. A yield of 200 ml or more may be obtained although withdrawal of less than this can be enough to relieve intrapericardial pressure. Subsequently, if signs of tamponade recur, as they may do within a few days, further aspiration is indicated.

Steroid may be injected while the needle tip is within the pericardium. Long-acting preparations are used in doses similar to those injected into a large joint such as the knee, e.g. prednisolone acetate 25 mg or triamcinolone hexacetonide 20 mg. This appears to promote the absorption of any remaining fluid and to encourage resolution of the pericarditis.

Complications of Pericarditis

Haemopericardium. Frank haemorrhage into the pericardium, as distinct from blood-staining of pericardial fluid, is not characteristic. A few cases are on record of spontaneous haemopericardium apparently originating from vessels in the inflamed pericardium. The presence of blood in the pericardial cavity, whatever the underlying pathology, promotes a fibrous reaction and can be a factor in the progression to constrictive pericarditis and later calcification (Handforth and Woodbury 1959).

Infection. Although purulent pericarditis is seen with a variety of causative organisms (Klacsmann et al. 1977) infection normally plays no part in rheumatoid pericarditis. There are a few reports of secondary infection, apparently blood-borne and usually staphylococcal, complicating pre-existing rheumatoid pericarditis (Gallagher and Gresham 1973; Marshall et al. 1979). This situation is analogous to septic arthritis occurring as a complication of rheumatoid arthritis, usually associated with septicaemia. In either case the patient is often frail and debilitated, with long-standing rheumatoid arthritis, and has a poor prognosis in spite of antibiotic treatment.

Constrictive Pericarditis. This is a rare sequel to rheumatoid pericarditis, but is of relatively more significance today than formerly owing to the virtual disappearance of the previously leading cause of constrictive pericarditis, tuberculosis (Editorial BMJ 1979). Among 32 patients operated on for constrictive pericarditis over a 15-year-period in Dublin, four were attributed to rheumatoid disease and four to tuberculosis, but in the majority, 21, the pathology was uncertain (Blake et al. 1983). The incidence of rheumatoid constrictive pericarditis is certainly very low; only one case has arisen in a series of 100 rheumatoid patients followed from the onset of their disease for 25 years (Reilly et al. 1989). This represents one case in some 1800 patient-years. Thould (1986) found five cases among a total of 2203 patients with rheumatoid arthritis referred to hospital.

In constrictive pericarditis, unlike the situation with simple obliterative adhesions, the pericardium is up to 5 mm thick, sometimes enclosing a quantity of loculated fluid. It is tough enough to prevent effective ventricular filling in diastole. There may also be an intermediate condition of chronic tamponade which is peculiar to rheumatoid pericarditis. In this there is a mixture of chronic fibrous thickening and much deposition of fibrin with inspissated fluid causing persistent tamponade. At operation the thickened pericardium is found to contain a quantity of semifluid sterile fibrinous mush, at first sight suggesting pus (Case History 5.2) (Kennedy et al. 1966; Thadani et al. 1975).

Case History 5.2
Rheumatoid pericarditis
Chronic tamponade: Pericardectomy

Mrs. M.D., Housewife, born 1935

1960	Onset of seropositive rheumatoid arthritis
1964	Thyrotoxicosis. Treated with propyl thiouracil, later with radio-iodine
1966	Transient pericarditis noted
1971	Pericardial rub, pleural effusion Minor increase in jugular venous pressure L hip arthroplasty
1972	Still signs of minor tamponade R hip arthroplasty
1975	Duodenal ulcer. Course of myocrysin
1975–8	Variable degree of mild tamponade
1977	Bilateral ankle arthroplasties
1978 Aug	Increasing signs of tamponade

1978 Nov	*Pericardectomy*: thickened pericardium removed from front of heart and 400 ml mushy fibrinous fluid released
1980	Good progress
Comment	Signs of pericarditis and minor tamponade present intermittently for 12 years with few symptoms. Priority given to hip and ankle surgery. Increasing tamponade necessitated relief

Rheumatoid constrictive pericarditis is commoner in men than in women by about 2:1. This unexplained male predominance is characteristic of constrictive pericarditis in general and also of rheumatoid pleural and pulmonary lesions. Constriction may develop at any stage of rheumatoid arthritis. In one series of 24 cases the average duration of arthritis was 8 years and the average age of the patients was 54 years. Three of the 24 had rheumatoid aortic valve lesions and one had heart block (Cosh and Iveson 1979).

The clinical presentation of constrictive pericarditis suggests congestive heart failure. As with tamponade, there is dyspnoea, congestion of neck veins, engorgement of the liver sometimes with ascites, and oedema of the lower limbs. The jugular venous pressure may be seen to rise with inspiration (Kussmaul's sign) and there may be pulsus paradoxus. Pericardial friction is absent but there is usually a third heart sound in diastole. Apart from the absence of a friction rub the signs are the same as those seen with tamponade. But while tamponade may develop over a matter of days and call for rapid relief by paracentesis, constrictive pericarditis develops slowly and is initially less urgent but eventually will need surgery. Case History 5.3 describes a patient in whom the interval between the development of a pericardial effusion and constriction was 10 months.

Case History 5.3

Rheumatoid arthritis
Constrictive pericarditis: Pericardectomy

Mrs. L.F., Housewife, born 1905

1958	Onset of seropositive rheumatoid arthritis
1959	Deterioration. Steroid treatment started
1964	Fractured fibula, osteoporosis Haematemesis for gastric ulcer
1965 Jan	R pleural and pericardial effusions
July	Tamponade with dyspnoea, hepatomegaly, oedema
Oct	Increasing jugular venous pressure Pulsus paradoxus. Triple rhythm
Nov	Cardiac catheter confirmed diagnosis of constrictive pericarditis

Dec   *Pericardectomy* Initially successful
Fatal pulmonary embolus post-operatively

Comment   Progression from development of pericardial effusion to
proven constriction took 10 months. Thickened pericardium
was removed effectively but death from pulmonary embolus
followed next day

The diagnosis is confirmed by cardiac catheterisation: the right ventricular pressure trace is seen to have a sharp step up in the latter half of diastole (Fig. 5.18). This is due to the constrictive effect of the thickened pericardium on the ventricle as it fills in diastole (Editorial *Lancet* 1987).

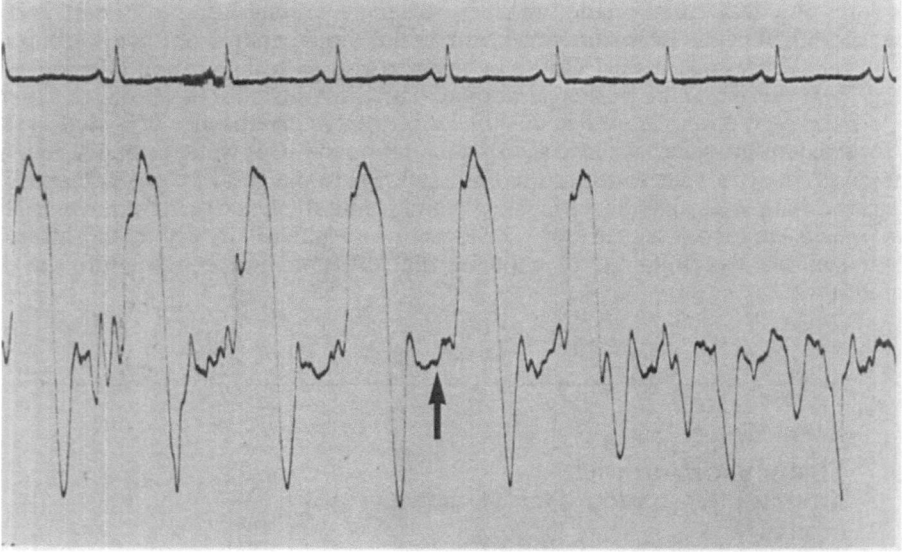

Fig. 5.18. Pressure recording from the right ventricle (*on left*) and right atrium (*on right*) in a patient with constrictive pericarditis. Note the sharp step up in diastolic pressure to a "plateau" in the latter part of the diastole in the right ventricle (*arrowed*). This is due to the constricting effect of the thickened pericardium checking the expansion of the ventricle as it fills in diastole. (By courtesy of Dr. DW Barritt.)

Surgery. Pericardectomy is indicated for relief of chronic tamponade (Case History 5.2) or of constrictive pericarditis (Case History 5.3). Once the decision has been taken to seek surgical advice action should be taken without delay, as a few days may be needed for preliminary investigation and the patient's condition may deteriorate. The diagnosis is first confirmed by cardiac catheterisation and intracardiac pressure recording. An estimation of the thickness of the pericardium may be obtained from echocardiography or angiocardiography.

The usual surgical approach is by mid-line sternal splitting incision. The aim is to remove as much as possible of the thickened pericardium, particularly over the ventricles and if possible an attempt should be made to remove the thickened epicardium.

The patient's response to an effective pericardectomy is prompt and very satisfactory. A successful result from pericardectomy was achieved in 21 out of 24 patients reviewed by Cosh and Iveson (1979), the causes of failure being other cardiac pathology, such as rheumatoid valve lesions or coronary disease. In the absence of such complications, the patient, arthritis permitting, is able to resume an active life once again (John et al. 1979).

References

Bacon PA, Gibson DG (1974) Cardiac involvement in rheumatoid arthritis. Echocardiographic study of 22 rheumatoid arthritis patients with nodules and 22 without. Ann Rheum Dis 33: 20–24

Baggenstoss AH, Rosenberg EF (1941) Cardiac lesions associated with chronic infectious (rheumatoid) arthritis. Arch Intern Med 67: 241–248

Baggenstoss AH, Rosenberg EF (1944) Unusual cardiac lesions associated with chronic multiple rheumatoid arthritis. Arch Pathol Chicago 37: 54–60

Ball GV, Schrohenloher R, Hester R (1975) Gamma globulin complexes in rheumatoid pericardial fluid. Am J Med 58: 122–128

Blake S, Bonar S, O'Neill H et al. (1983) Aetiology of chronic constrictive pericarditis. Br Heart J 50: 273–276

Boddington MM, Spriggs AI, Morton JA, Mowat AG (1971) Cytodiagnosis of rheumatoid pleural effusions. J Clin Pathol 24: 95–106

Bywaters EGL (1950) The relation between heart and joint disease including "rheumatoid heart disease" and chronic post-rheumatic arthritis (Type Jaccoud). Br Heart J 12: 101–131

Calin A, Marks SH (1981) The case against seronegative rheumatoid arthritis. Am J Med 70: 992–994

Carson DA (1982) Antiglobulin antibodies. In: Panayi GS (ed) The scientific basis of rheumatology. Churchill Livingstone, London, pp 114–130

Cathcart ES, Spodick DH (1962) Rheumatoid heart disease. N Engl J Med 266: 959–964

Charcot JM (1881) Clinical lectures on senile and chronic diseases. Translated into English by Tuke WS. The New Sydenham Society, London.

Cosh JA, Iveson M (1979) Constrictive pericarditis and rheumatoid arthritis. Ann Rheum Dis 38: 490–491

Decker JL, Malone DG, Haraoui B et al. (1984) Rheumatoid arthritis: evolving concepts of pathogenesis and treatment. Ann Intern Med 101: 810–824

Dodson WH, Hollingsworth JW (1966) Pleural effusion in rheumatoid arthritis. Impaired transport of glucose. N Engl J Med 275: 1337–1342

Editorial (1979) Rheumatoid constrictive pericarditis. Br Med J 2: 755

Editorial (1987) Restrictive cardiomyopathy or constrictive pericarditis? Lancet II: 372–374

Ellman P, Ball RE (1948) Rheumatoid disease with joint and pulmonary manifestations. Br Med J 2: 816–820

Fowler NO (1978) Physiology of cardiac tamponade and pulsus paradoxus. Mod Concepts Cardiovasc Dis 47: 109–118

Franco AE, Levine HD, Hall AP (1972) Rheumatoid pericarditis: report of 17 cases diagnosed clinically. Ann Intern Med 77: 837–844

Gallagher PJ, Gresham GA (1973) Heart block with infected rheumatoid granulomas. Br Heart J 35: 110–112

Handforth CP, Woodbury JFL (1959) Cardiovascular manifestations of rheumatoid arthritis. Can Med Assoc J 80: 86–90

Jacoby RK, Jayson MIV, Cosh JA (1973) Onset, early stages of prognosis of rheumatoid arthritis; a clinical study of 100 patients with 11 year follow up. Br Med J 1: 96–100

Jaraquemada D, Ollier W, Awad J et al. (1986) HLA and rheumatoid arthritis: a combined analysis of 440 British patients. Ann Rheum Dis 45: 627–636

John JT, Hough A, Sergent JS (1979) Pericardial disease in rheumatoid arthritis. Am J Med 66: 385–390

Jurik AG, Graudal H (1986) Pericarditis in rheumatoid arthritis: a clinical and radiographic study. Rheumatol Int 6: 37–42

Kennedy WPU, Partridge REH, Matthews MB (1966) Rheumatoid pericarditis with cardiac failure treated by pericardectomy. Br Heart J 28: 602–608

Kirk JA, Cosh JA (1969) The pericarditis of rheumatoid arthritis. Q J Med 38: 397–423

Klacsmann PG, Bulkley BH, Hutchins GM (1977) The changed spectrum of purulent pericarditis. Am J Med 63: 666–673

Krane SM, Simon LS (1986) Rheumatoid arthritis: clinical features and pathogenetic mechanisms. Med Clin North Am 70: 263–284

MacDonald WJ, Crawford MH, Klippel JH et al. (1977) Echocardiographic assessment of cardiac structure and function in patients with rheumatoid arthritis. Am J Med 63: 890–896

Marshall AJ, Brownlee WC, Keen G (1979) Constrictive pericarditis, pyopericardium and tamponade with rheumatoid arthritis. Ann Rheum Dis 38: 387–389

McDermott M, Molloy M, Cashin P et al. (1986) A multicase family study of rheumatoid arthritis in SW Ireland. Disease Markers 4: 103–111

Michet CJ, Hunder GG (1984) Pericarditis. In: Ansell BM, Simkin PA (eds). The heart and rheumatic disease. Butterworths, London, pp 1–26

Nomeir AM, Turner RA, Watts LE (1976) Cardiac involvement in rheumatoid arthritis. Arthritis Rheum 22: 561–564

Rasker JJ, Cosh JA (1981) Cause and age at death in a prospective study of one hundred patients with rheumatoid arthritis. Ann Rheum Dis 40: 115–120

Rasker JJ, Kuipers FC (1983) Are rheumatoid nodules caused by vasculitis? A study of 13 early cases. Ann Rheum Dis 42: 384–388

Reilly PA, Cosh JA, Rasker JJ, Maddison PJ (1989) A 25 year prospective study of 100 patients with rheumatoid arthritis. Ann Rheum Dis 48: in press.

Richards AJ, Koehler BE, Broder I, Gordon DA (1976) Rheumatoid pericarditis: a comparison of immunologic characteristics of pericardial fluid, synovial fluid and serum. J Rheumatol 3: 275–278

Ropes MW, Bennett GA, Cobb S et al. (1958) Revised diagnostic criteria for rheumatoid arthritis. Bull Rheum Dis 9: 175–176

Schorn D, Hough IP, Anderson IF (1976) The heart in rheumatoid arthritis. S Afr Med J 50: 8–10

Scott DGI, Bacon PA, Tribe CR (1981) Systemic rheumatoid vasculitis: a clinical and laboratory study of 50 cases. Medicine (Baltimore) 60: 288–297

Sinclair RJG, Cruickshank B (1956) A clinical and pathological study of 16 cases of rheumatoid arthritis with extensive visceral involvement ("Rheumatoid disease"). Q J Med 25: 313–332

Sokoloff L (1953) The heart in rheumatoid arthritis. Am Heart J 45: 635–643

Sokoloff L (1964) Cardiac involvement in rheumatoid arthritis and allied disorders: current concepts. Mod Concepts Cardiovasc Dis 33: 847–850

Stastny P (1978) Association of the B cell alloantigen HLA–DRw4 with rheumatoid arthritis. N Engl J Med 298: 869–871

Thadani U, Iveson JMI, Wright V (1975) Cardiac tamponade, constrictive pericarditis and pericardial resection in rheumatoid pericarditis. Medicine (Baltimore) 54: 261–270

Thould AK (1986) Constrictive pericarditis in rheumatoid arthritis. Ann Rheum Dis 45: 89–94

Walker DJ, Griffiths ID (1986) HLA associations are with severe rheumatoid arthritis. Disease Markers 4: 121–132

Chapter 6

Rheumatoid Heart Disease II: Valve Lesions, Heart Block, Juvenile Arthritis

Valve Lesions

Rheumatoid heart valve lesions are uncommon, but when they do occur they are serious and potentially life-threatening. Aortic incompetence is the most important, capable of causing progressive, sometimes rapid, deterioration in valve function likely to require surgery. The other main lesion, mitral incompetence, is rather less serious. No significant stenosis occurs at these valves. Minor pathological changes are relatively common autopsy findings at any of the four valves, but are of little clinical significance.

Incidence

As with rheumatoid pericarditis, there is a considerable difference between the frequency of rheumatoid valve lesions found at autopsy and their frequency on clinical observation.

Autopsy Studies. In his classical report on 100 hearts examined at autopsies on rheumatoid patients, Cruickshank (1958) noted five examples of granulomas in relation to the aortic and mitral valves, all small and previously undetected. Only one was large enough to be visible by the naked eye and the remainder were only identified on microscopy. In addition he found nine examples of non-specific endocardial lesions. Sokoloff (1964) gave an estimate of 10% for granulomatous lesions, based on a number of published reports, including Cruickshank's.

In a later review of autopsy findings Iveson and Pomerance (1977) concluded that cardiac rheumatoid granulomas occurred in 3% and non-specific lesions in a further 10%. They suggested that the latter represented the late, healing stage of earlier granulomas.

Clinical Studies. To the rheumatologist, rheumatoid aortic or mitral valve lesions are a rarity, with a frequency of under 1% of patients with rheumatoid arthritis.

In a 25-year prospective study of 100 rheumatoid patients, during which time 63 died, there were no examples of valve lesions, although three patients died as a result of other forms of rheumatoid heart disease. Two had heart block (one is described in Case History 6.4) and one had constrictive pericarditis (Case History 5.3) (Rasker and Cosh 1981; Reilly et al. 1989).

The cardiac surgeon sees a more selected group of patients. In the Leeds Cardiothoracic Unit five examples of rheumatoid aortic incompetence were seen over a period of 5 years; four had successful valve replacements. During that time 150 aortic replacements were carried out in all, giving an incidence of 3% for rheumatoid lesions (Iveson et al. 1975). A similar incidence of 3% was given in a report by Qaiyumi et al. (1984). They reviewed 100 patients with aortic incompetence (96 men, 3 women) referred to a veteran's hospital for assessment and possible heart surgery; they found three with rheumatoid and seven with spondylitic valve lesions.

Echocardiography may reveal a valve abnormality that is otherwise unsuspected, particularly of the mitral valve. Slowing of the rate of mitral cusp closure was noted in up to 25% of rheumatoid patients examined in this way and was thought to indicate chronic inflammatory changes in the valve (MacDonald et al. 1977; Mody et al. 1987; Nomeir et al. 1979; Schorn et al. 1976). The occasional finding of extreme slowing of mitral cusp movement was thought by Bacon and Gibson (1974) to indicate the presence of a major granulomatous lesion, although this could not be confirmed.

Pathology

Both specific and non-specific pathological lesions may occur in the valve ring or cusps of the aortic or mitral valves. The bigger lesions cause valvular incompetence, but many of the smaller ones are undetectable clinically.

The specific lesion is a granuloma of the same basic formation as a rheumatoid nodule, i.e. a central core of necrotic fibrinoid material surrounded by epithelioid cells in a rough palisade pattern, beyond which is an area of round cell infiltration and fibroblasts (Fig. 6.1). Granulomas in the heart are often multiple, being found in the myocardium, pericardium, valve rings and cusps and occasionally in the aortic wall (Carpenter et al. 1967; Goehrs et al. 1960; Reimer et al. 1976; Roberts et al. 1968). They range in diameter from 1 mm to 10 mm or more. Figure 6.2 shows a granuloma in the base of an aortic valve cusp, which is thickened, distorted and incompetent as a result. The mitral valve may be affected in the same way; both valves were involved in the heart shown in Fig. 6.2 and 6.3. Smaller granulomas within the cusp itself produce diffuse thickening and incompetence (Fig. 6.4). Occasionally such a lesion may perforate through the cusp producing fenestration with worsened incompetence (Fig. 6.5). Rupture of a granulomatous lesion has also been known to produce a fistula between a sinus of Valsalva and the right atrium (Howell et al. 1972).

Non-specific lesions are commoner, possibly representing the final, healed stage of a granuloma. They also produce cusp thickening with irregular fibrosis, a variable degree of round cell infiltration and some increase in vascularity (Fig. 6.6). Calcification may follow later on in long standing lesions (Case History 6.1).

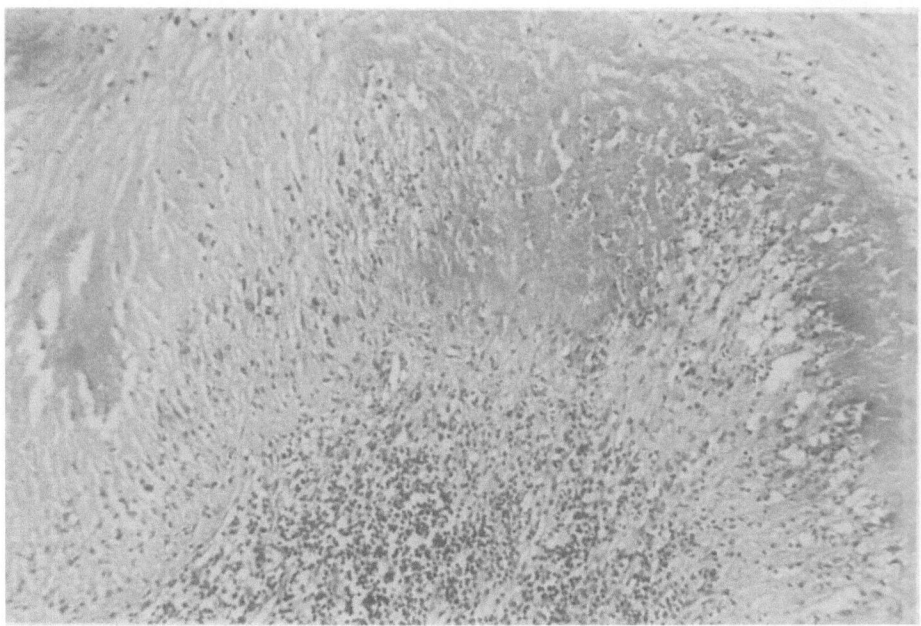

Fig. 6.1.   Rheumatoid granuloma in aortic valve cusp. Histology of a granuloma within a thickened aortic valve cusp in a patient with severe aortic regurgitation (Case History 6.2) showing the necrotic centre. ($\times$ 40)

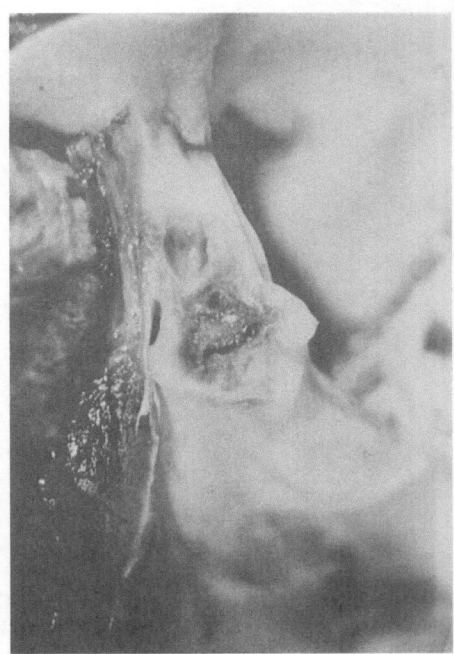

Fig. 6.2.   Rheumatoid granuloma in aortic valve cusp. Close-up view of a granuloma 10 mm in diameter lying at the base of an aortic valve cusp: see Fig. 6.3 and Case History 6.1.

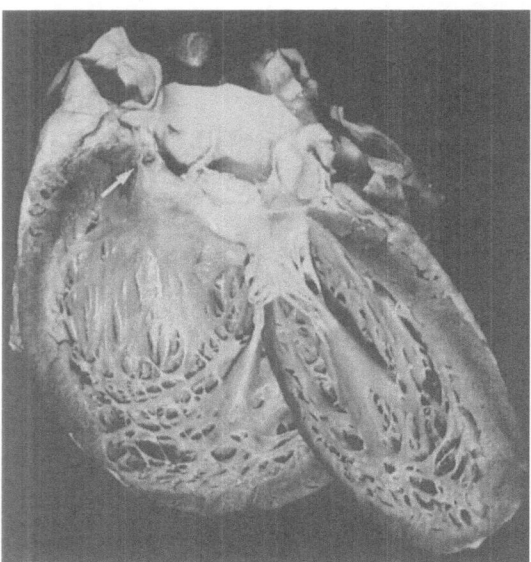

Fig. 6.3. Left ventricle and aortic valve as seen at autopsy in the patient described in Case History 6.1. The ventricle is dilated and hypertrophied as a result of gross aortic regurgitation; the aortic valve cusps are thickened and incompetent and there is a granuloma (*arrowed*) at the base of one cusp (see Fig. 6.2). The mitral valve is also thickened and incompetent.

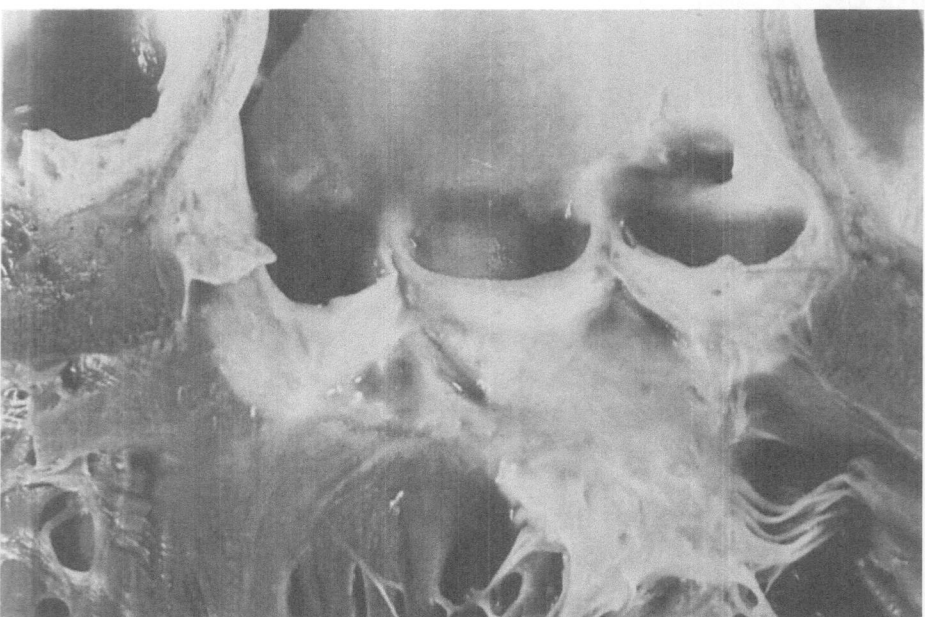

Fig. 6.4. Rheumatoid aortic valve lesion. Diffuse granulomatous infiltration has produced thickening of the cusps with incompetence, and there is a well-marked endocardial jet lesion below the valve. This patient also had florid pericarditis, shown in Fig. 5.10.

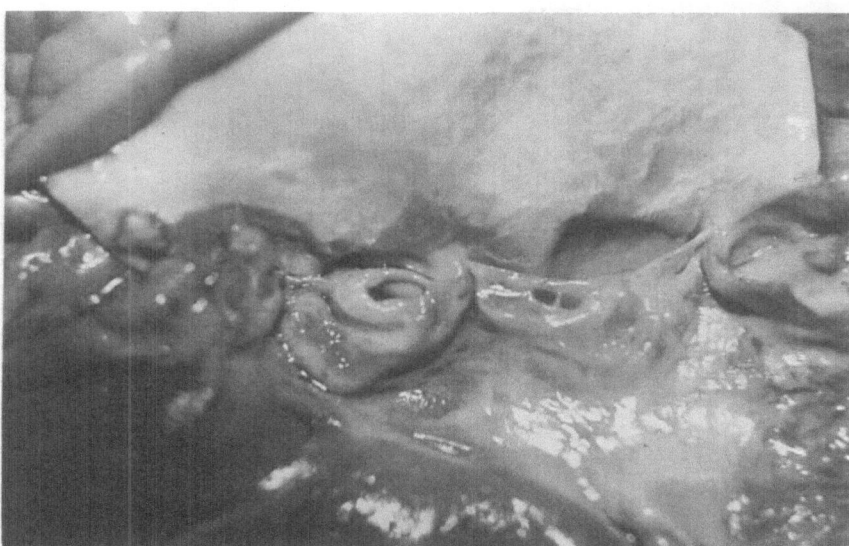

Fig. 6.5. Aortic valve from a patient with rheumatoid arthritis. There is thickening and perforation of two cusps (fenestration), adding to the valvular incompetence. Note the regurgitant jet lesion below the valve.

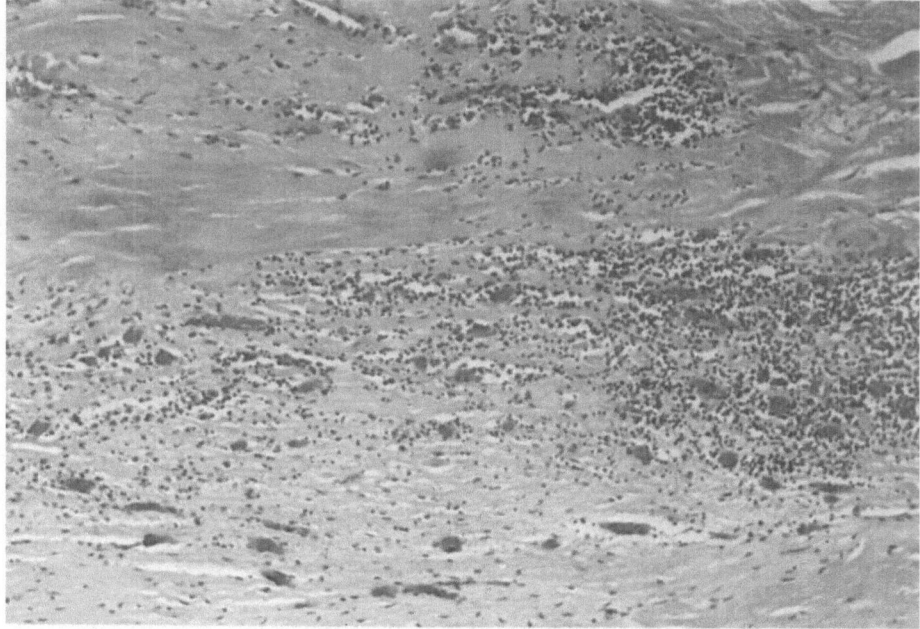

Fig. 6.6. Non-specific rheumatoid valve lesion. Histology of tissue at the base of an incompetent aortic valve showing increased vascularity, diffuse round cell infiltration and fibrosis (× 50).

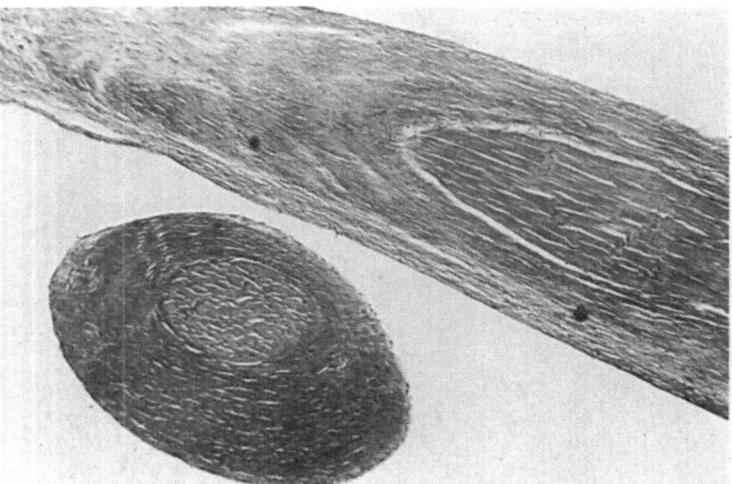

Fig. 6.7. Chordae tendineae from the mitral valve of the patient described in Case History 6.1. Cross-section of the two chordae (× 40) shows the thick layer of laminated fibrin deposited on the surface of each, associated with mitral regurgitation.

Case History 6.1
Rheumatoid arthritis
Aortic and mitral valve lesions

Mr. W.P., Engineer, born 1906

1949	Onset of seropositive RA
1953	Arthritis disabling, hands, feet, knees . Gold therapy started
1959	Aortic systolic and diastolic murmurs Mitral presystolic and mid-diastolic murmurs No cardiomegaly
1963 Aug	Attacks of LV failure
1963 Dec	Hospital admission with congestive failure Free aortic regurgitation Mitral pansystolic murmur
1964 Jan	Died
Autopsy	Heart much enlarged: 710 g LV dilated and hypertrophied (Fig. 6.3) Aortic valve cusps thickened, rolled margins, slight adhesions at commissures. Large granuloma at base of R coronary cusp (Fig. 6.2) Mitral valve cusps and chordae thickened (Fig. 6.7) Some adhesion at commissures. Scattered areas of calcification in both aortic and mitral valve rings

Clinical Features

Rheumatoid valve lesions are found in either sex, with a female preponderance reflecting the sex incidence of rheumatoid arthritis as a whole. All patients are seropositive with definite or classical rheumatoid arthritis and there are nodules and other extra-articular lesions in most. Disability due to the arthritis is usually considerable, but this is not always so, and aortic valve lesions have been recorded in patients with minimal arthritis (Good et al. 1970; Lefkowitz et al. 1968).

Patients may be of any age from childhood up to 70 years or more, and the duration of arthritis at the time of discovery of the valve lesions ranges from 1 year to over 30 years.

Most clinical reports are of aortic incompetence and less often mitral incompetence or combined aortic and mitral lesions. Occasionally other rheumatoid heart lesions are also present, such as pericarditis or heart block. At least 40 examples of aortic incompetence due to rheumatoid disease are on record. Twenty-two are summarised by Iveson et al. (1975), 14 of the 22 having mitral incompetence also, 2 more were added by Iveson and Pomerance (1977) and a further 16 cases are known to the authors.

The clinical effects of rheumatoid aortic or mitral incompetence are similar to the equivalent lesions found in rheumatic heart disease, but differ in not being associated with any degree of stenosis at either valve. The rate of deterioration is on the whole faster with rheumatoid valve lesions. Case History 6.2 describes an unusually rapid deterioration over the course of a few months.

Case History 6.2

Rheumatoid arthritis
Aortic incompetence

Mr. A.H., Warehouseman, born 1922

1974	Onset of seropositive RA
1978 Sept	Aortic diastolic murmur first heard No cardiac symptoms
1978 Nov	LV failure, progressing to congestive failure
1978 Dec	Transferred for emergency cardiac surgery Haematemesis from duodenal ulcer Perforation of duodenal ulcer Died before cardiac surgery undertaken
Autopsy	LV dilated Aortic valve cusps grossly thickened Granuloma in one cusp with central necrosis Histology shown in Figs. 6.1 and 6.6 Two ulcers in duodenum, one penetrating the pancreas, the other, anterior, perforated
Comment	Rapid deterioration due to destructive effect of granuloma in aortic valve cusp

---

Aortic Incompetence. The haemodynamic effects and symptoms are given in detail under the sections on rheumatic heart disease (Chap. 2, pp. 35–37). Essentially there is an increased pulse pressure and an aortic diastolic murmur, and if the lesion progresses, left ventricular dilatation and hypertrophy follow. The symptoms are effort dyspnoea, sometimes with angina, with the possibility of progression to left ventricular failure, pulmonary oedema and congestive failure. A change of rhythm to atrial fibrillation, or rapidly advancing damage to the valve will add to the clincial deterioration. As well as the aortic diastolic murmur there is usually a soft aortic systolic murmur due to the ejection of blood past the abnormal thickened valve cusps; this is very different from the much louder systolic murmur of aortic stenosis. When there is free aortic regurgitation, the short mid-diastolic murmur of Austin Flint may be heard at the cardiac apex.

Mitral Incompetence. The haemodynamic effects and symptoms are given in detail for rheumatic heart disease (Chap. 2, pp. 33–34). Systolic regurgitation at the mitral valve causes raised pressure in the left atrium and pulmonary veins, and the characteristic holosystolic murmur is heard at the cardiac apex. It may be loud and accompanied by a thrill. Dyspnoea and fatigue are the main symptoms and in due course pulmonary oedema and congestive failure may follow. Sudden deterioration may be caused by a ruptured chorda, and rupture of a papillary muscle due to granulomatous infiltration has been reported (Mallee et al. 1979). Signs of combined aortic and mitral incompetence will be found if both valves are affected (Case History 6.1).

Diagnosis

The diagnosis of a rheumatoid valve lesion is based on the clinical findings of aortic or mitral incompetence in the presence of seropositive rheumatoid arthritis, supported by investigational findings as follows. These findings are very much as described under rheumatic heart disease (pp. 46–57), but there are usually certain differences.

Radiology. Chest films will show evidence of left ventricular enlargement in the presence of significant aortic regurgitation, and left ventricular and left atrial enlargement when there is significant mitral regurgitation. With either lesion there may be pulmonary vascular congestion and possibly the "batswing" shadowing of pulmonary oedema in the lung fields. Calcification is occasionally found in the aortic or mitral valve ring if the valve lesion is long-standing. On fluoroscopy an increased excursion of left ventricular movement and increased aortic pulsation will be seen with significant aortic regurgitation. If valve surgery is being planned, cardioangiography may be indicated to give additional information on the size of individual cardiac chambers and the degree of regurgitation.

Electrocardiography. Evidence of left ventricular hypertrophy may be seen with aortic or, less often, with mitral regurgitation. Marked changes such as ST depression and T inversion, or left bundle branch block are only likely when there is major aortic regurgitation with clinical and radiological signs of left ventricular hypertrophy. There is no close parallel between the degree of the ECG changes and the severity of the valve lesion, particularly when the lesion is of recent development, for the ECG changes take time to evolve. Arrhythmias may be seen, ranging from atrial or ventricular ectopic beats to atrial fibrillation or flutter, or ventricular paroxysmal tachycardia. Other possible findings include ST depressions in patients treated with digitalis, and various grades of heart block if there are rheumatoid lesions affecting conducting tissue.

Echocardiography. Echocardiography is a valuable further investigation, often more informative than X-ray films or ECG. The diameter of the aortic orifice can be measured (Fig. 5.16) to give evidence of widening of the valve ring, more likely to be found with aortic atherosclerosis or with the aortic valve lesion of spondylitis. Abnormal echoes may be given by the aortic valve cusps if they are distorted or thickened. At the mitral valve, thickening or abnormal movement of the cusps may be identified in advance of any other evidence (Fig. 3.6). "Fluttering" of the anterior mitral cusp can be seen if there is free aortic regurgitation (Fig. 3.7). In addition, pericardial thickening or effusion may be found, often unsuspected clinically; this is of practical importance to the surgeon who may find that he has to resect a thickened pericardium before carrying out a valve replacement (Case History 6.3).

Case History 6.3

Rheumatoid arthritis
Aortic incompetence
Aortic valve replacement, Pericardectomy

Mrs. L.P., Housewife, born 1915

1953	Onset of seropositive RA
1968	Moderately severe disability: corticosteroid treatment started
1969	Aortic diastolic murmur heard
	Transfusion provoked LV failure
1970	Worsening LV failure
	Cardiomegaly, BP 140/60
1970 Oct	*Aortic valve replacement: Starr valve*
	Partial anterior pericardectomy
1976	Cardiac condition good
	Arthritis disabling: still on steroid
Comment	The thickened pericardium was not recognised pre-operatively; 450 ml pericardial fluid released. Aortic valve cusps thickened with rolled margins. Histology non-specific

---

Cardiac Catheter Studies. These may be advisable prior to valve surgery if further information is needed on pressures in the right side of the heart, or to assess pulmonary wedge pressure.

Differential Diagnosis

It is often difficult to distinguish specific rheumatoid valve lesions from similar valve lesions of different pathology, particularly rheumatic heart disease, which might arise by coincidence in a patient with rheumatoid arthritis. The distinction may only be possible when surgical valve replacement is carried out and the valve itself can be inspected.

Rheumatic Heart Disease. Points in favour of this would be the presence of signs of stenosis at either valve, of pulmonary hypertension, of well-established calcification at the valves, or of a long history of known valve disease, e.g. 10 years. The presence or absence of a past history of rheumatic fever cannot be relied on as an indicator of diagnosis.

Isolated Aortic Incompetence of Other Origin. This may be found in a rheumatoid patient by coincidence. Without an associated mitral lesion rheumatic heart disease is unlikely. A cause noted with increasing frequency (Olson et al. 1984) is aortic dilatation due to atherosclerosis combined with aortic incompetence; there may be hypertension and scattered calcification in the aortic wall also. Figure 6.8 a, b illustrates such a patient, who also had severe rheumatoid arthritis: at autopsy the aortic lesions were seen to be purely atherosclerotic.

Aortic Stenosis with Incompetence. Without a mitral lesion this may be due to congenital aortic stenosis, developing incompetence in later years. Alternatively the aortic valve may be congenitally bicuspid, developing rigidity, calcification

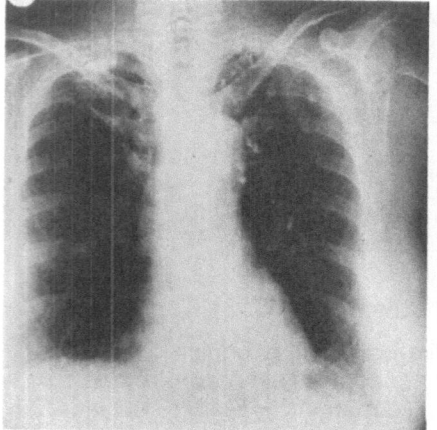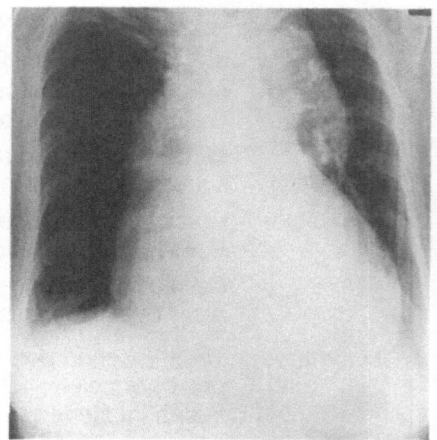

a   b

Fig. 6.8. **a** Chest X-ray film of a woman patient with chronic rheumatoid arthritis. The heart is normal in size with slight aortic unfolding. Calcified lesions at the apex of each lung and the basal pleural adhesion are the result of old healed tuberculosis. **b** Chest X-ray film of the same patient nine years later. There is marked aortic dilatation with mural calcification and the heart is grossly enlarged due to severe aortic regurgitation. At autopsy the cause was found to be aortic atherosclerosis unrelated to her rheumatoid arthritis.

and incompetence in later adult life (Cosh and Lever 1984; Subramanian et al. 1985). With such a lesion the aortic systolic murmur is much louder than with a rheumatoid aortic valve lesion, and may be accompanied by a thrill, with an aortic second sound in which the aortic element is soft or absent. Calcification at the valve may be florid as the lesion will have been present for many years, while in a rheumatoid aortic valve lesion calcification, if present at all, is likely to be scanty.

Infective Endocarditis. Infective endocarditis must always be considered where there is a progressive valve lesion. Close observation is required, seeking signs of infection, peripheral embolism or changing murmurs, and blood cultures must be made as required.

Systemic Lupus Erythematosus. There are a number of features in common with rheumatoid arthritis, and systemic lupus erythematosus too may cause aortic or mitral valve lesions. Other autoimmune lesions will be present, of the skin, kidney, nervous system or viscera. Tests for antinuclear factor will be positive.

Treatment

Rheumatoid Disease

The presence of a significant extra-articular lesion such as a rheumatoid valve lesion calls for a review of the management of the rheumatoid disease itself. While it is uncertain whether such treatment can promote healing in a valve lesion, it is probable that for every lesion that is clinically apparent there will be others too small to be detected which might be prevented from advancing. Quite apart from lesions in the heart there may be others elsewhere in the body. Even if the arthritis itself is not particularly serious, systemic treatment is indicated with a disease-modifying drug such as gold, penicillamine or an immunosuppressive drug. This is in addition to analgesics and anti-inflammatory drugs for the control of symptoms (see also Chap. 5, p. 97 on the treatment of pericarditis). If anaemia is present this should be corrected as far as possible to reduce the circulatory demands on the heart.

Valve lesions that do not give rise to symptoms require no particular therapy, but the patient should be kept under review periodically. He or she should be asked to report any newly developing symptoms of dyspnoea, angina, oedema or fever. Advice should be given about prophylaxis against infective endocarditis (Table 4.1).

Medical Treatment. This is indicated for valve lesions giving rise to symptoms. A regular oral diuretic is indicated if there are any signs of congestive failure. Frank left ventricular failure or pulmonary oedema requires an intravenous diuretic and, if severe, morphine and oxygen. Digitalisation is advisable if there is atrial fibrillation with evidence of congestive failure. In an emergency intravenous digoxin 0.75 or 1 mg is given, but if there is no urgency it is given orally, beginning with a loading dose of 0.75 or 1 mg, followed by 0.25 mg daily or less depending on the response of the pulse rate. Care should be taken to avoid overdosage in older patients, especially if digitalis is combined with diuretics giving a risk of potassium deficiency. Angina is an indication for glyceryl trinitrate, isosorbide or nifedipine. Beta-blocking drugs should be used with caution if there has been previous evidence of congestive failure, and they should be avoided altogether if there is any degree of heart block.

Cardiac Surgery. Surgical valve replacement must be considered when a valve lesion has become disabling or is deteriorating, and the presence of rheumatoid arthritis need be no bar to this. With cardiac function improved or restored to normal the scope for effective treatment for the arthritis, medical or surgical, is itself improved.

The indication for aortic or mitral valve replacement is the progression of cardiac symptoms beyond their control by medical means. The development of left ventricular failure, or sudden deterioration due to arrhythmia or to a ruptured chorda adds urgency. Many examples of successful aortic valve replacement for rheumatoid valve disease are on record (Case History 6.3) (Iveson et al. 1975; Newman and Cooney 1980) and even of replacement of both aortic and mitral valves together (Bortolotti et al. 1978). The presence of an active vasculitis, at one time considered a contra-indication for surgery is no longer so (Liew et al. 1979). In the choice of a prosthetic valve preference should be given to a type not requiring long-term subsequent anticoagulant treatment, so as to reduce the risk of drug interaction with the analgesic and anti-inflammatory drugs needed by the patient with rheumatoid arthritis.

Heart Block

Heart block is a rare complication of rheumatoid arthritis, arising in patients with long-standing seropositive nodular disease. Other extra-articular lesions are usually also present, both in the heart and elsewhere, and these may include pericarditis and aortic or mitral incompetence.

Incidence

Incidence is difficult to assess in so uncommon a condition. Many of the reports are of individual case histories, the first being that of Handforth and Woodbury (1959). David-Chaussé et al. reported 12 cases in 1976, ten of complete and two of first degree block. These arose over the course of 18 years among over 1800 patients attending hospital with rheumatoid arthritis. Ahern et al. (1983) described 8 cases of complete block among 7500 hospital in-patients admitted over the course of 15 years; this gives an incidence of 1 case in approximately 1000 patients with sufficiently severe arthritis to be admitted to hospital.

In their 25-year prospective study of 100 patients with rheumatoid arthritis Reilly et al. (1989) found 1 case of complete heart block, of suggestive but unproven rheumatoid pathology, and 1 case of first degree heart block, with autopsy confirmation of the pathology (Case History 6.4). Taking an average survival for the 100 patients of 18 years gives an incidence for complete block of one in 1800 patient-years or, for all forms of block, 1 case in 900 patient-years. This is probably an underestimate, as first degree block is symptomless and may well have been present unnoticed in other patients among the 100 in the series.

Case History 6.4

Rheumatoid arthritis
Heart block, first degree
Myocardial granulomata, Myocarditis

Mrs. N.D., Housewife, born 1898

1960	Onset seropositive RA
1963	Disabling arthritis, nodules
	Started steroid therapy
1965	L pleural effusion
	ECG evidence of pericarditis
1967	Paroxysmal nocturnal dyspnoea
	Cardiomegaly, gallop rhythm
	First degree heart block
	PR 0.28 sec (Fig. 6.9)
1968 Jan	Congestive heart failure
	Died with terminal bronchopneumonia
Autopsy	Mild adhesive pericarditis
	Many granulomas in myocardium, mainly between roots of great vessels and one in septum near AV node (Figs. 6.10, 6.11)
	Also diffuse myocardial cellular infiltration
Comment	First degree block due to granuloma near AV node. LV failure and finally congestive failure due to myocarditis

---

Pathology

In most cases heart block is due to the presence of a rheumatoid granuloma in or near the atrio-ventricular node or conducting tissue. Sometimes there is merely a simple infiltration of the AV node with lymphocytes, plasma cells and histiocytes without frank granuloma formation (Ahern et al. 1983; Davies 1984; Gowans 1960; Harris 1970). Additional granulomas may be present elsewhere in the heart or there may be, in addition, pericarditis or a rheumatoid valve lesion (Gelson et al. 1977). Bacterial infection has been known to develop as a secondary complication in a granuloma that has caused heart block (Gallagher and Gresham 1973). In a few reported instances heart block has been caused by amyloid disease secondary to the rheumatoid arthritis, the AV node being the site of deposits of amyloid tissue (Cathcart and Spodick 1962; Thery et al. 1974).

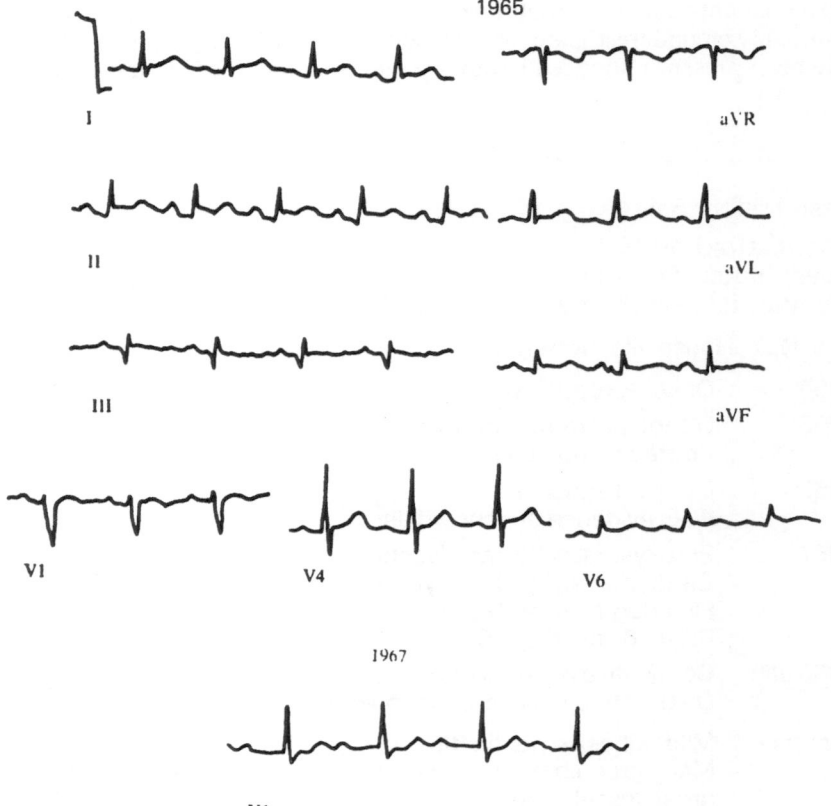

1965

I   aVR

II   aVL

III   aVF

V1   V4   V6

1967

V6

Fig. 6.9. Electrocardiograms from the patient in Case History 6.4. In the upper recording (of 9 leads) there are minor changes consistent with pericarditis – ST elevation in leads I, II, aVF and V6; the PR interval is normal. In the lowest strip, recorded shortly before death, there is first degree heart block with PR 0.28 second.

Clinical Features

Heart block usually presents in its complete form, diagnosed following the discovery of fixed bradycardia associated with syncope, or less dramatic symptoms such as weakness, dizziness or breathlessness. Rheumatoid disease may also cause lesser degrees of block – first or second degree or bundle branch block which, being symptomless, may go unobserved. Rheumatoid heart block is associated with long-established seropositive nodular arthritis, and so is found mainly in middle-aged or older patients or either sex.

In a review of 20 cases of complete block from the literature with another 8 known to the authors, Ahern et al. (1983) found the following. There is a female to male ratio of 2:1, an average age on diagnosis of 60 years (range 36 to 79) and an average duration of arthritis of 12 years (range 2 to 49) when block is diagnosed.

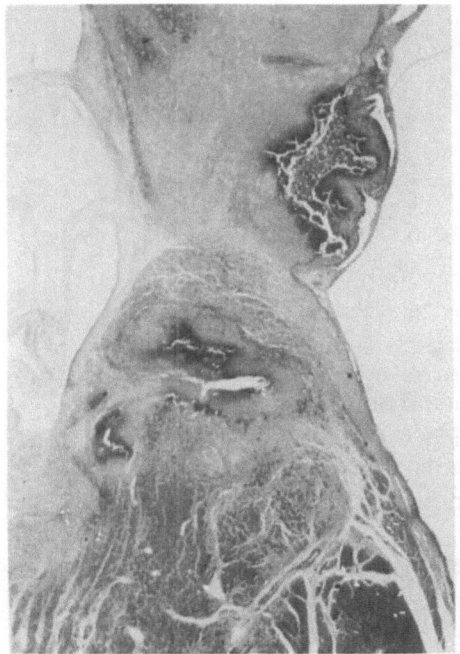 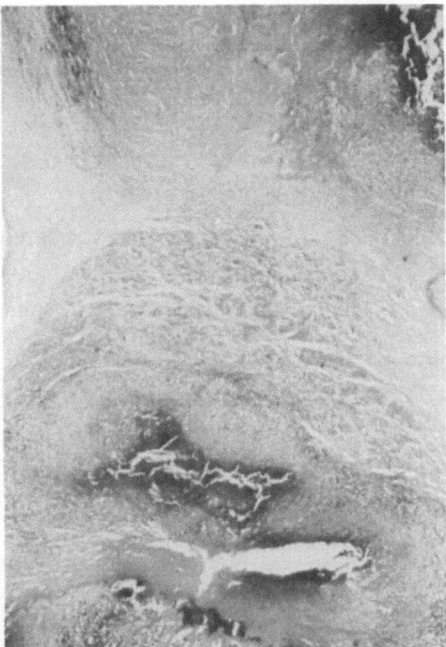

Fig. 6.10.   Fig. 6.11.

Fig. 6.10. Rheumatoid granulomas in septum. A section (× 15) through the interventricular septum from the patient in Case History 6.4. There is a large granuloma beneath the left ventricular endocardium (right) and another in the region of the AV node (centre) with cellular infiltration in the adjoining septal myocardium and in the atrial myocardium (above). Part of the tricuspid valve is seen on the left.

Fig. 6.11. Rheumatoid granuloma. Higher magnification (× 250) of the central portion of the preceding figure, showing the granuloma in the region of the AV node. (Figs. 6.9, 6.10 and 6.11 are reproduced with permission from the *Quarterly Journal of Medicine*).

Complete heart block does not necessarily develop as a sudden change from sinus rhythm. Some patients have been observed to progress from first to second degree block and then to complete block. Alternatively, block of any degree may occasionally revert to a lesser degree of block or to sinus rhythm (Case History 6.5). However, the usual pattern appears to be one of progression to complete block and for this to be permanent (Case History 6.6). Lesser degrees of block may be apparently permanent as in Case History 6.4, which describes a patient with first degree block and proven rheumatoid pathology (Fig. 6.9, 6.10, 6.11).

Once the threat of syncope or sudden death has been removed by implantation of a pacemaker the patient's prognosis is good unless there are other pathological lesions; the patient in Case History 6.6 did well until she developed aortic incompetence from which she eventually died.

Case History 6.5

Rheumatoid arthritis
Complete heart block
Spontaneous recovery

Miss E.S., Civil servant, born 1910

1972	Onset of seropositive RA
1978 June	Admitted to hospital for therapy
June 13	Normal heart; regular pulse, 80/min
June 14	Dyspnoea, pulmonary basal rales Jugular venous pressure raised ECG: complete block and R bbb
June 17	Second degree block (Fig. 6.12) Changed to first degree block, same day
June 19	Returned to normal conduction
1980	Remains well Normal heart and pulse

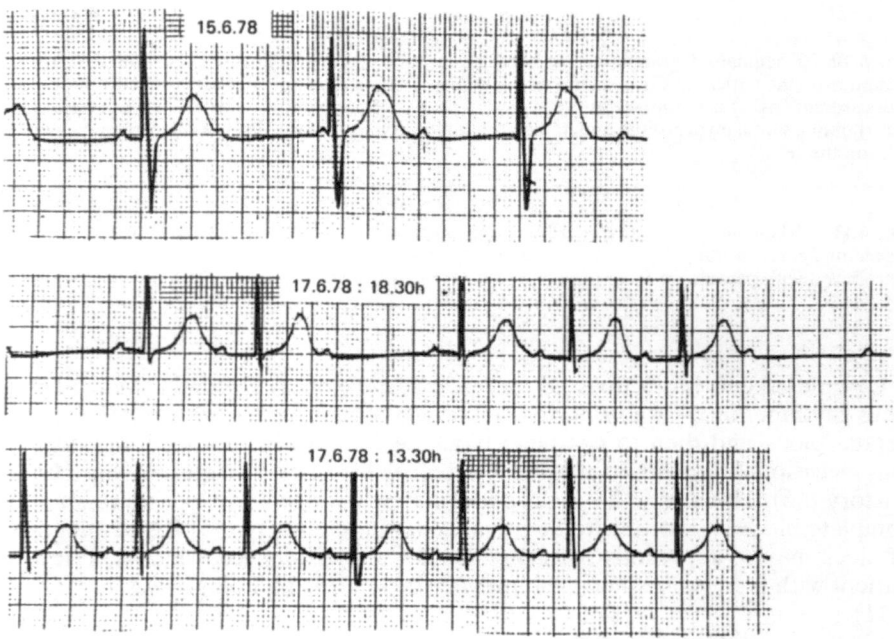

Fig. 6.12. Successive electrocardiograms from the patient described in Case History 6.5. In the upper tracing there is total AV dissociation. Two days later (*middle strip*) she has second degree block with Wenckebach periods. Earlier in that day (*lowest strip*) she had first degree block with PR 0.24 second.

Comment Temporary complete heart block developing in a patient with moderately active RA, recovering spontaneously within 5 days. The reason for heart block is uncertain. Vasculitis is a possibility, but she had no other signs of this

With acknowledgement to Professor Derek Brewerton

Case History 6.6

Rheumatoid arthritis
Complete heart block
Aortic incompetence

Mrs P.P., Housewife, born 1919

1957	Onset of seropositive RA
1958–77	14 hospital admissions 1967 synovectomy R knee 1974 arthroplasty R knee 1975/6 arthroplasties both hips
1977	Dyspnoea and bradycardia ECG: 2:1 AV block (Fig. 6.13) Returned to sinus rhythm
1977 Oct	Variable degree of heart block Recovered sinus rhythm on isoprenaline
1977 Nov	Complete heart block *Pacemaker implanted*, improved
1980	Aortic incompetence developed
1981	Died in congestive failure
Comment	A period of 2 months unstable conduction culminating in complete block successfully treated with pacemaker. Later developed aortic valve lesion, almost certainly of rheumatoid pathology. Refused cardiac surgery

---

Symptoms. First degree block is symptomless, and can only be shown by ECG demonstration of a prolonged PR interval of 0.20 to 0.30 seconds. For this reason its true incidence may be higher than is realised.

Second degree block is also usually symptomless, producing only a minor irregularity of the pulse or bradycardia which may not be noticed. In Type I (Wenckebach) the PR interval lengthens progressively over a number of cycles until a ventricular beat is missed – the Wenckebach period. After this the process is repeated (Fig. 1.7 and 6.12). Type II (Mobitz) gives rise to bradycardia with a fixed ratio between the atrial and ventricular rates e.g. 2:1 or

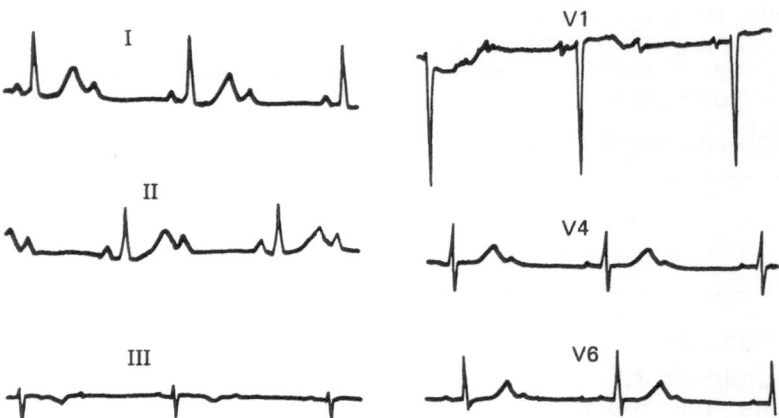

Fig. 6.13. Second degree heart block (Mobitz type) with 2:1 AV conduction, in the patient described in Case History 6.6. She later developed complete block.

4:1 or less often 3:1 (Fig. 6.13). The PR interval is usually normal. Close observation of the jugular venous pulse will reveal the atrial rate as being faster than the ventricular rate. Either form of second degree block is likely to be transitional, changing unpredictably back to normal, or to first degree or to complete block. The latter is more likely in the case of Type II. A simple exercise test, by increasing the atrial rate, or carotid pressure, may cause a temporary increase in the degree of block.

Complete block also may be symptomless, only being recognised when a bradycardia of the order of 40/minute is discovered. This can well happen with a patient whose physical activity is limited by arthritis. Symptoms that may be reported are weakness and fatigue or, on exertion, dyspnoea, faintness or syncope. Spontaneous syncope at rest will occur if the idioventricular rhythm fails giving a period of ventricular standstill of more than 15 seconds (Stokes-Adams attack). More prolonged periods of standstill will cause profound loss of consciousness, convulsions or death. The mechanism in fatal cases may be by ventricular fibrillation or ventricular asystole. Complete block may be recognised clinically by observation of the jugular venous pulse, with dissociation between atrial and ventricular rhythm and "cannon" waves when atrial and ventricular systole happen to coincide. The blood pressure shows a characteristically wide pulse pressure due to the fall in diastolic pressure during the abnormally prolonged diastolic period and the compensatory high peak of pressure achieved in systole, e.g. 200/50 mmHg.

Diagnosis

Heart block is diagnosed by the electrocardiogram. This will identify the degree of block, which in most cases is complete block, often combined with right or left bundle branch block (Fig. 6.14). In patients with intermittent block or with unstable degrees of block prolonged ECG monitoring is helpful, e.g. with a 24-hour ambulatory monitoring system.

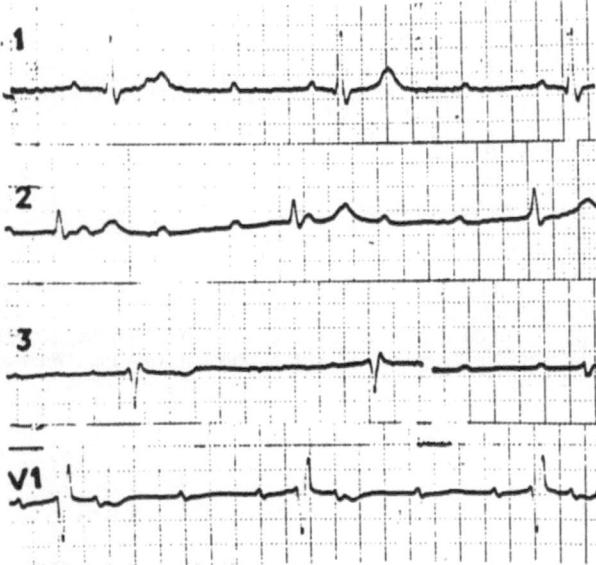

Fig. 6.14. Complete heart block with right bundle branch block in a man of 63 who died in a Stokes-Adams attack. He had a 3-year history of progressive seropositive arthritis with vasculitis and peripheral neuritis.

The technique of His bundle electrography enables the diagnosis and analysis of heart block to be carried one stage further, although this is of little practical relevance in terms of clinical management. The His bundle electrogram (Fig. 6.15) indicates the site of the conduction delay. If this is at the AV node the time interval between atrial activation and His bundle activation (A–H) is prolonged. If at the His bundle itself, or the distal part of the bundle and Purkinje system, the H–V time is prolonged (Narula et al. 1971; Puech 1975).

In one of the few reported studies made of rheumatoid heart block (Gelson et al. 1977) the delay was seen to be in the H–V section. In first degree block, as in Case History 6.4, the delay would be in the A–H section. If the pathological lesion were a diffuse one, electrical delay could affect all three sections – proximal to, within, or distal to the bundle of His.

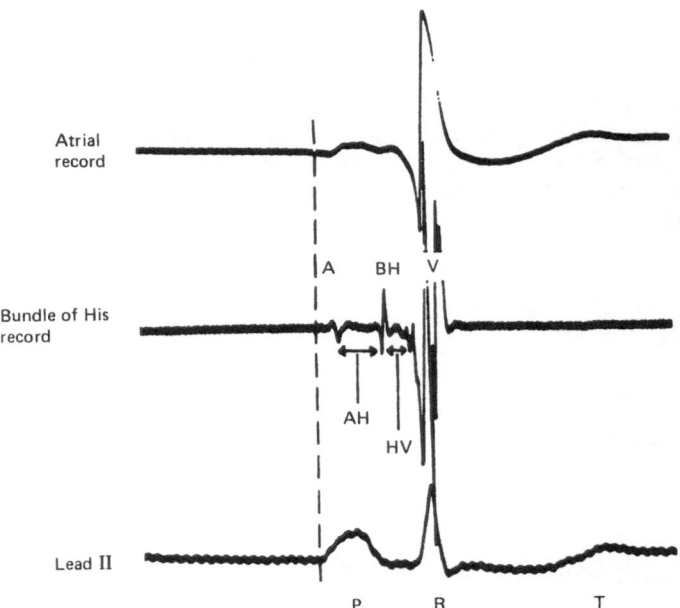

Fig. 6.15. His bundle electrogram from a normal subject. The middle trace is from an electrode placed over the bundle of His. The passage of the impulse down the bundle is marked *BH*; *AH* represents the time being taken for passage of the impulse from the AV node to the bundle, and *HV* the further time taken to pass to the ventricle. (Reproduced with permission from the *American Journal of Medicine*.)

Differential Diagnosis

Heart block may arise from a cause unrelated to rheumatoid arthritis, present by coincidence.

Degenerative disease of the conducting system is the most likely such cause (Davies 1971). This occurs in late adult life and is not necessarily associated with other pathology such as atherosclerosis. This would be suggested if the patient had seronegative polyarthritis, without nodules or extra-articular manifestations, whereas seropositive disease with nodules and extra-articular lesions is compatible with rheumatoid disease as the cause.

Myocardial infarction is a common cause of complete block. It is most likely to arise with, or shortly after, an inferior infarct and often recovers spontaneously within a week or two. Block may also accompany an anterior infarct in which case it carries a poor prognosis. Block following infarction is unlikely to be confused with rheumatoid block, which causes neither pain nor shock.

Ankylosing spondylitis is a potential cause of heart block through damage to the conducting system which is usually associated with a proximal aortitis and aortic incompetence (pp. 182–188). The obvious presence of spondylitis, generally of some years duration when block develops, and its seronegativity will clearly differentiate it from rheumatoid heart block.

Amyloid disease with intracardiac deposits of amyloid tissue has on rare occasions caused heart block (Cathcart and Spodick 1962; Thery et al. 1974). One of the possible causes of amyloid disease is chronic rheumatoid arthritis; there were four examples in the 100 patients followed up by Reilly et al. (1989). Amyloid disease is usually recognised as a result of renal involvement and confirmed by renal or rectal biopsy.

Sino-atrial disease (the "sick sinus syndrome") gives rise to a marked but variable sinus bradycardia, sometimes with intermittent atrial arrhythmias. Atrio-ventricular dissociation is not a feature. The condition is due to degenerative changes in the region of the S–A node and there is no known association with any disorder of connective tissue.

Treatment

Established complete heart block is best treated with an implanted demand-type pacemaker. However, in the short term, if complete block has just developed, or might possibly be a temporary phenomenon, the alternatives of corticosteroid or isoprenaline may be considered.

Corticosteroid treatment may be given a trial on a temporary basis while waiting to see whether complete block persists, the rationale being that an inflammatory lesion in the region of the conducting tissue might thereby be suppressed. An appropriate dose would be hydrocortisone 100 mg 8-hourly by intramuscular injection followed within three days by a change to prednisone 20 mg 8-hourly, reducing to a maintenance dose of 10 mg daily or less. If ineffective, prednisone should be withdrawn and arrangements made for pacing. If effective, the dose should be gradually reduced to a minimum effective level, with frequent checks on cardiac rhythm and conduction, bearing in mind that a reversion to sinus rhythm may be transient.

During a period of assessment or while awaiting pacemaker implantation, isoprenaline may be effective, and 5 mg may be given by slow intravenous infusion under continuous ECG monitoring. This may be followed by the slow release form of isoprenaline, 15 or 30 mg orally 8-hourly or more frequently, increasing if necessary up to a daily total of 600 mg. The drug increases the idioventricular rate but there is some risk of inducing ventricular ectopic beats or even ventricular tachycardia.

When it has become clear that complete block is likely to be permanent, an implanted pacemaker is the safest treatment. Finally, when cardiac rhythm is safely controlled, the general management of the rheumatoid arthritis must be reviewed as described above.

Myocarditis

Myocardial involvement is not uncommon as an autopsy finding in the presence of chronic seropositive nodular rheumatoid arthritis. It may take the form of one or more granulomas scattered throughout the myocardium, associated with others in the valve rings or the conducting tissue. It may also be seen as a more

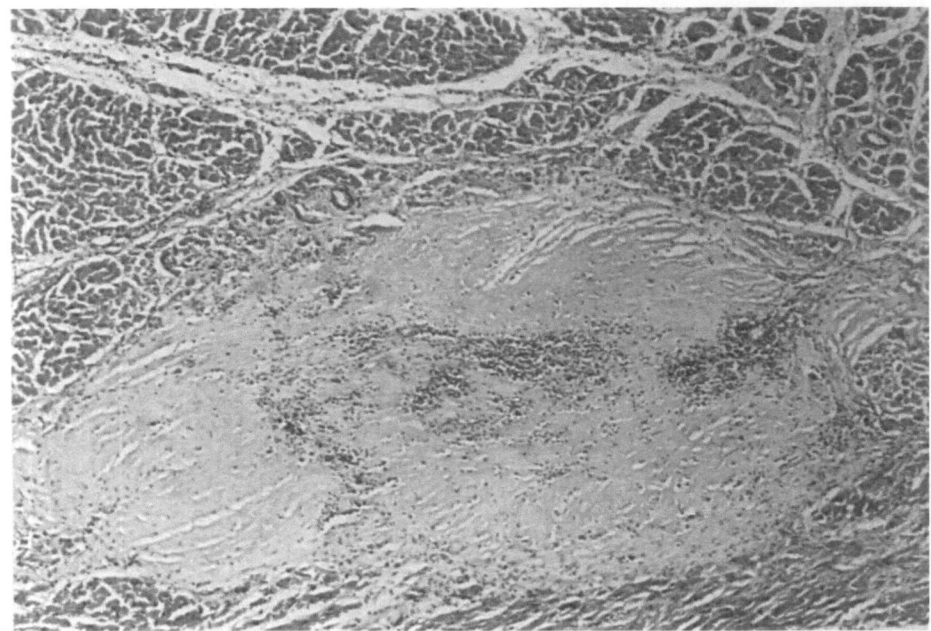

Fig. 6.16. Myocardium. Histology of a fibrous nodule in the myocardium of a patient with rheumatoid arthritis showing mononuclear cellular infiltration within and around the nodule ($\times$ 50)

diffuse cellular infiltration of lymphocytes, plasma cells and histiocytes adjoining a myocardial blood vessel (Fig. 6.16) (Bennett 1984; Bonfiglio and Atwater 1969; Sokoloff 1964). Cruickshank (1958) found such evidence of myocarditis in 11 of the 100 hearts from rheumatoid patients that he examined in detail. Lesions were seen most often in the left ventricular muscle near the mitral valve ring.

Clinical evidence of myocarditis is usually scanty and indirect. It may be suspected if left ventricular or congestive failure develop without any overt cause such as a valve lesion, arrhythmia, hypertension or coronary disease. There is generalised cardiac enlargement and gallop rhythm. The electrocardiogram shows ST-T depressions and possibly ectopic beats or other arrhythmias, although these changes are non-specific. The presence of any degree of heart block is consistent with myocarditis as the granuloma causing the block may be accompanied by others elsewhere in the myocardium.

Echocardiography may reveal abnormal myocardial function in the form of reduced ejection fraction and impaired ventricular wall movement in systole. However, published studies have given uncertain evidence of abnormal myocardial function due to rheumatoid disease (Bacon and Gibson 1974; MacDonald et al. 1977).

If myocarditis is suspected, the treatment is essentially the treatment of the resulting physical state, whether of cardiac failure, heart block, valve lesion or arrhythmia. In addition attention must be given to the management of the associated rheumatoid arthritis.

Coronary Arteritis

The vasculitis associated with seropositive erosive rheumatoid arthritis mainly affects small vessels, and a common skin manifestation is the characteristic nailfold lesion (Fig. 5.5). These tiny infarcts quickly heal. Vasculitis in rather larger arteries, such as distal branches of the digital arteries, can cause bigger and more obvious infarcts, as in Fig. 5.7, as well as lesions of peripheral nerves, the gastro-intestinal tract and other viscera. The coronary vessels are not immune from similar small lesions, but they are usually clinically silent and are only likely to be identified on a careful search at autopsy (Cruickshank 1958; Lebowitz 1963; Sokoloff 1964).

Occasionally arteritis involves a larger coronary vessel and the partial or total occlusion of the artery resulting from the inflammatory reaction in its wall can cause cardiac pain or frank infarction (Rudge et al. 1981; Karten 1969; Parrillo and Fauci 1984). Death from this form of cardiac infarction has been reported but is rare.

The nature of the inflammatory changes seen in the artery wall varies, depending in part on the stage of evolution or of healing of the individual lesion. Karten (1969) reported lesions ranging from "a mild subacute adventitial inflammation to widespread necrosis of the entire artery wall with mononuclear and polymorphonuclear cellular exudation".

Mortality from coronary disease does not appear to be increased in patients with rheumatoid arthritis (Monson and Hall 1976; Mutru et al. 1976) although not all reports are in agreement. In spite of the occasional case report it is unlikely that coronary arteritis contributes significantly to morbidity or mortality in rheumatoid arthritis (Editorial *(BMJ)* 1970). In a careful review of the available coronary artery histology from 7 rheumatoid patients dying from myocardial infarction Karten (1969) could find no sign of arteritis, and death was attributed to coincidental coronary atherosclerosis.

It appears therefore that coronary arteritis does occur as part of a generalised arteritis in rheumatoid patients, but it is almost always clinically silent. Figure 6.17 shows the ECG of a woman patient with severe rheumatoid arthritis. The tracings suggest a partial thickness anterior infarct, subsequently returning to normal. She had no relevant symptoms, and the ECG was a routine recording. As she had clinical evidence of arteritis elsewhere, the presumptive diagnosis was of coronary arteritis and myocardial infarction with subsequent healing.

Juvenile Arthritis

Chronic arthritis in childhood differs in a number of respects from arthritis in adults. Although some subgroups of juvenile arthritis may be recognised as corresponding to adult forms, most cases have no precise adult counterpart, and are classed as juvenile chronic arthritis (JCA). Consequently the blanket terms Still's disease and juvenile rheumatoid arthritis have been dropped in favour of the more specific names for the individual childhood forms of arthritis.

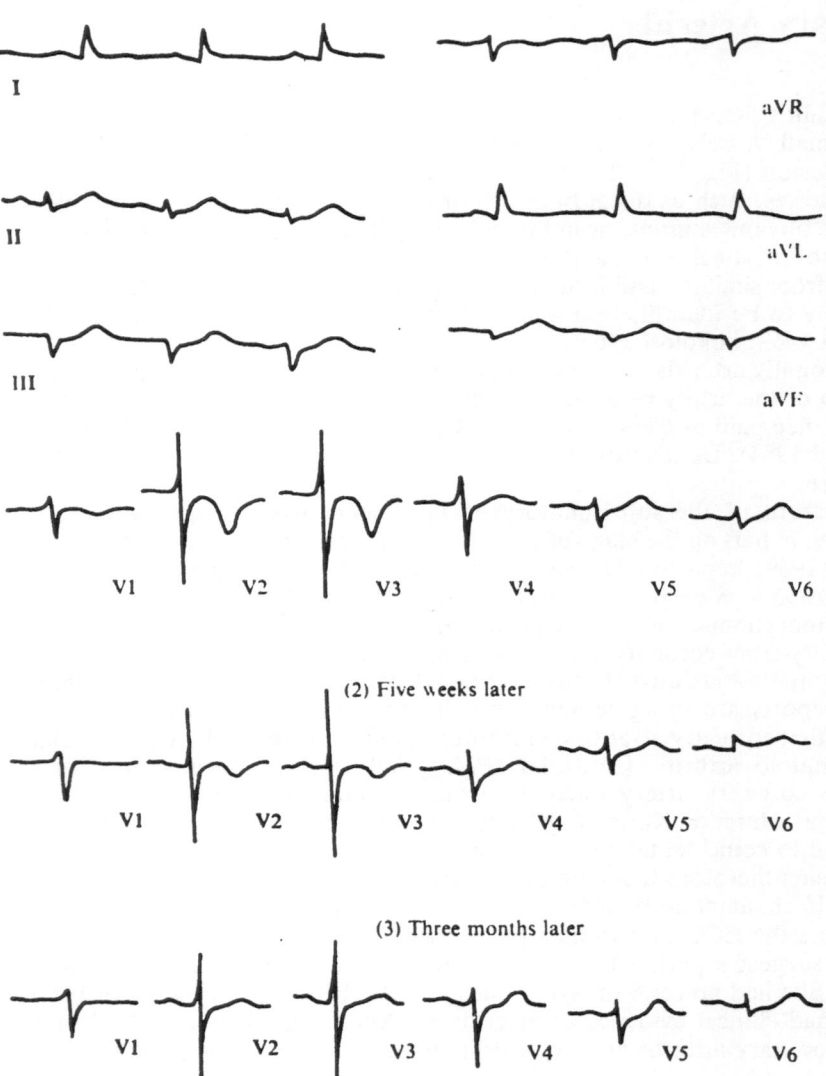

Fig. 6.17. Possible coronary arteritis. Electrocardiograms from a woman patient with rheumatoid arthritis and vasculitis. The 12-lead recording (*above*) shows deep T wave inversions suggesting a partial thickness antero-medial infarct, which may have been due to coronary arteritis. No proof was available. Subsequent recordings 5 weeks and 3 months later showed a return to normal. (Reproduced with permission from the Quarterly Journal of Medicine).

The biggest group is the pauci-articular form of JCA, in which four or fewer joints are affected, mainly seen in girls under 5 years of age with a positive test for antinuclear antibodies and a risk of developing iridocyclitis. Systemic JCA typically affects infants and younger children and corresponds to the original description of Still, having fever, lymphadenopathy and rash for weeks or months before developing polyarthritis. Polyarticular JCA affects younger girls, and is a seronegative symmetrical polyarthritis with few if any systemic symptoms. Other groups are the juvenile form of rheumatoid arthritis, in older girls, with positive Rose Waaler tests, nodule formation and bony erosions; juvenile ankylosing spondylitis, mainly in boys, with peripheral arthritis and little spinal involvement in the early years, but positive for HLA–B27; and juvenile psoriatic arthritis (Ansell 1980).

Pericarditis

Pericarditis is found mainly with arthritis associated with considerable systemic illness i.e. the group referred to as systemic JCA. This group corresponds most closely to the original description given by Still in 1897, and pericarditis was one of the features that he noted.

Incidence. Among the 285 cases of juvenile arthritis studied at Taplow over a 15-year period by Lietman and Bywaters (1963), pericarditis was diagnosed clinically in 20 children, i.e. 7%. On the other hand, among the 11 who died and came to autopsy 5 cases had evidence of current or previous pericarditis i.e. 45%. This difference between the frequency of pericarditis as a pathological finding and its infrequency as a clinical finding mirrors the situation in adult patients with rheumatoid arthritis, and, indeed, other forms of arthritis. It suggests that pericarditis occurs more often than is recognised in childhood arthritis. This is borne out by echocardiographic studies: Bernstein (1977) found evidence of pericarditis in 20 out of 55 children (36%) with juvenile arthritis.

Clinical Features. Pericarditis may develop at any time during the course of juvenile arthritis, predominantly in the group of systemic JCA while systemic features are prominent. This may be at the onset of the arthritis or at any time up to 5 years after the onset. It is found in both boys and girls, at any age from 2 years upwards, though rather commoner in older children. It is uncommon in children with mild, afebrile, pauci-articular arthritis, and is essentially a part of the systemic manifestations of arthritis in childhood.

   Pericarditis is diagnosed clinically by the finding of a pericardial friction rub, often with tachycardia and tachypnoea, and there may be central chest pain which tends to be influenced by respiration and by change in posture. Chest X-ray films show enlargement of the cardiac shadow. Electrocardiographic changes are usually limited to T wave flattening or inversion which may persist for some weeks after the pain and friction rub have subsided, and the ECG finally returns to normal. The most sensitive diagnostic test is echocardiography, which may provide the only evidence of pericarditis (Bernstein et al. 1974; Bernstein 1977). The blood picture shows a leucocytosis and a raised ESR, and the Rose Waaler test is usually negative. The subsequent clinical course of the arthritis and the degree of residual joint damage are not necessarily worse in the child who has had pericarditis. The effusion is usually small and disappears as the child's general condition improves. The mean duration of signs of pericarditis in one study was 7 weeks; recurrent episodes of pericarditis may occur while the arthritis is still in an active phase (Ansell and Bywaters 1983; Brewer 1977; Lietman and Bywaters 1963; Michet and Hunder 1984).

Large pericardial effusions or signs of tamponade are uncommon, but if they do occur pericardial aspiration is necessary and brings immediate relief (Majeed and Kvastnicka 1978; Scharf et al. 1976). The fluid is clear or lightly blood-stained and is characteristic of an inflammatory exudate, containing protein, fibrin and white cells which are mainly polymorphs. The levels of glucose and of complement are reduced.

Treatment. Treatment is on conservative lines, with aspirin or non-steroidal anti-inflammatory drugs for pain relief. Corticosteroids are not usually indicated, although they have been given in good effect in resistant cases and, if pericardial aspiration is indicated, it is probably helpful for steroid to be injected intra-pericardially.

Valve Lesions

The only heart valve lesion known to be associated with juvenile arthritis is aortic incompetence, and this is rare.

One report describes 4 girls with juvenile rheumatoid arthritis, seropositive, who were aged between 8 and 10 years at the onset of the arthritis. Over the course of 4 years each of them developed aortic incompetence. The lesion was progressive in 3: 2 had successful valve replacements but the third deteriorated and died before surgery could be undertaken (Leak et al. 1981).

Another report is of a young woman who had had seronegative juvenile chronic arthritis beginning as a systemic illness at the age of 2 years. At the age of 22 years she had widespread joint damage and a normal heart; she was seronegative. In the following 5 years she developed progressive aortic incompetence culminating in surgical valve replacement at the age of 27 years. Her subsequent progress was good (Kramer et al. 1983).

Adult Still's Disease

The pattern of severe systemic illness followed by polyarthritis as described by Still occasionally develops in an adult of either sex (Bywaters 1971; Esdaile et al. 1980). The presenting feature is of persistent unexplained fever, with a macular rash; after an interval, which may be of weeks or months, polyarthritis develops. Lymph node enlargement and splenomegaly are common and about one quarter of patients have pericarditis or pleurisy. Most are seronegative. After a variable course, the illness subsides and the arthritis settles with little residual damage (Bujak et al. 1973; Esdaile et al. 1980).

Instances are on record of cardiac tamponade due to large pericardial effusions in adult Still's disease, requiring aspiration or surgical relief, but as a rule the pericarditis settles spontaneously without difficulty (Jamieson 1983; Vukman and Fay 1981).

References

Ahern M, Lever JV, Cosh JA (1983) Complete heart block in rheumatoid arthritis. Ann Rheum Dis 42: 389–397

Ansell BM (1980) Rheumatic disorders in childhood. Butterworths, London

Ansell BM, Bywaters EGL (1983) Juvenile chronic arthritis. In: Scott JT (ed) Copeman's textbook of the rheumatic diseases, 6th edition. Churchill Livingstone, London

Bacon PS, Gibson DG (1974) Cardiac involvement in rheumatoid arthritis. Echocardiographic study of 22 rheumatoid arthritis patients with nodules and 22 without. Ann Rheum Dis 33: 20–24

Bennett RM (1984) Myocardial involvement in rheumatoid arthritis. In: Ansell BM, Simkin PA (eds) The heart and rheumatic disease. Butterworths, London, pp 36–39

Bernstein B (1977) Pericarditis in juvenile rheumatoid arthritis. Arthritis Rheum 20: 241–245

Bernstein B, Takahashi M, Hanson V (1974) Cardiac involvement in juvenile rheumatoid arthritis. J Pediatr 85: 313–317

Bonfiglio T, Atwater EC (1969) Heart disease in patients with seropositive rheumatoid arthritis. Arch Intern Med 124: 714–719

Bortolotti V, Casarotto D, Galucci V et al. (1978) Mitral and aortic valve replacement in valvular rheumatoid heart disease. Chest 73: 427–429

Brewer EJ (1977) Juvenile rheumatoid arthritis – cardiac involvement. Arthritis Rheum 20: 231–236

Bujak JS, Aptekar RG, Decker JL, Wolff SM (1973) Juvenile rheumatoid arthritis presenting in the adult as fever of unknown origin. Medicine (Baltimore) 52: 431–444

Bywaters EGL (1971) Still's disease in the adult. Ann Rheum Dis 30: 121–133

Carpenter DF, Golden A, Roberts WC (1967) Quadrivalvular rheumatoid heart disease associated with left bundle branch block. Am J Med 43: 922–929

Cathcart ES, Spodick DH (1962) Rheumatoid heart disease. N Engl J Med 266: 959–964

Cosh JA, Lever JV (1984) The aortic valve. In Ansell BM, Simkin PA (eds) The heart and rheumatic disease. Butterworths, London, pp 83–119

Cruickshank B (1958) Heart lesions in rheumatoid disease. J Path Bact 76: 223–240

David-Chaussé J, Blanchot P, Warin J, Dehais J, Bullier R, Texier JM (1976) Atrio-ventricular block in rheumatoid arthritis. Rev Rhum Mal Osteoartic 43: 177–183

Davies MJ (1971) Pathology of conducting tissue of the heart. Butterworths, London, pp 77–95

Davies MJ (1984) The conduction system in rheumatoid arthritis. In Ansell BM, Simkin PA (eds) The heart and rheumatic disease. Butterworths, London, pp 74–76

Editorial (1970) Coronary occlusion in rheumatoid arthritis. Br Med J 1: 707

Esdaile JM, Tannenbaum H, Hawkins D (1980) Adult Still's disease. Am J Med 68: 825–830

Gallagher PJ, Gresham GA (1973) Heart block with infected rheumatoid granulomas. Br Heart J 35: 110–112

Gelson A, Sanderson JM, Carson P (1977) Rheumatoid pericardial effusion with heart block treated by pericardectomy and implantation of permanent pacemaker. Br Heart J 39: 113–115

Goehrs HR, Baggenstoss AH, Slocumb CH (1960) Cardiac lesions in rheumatoid arthritis. Arthritis Rheum 3: 298–308

Good AE, Lang K, Olsen JR, Frishette WA (1970) Cardiac necrobiotic (rheumatoid) granulomas without arthritis. Arthritis Rheum 13: 166–174

Gowans JDC (1960) Complete heart block with Stokes Adams syndrome due to rheumatoid heart disease. N Engl J Med 262: 1012–1014

Handforth CP, Woodbury JFL (1959) Cardiovascular manifestations of rheumatoid arthritis. Canad Med Ass J 80: 86–90

Harris M (1970) Rheumatoid heart disease with complete heart block. J Clin Path 23: 623–626

Howell A, Say J, Hedworth-Whitty R (1972) Rupture of the sinus of Valsalva due to severe rheumatoid heart disease. Br Heart J 34: 537–540

Iveson JMI, Pomerance A (1977) Cardiac involvement in rheumatoid disease. Clin Rheum Dis 3: 467–500

Iveson JMI, Thadani U, Ionescu M, Wright V (1975) Aortic valve incompetence and replacement in rheumatoid arthritis. Ann Rheum Dis 34: 312–320

Jamieson TW (1983) Adult Still's disease complicated by cardiac tamponade. JAMA 249: 2065–2066

Karten I (1969) Arteritis, myocardial infarction and rheumatoid arthritis. JAMA 210: 1717–1720

Kramer PH, Imboden JB, Waldman FM, Turley K, Ports TA (1983) Severe aortic insufficiency in juvenile chronic arthritis. Am J Med 74: 1088–1091

Leak AM, Millar-Craig MW, Ansell BM (1981) Aortic regurgitation in seropositive juvenile
    arthritis. Ann Rheum Dis 40: 229–234
Lebowitz WB (1963) The heart in rheumatoid arthritis (rheumatoid disease). Ann Intern Med 58:
    102–123
Lefkowitz A, Kaplan SB, Young JM (1968) Rheumatoid granuloma in aortic valve ring causing fatal
    aortic insufficiency in a patient with minimal arthritis. Arthritis Rheum 11: 494–496
Lietman PS, Bywaters EGL (1963) Pericarditis in juvenile rheumatoid arthritis. Pediatrics 32: 855–
    860
Liew M, Wilson D, Horton D, Fleming A (1979) Successful valve replacement for aortic
    incompetence in rheumatoid arthritis with vasculitis. Ann Rheum Dis 38: 483–484
MacDonald WJ, Crawford MH, Klippel JH, Zvaifler NJ, O'Rourke RA (1977) Echocardiographic
    assessment of cardiac structure and function in patients with rheumatoid arthritis. Am J Med 63:
    890–896
Majeed HA, Kvastnicka J (1978) Juvenile rheumatoid arthritis with cardiac tamponade. Ann
    Rheum Dis 37: 273–276
Mallee C, Wegener RP, Rasker JJ (1979) An unusual complication in a patient with rheumatoid
    heart disease. Neth J Med 22: 77–79
Michet CJ, Hunder GG (1984) Pericarditis. In: Ansell BM, Simkin PA (eds) The heart and
    rheumatic disease. Butterworths, London, pp 1–26
Mody GM, Stevens JE, Meyers OL (1987) The heart in rheumatoid arthritis – a clinical and
    echocardiographic study. Q J Med 65: 921–928
Monson RR, Hall AP (1976) Mortality among arthritics. J Chronic Dis 29: 459–467
Mutru O, Koota K, Isomaki H (1976) Causes of death in autopsied rheumatoid arthritis patients.
    Scand J Rheum 5: 239–240
Narula OS, Scherlag BJ, Samet P, Javier RP (1971) Atrioventricular block: localisation and
    classification by His bundle recordings. Am J Med 50: 146–165
Newman JH, Cooney LM (1980) Cardiac abnormalities associated with rheumatoid arthritis: aortic
    insufficiency requiring valve replacement. J Rheumatol 7: 375–378
Nomeir AM, Turner RA, Watts LE (1979) Cardiac involvement in rheumatoid arthritis. Arthritis
    Rheum 22: 561–564
Olson LJ, Subramanian R, Edwards WD (1984) Surgical pathology of pure aortic insufficiency: a
    study of 225 cases. Mayo Clin Proc 59: 835–841
Parrillo JE, Fauci AS (1984) Coronary vasculitis. In: Ansell BM, Simkin PA (eds) The heart in
    rheumatic disease. Butterworths, London, pp 222–223
Puech P (1975) Atrioventricular block: the value of intracardiac recordings. In: Krikler D, Goodwin
    JF (eds) Cardiac arrhythmias. Saunders, London, pp 81–115
Qaiyumi S, Hassan ZU, Toone E (1984) Seronegative arthropathies in lone aortic insufficiency.
    Arch Intern Med 145: 822–824
Rasker JJ, Cosh JA (1981) Cause and age at death in a prospective study of one hundred patients
    with rheumatoid arthritis. Ann Rheum Dis 40: 115–120
Reilly PA, Cosh JA, Rasker JJ, Maddison PJ (1989) A 25 year prospective study of 100 patients with
    rheumatoid arthritis. Ann Rheum Dis 48: in press
Reimer KA, Rodgers RF, Oyasu R (1976) Rheumatoid aortitis with rheumatoid heart disease and
    granulomatous aortitis. JAMA 235: 2510–2512
Roberts WC, Kehoe JA, Carpenter DF, Golden A (1968) Cardiac valvular lesions in rheumatoid
    arthritis. Arch Intern Med 122: 141–146
Rudge SR, Lloyd Jones JK, Macfarlane A (1981) Coronary and peripheral vascular occlusion due to
    rheumatoid arthritis. Postgrad Med J 57: 196–198
Scharf J, Levy J, Benderly A, Nahir M (1976) Pericardial tamponade in juvenile rheumatoid
    arthritis. Arthritis Rheum 19: 760–762
Schorn D, Hough IP, Anderson IF (1976) The heart in rheumatoid arthritis. S Afr Med J 50: 8–10
Sokoloff L (1964) Cardiac involvement in rheumatoid arthritis and allied disorders: current
    concepts. Mod Concepts Cardiovasc Dis 33: 847–850
Subramanian R, Olson LJ, Edwards WD (1985) Surgical pathology of combined aortic stenosis and
    insufficiency: a study of 213 cases. Mayo Clin Proc 60: 247–254
Thery C, Lekeffre J, Gosselin B, Warembourg H (1974) Le bloc auriculo-ventriculaire de la
    polyarthrite rhumatoide. Etude histologique de systeme de His Tawara. A propos de deux
    observations. Arch Mal Coeur 10: 1181–1191
Vukman RB, Fay GJ (1981) Juvenile rheumatoid arthritis with pericardial tamponade in an adult.
    Arch Intern Med 141: 1078–1079

Chapter 7

Systemic Lupus Erythematosus

Introduction

Systemic lupus erythematosus (SLE) is an autoimmune inflammatory disease of fluctuating severity in which the production of autoantibodies to cellular constituents, particularly DNA, is associated with a wide variety of systemic manifestations. It chiefly affects young women, particularly of black races. The increasing sensitivity of diagnostic methods has shown that it is by no means as rare as it was previously thought to be and its outcome is not necessarily serious.

The American Rheumatism Association's eleven diagnostic criteria are set out in Table 7.1 (Tan et al. 1982). The presence of any four of the eleven is, by convention, held to be diagnostic of SLE. However, as further aspects of the disease become clarified it appears that not all cases of SLE are covered by these criteria.

Table 7.1. The American Rheumatism Association revised criteria for the diagnosis of systemic lupus erythematosus (Tan et al. 1982)

1. Malar rash
2. Discoid rash
3. Photosensitivity
4. Oral ulcers
5. Arthritis (non-erosive, of 2 or more joints)
6. Serositis
7. Renal disorder (proteinuria or casts)
8. Neurological disorder
9. Haematological disorder
10. Immunological disorder (positive LE test; anti DNA and other antibodies)
11. Antinuclear antibody

The diagnosis of SLE is based on the presence of any four of the above, simultaneously or serially

Prevalence

The prevalence of systemic lupus erythematosus varies considerably in different countries and different races. As the disease is activated by sunlight it is found more frequently in tropical climates; racially it is more common among North American and West Indian blacks and in South East Asia. A San Francisco survey (Fessel 1974) found a prevalence in the general population of 1 in 2000. In girls and women aged between 15 and 64 years the prevalence was more than twice as high, and among black women higher still, 1 in 250.

In Britain, Wood (1977) found a much lower figure, 7 in 100 000. Hochberg (1987a) found a very similar figure for the general population of England and Wales; for the female population he found a prevalence of 12.5 in 100 000 and for girls and women aged from 15 to 64 years, 17.7 in 100 000. These rates are lower than for other Western countries.

By comparison with rheumatoid arthritis SLE is far less frequent, with a ratio of 1 to 150 for Britain (Wood 1977). By contrast, Fessel's figures for California give a ratio of 1 case of SLE to 5 or 10 of rheumatoid arthritis, while in the Caribbean and in South East Asia SLE is said to be more common than rheumatoid arthritis.

The total number of deaths from SLE in England and Wales in the decade 1974–83 was 1246, with a 4:1 female preponderance. In the age group 15 to 34 years the sex ratio was 7.5 to 1. During that decade the annual mortality declined from 4.5 to 3 per million persons per year (Hochberg 1987b).

Immunopathology

Autoantibodies

A number of non-organ-specific antibodies are produced in SLE against cell components, most importantly against nuclear DNA, but also against cytoplasmic and membrane components. The antibody against double-stranded (ds) DNA in high concentration is diagnostic of the disease, low concentrations being found rarely in other connective tissue diseases. It is demonstrated in the serum by the Farr radioimmunoassay or by immunofluorescent staining of the protozoan *Crithidia luciliae*; the kinetoplast of this organism is a particularly good source of dsDNA (Fig. 7.1). Quantitative estimation of the serum level of the antibody is made by radioimmunoassay and this estimate of "DNA binding" may be used to monitor the disease activity (Morgan and Hughes 1984).

Other antibodies found in SLE but without the same specificity for the disease include those against denatured single-stranded (ss) DNA, against nuclear ribonucleoprotein (RNP) and against histone. The latter, which formed the basis for the original LE cell test, is more characteristic of the drug-induced form of SLE than of the spontaneous form. Antibodies common to SLE and to Sjogren's syndrome are those against the nuclear antigen La (SSB) and the cytoplasmic antigen Ro (SSA). Antibodies to ssDNA and to Ro are often present in the minority of SLE patients who are antinuclear antibody negative (Maddison et al. 1981).

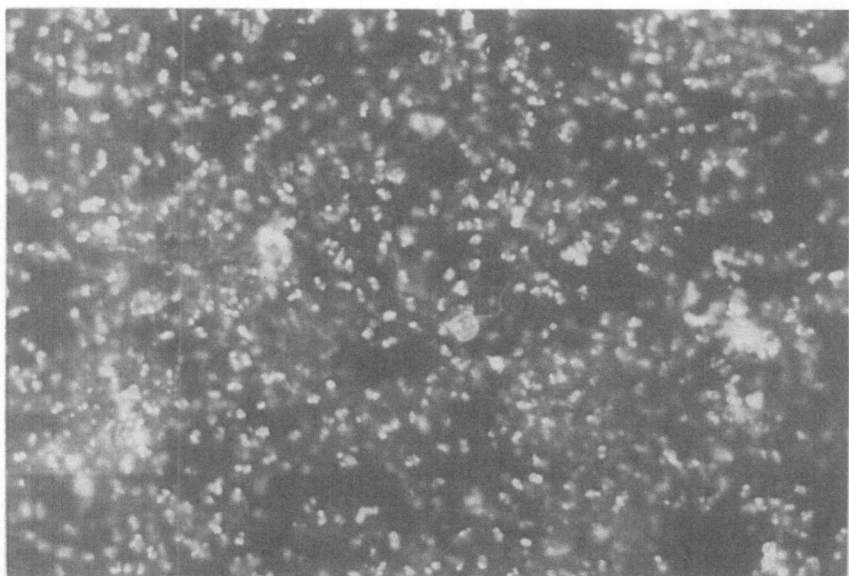

Fig. 7.1. Immunofluorescent staining of *Crithidia luciliae* indicating the presence of antinuclear dsDNA antibody in the test serum (× 600).

Antibodies against the phospholipid constituents of cell membranes have been shown to be associated with various thrombotic lesions in SLE, including recurrent abortion, which is attributed to thrombosis in placental vessels. The effects of this group of antibodies may be through their action on platelet cell membrane, thereby initiating the process of thrombosis, and in some circumstances causing thrombocytopenia (Hughes et al. 1986).

Aetiology

The essential cause of SLE is not known, but there are a number of factors which appear to contribute to the immunological disorder. The excessive generation of autoantibodies and of immunoglobulin is due to abnormal B cell activity associated with deficient control by T cell regulatory activity. Some aspects of this pattern suggest a possible viral causation, as has been identified in animal models of the disease (Bakke et al. 1983).

A genetic factor is apparent from the significant association of SLE with HLA antigens B8 and DR3, and also with complement deficiency, which arises from the inheritance of "null" alleles such as C2 and C4, being part of the major histocompatibility complex on the 6th chromosome. SLE, or syndromes very similar to it, are known to be found in the absence of the early components of complement, C2 and C4, whether the "null" allele is homozygous or heterozygous (Howard et al. 1986; Rynes 1982).

It is suggested that deficiency of one or other of these complement components influences the size of antigen/antibody complexes that the body normally forms. The deficiency leads to abnormally large complexes, interfering with their normal "solubilisation" and disposal from the blood by macrophage action as it passes through the sinusoids of the liver and spleen. In consequence the abnormally large complexes deposit instead at peripheral sites, in the small vessels of the kidney, skin or lung, or on serosal surfaces. Here they not only initiate an inflammatory reaction but also are responsible for liberation of fresh antigen and thereby help to maintain the disease process (Lachmann 1987).

A hormonal aetiological factor is indicated by the striking female:male predominance of 9 or 10 to 1, and the fact that new cases of SLE rarely arise after the menopause. Finally, sunlight is an important factor, acting through the effect of ultraviolet light on the skin in denaturing DNA and thereby releasing new antigenic material.

Vasculitis

The excessive formation of autoantibody leads to the formation of antigen/ antibody complexes which may gain access to the circulation and deposit peripherally on small vessel walls, usually capillaries and small arteries. They bind to complement and so initiate the chain reaction of complement breakdown with damaging effects on local tissues.

The most serious effect is the production of lupus nephritis following the deposition – or formation – of immune complexes with complement on the basement membrane of glomerular capillaries. The basement membrane becomes thickened (Fig. 7.2) and the presence of bound IgG can be shown by fluorescent staining (Fig. 7.3). On electron microscopy the immune complex deposits are seen as dense masses in contact with the basement membrane (Fig. 7.4).

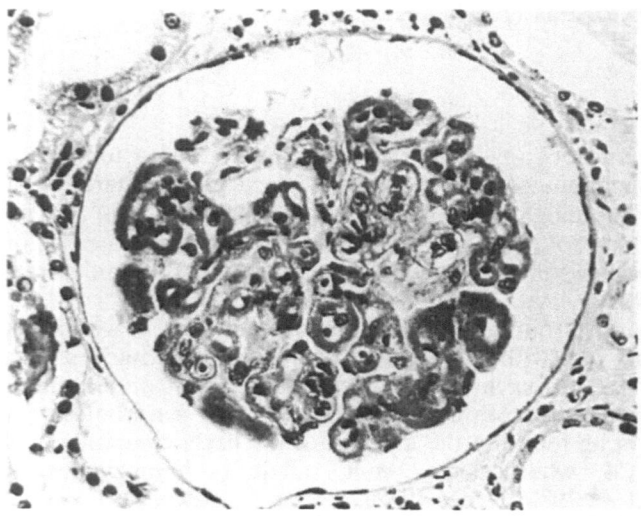

Fig. 7.2. Lupus nephritis. Renal glomerulus showing marked thickening of capillary basement membrane giving rise to the classical "wire loop" appearance (× 800).

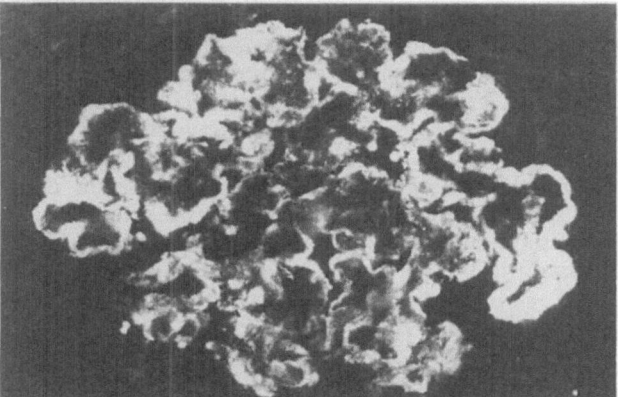

Fig. 7.3. Renal glomerulus showing deposits of IgG stained by immunofluorescent technique (× 690).

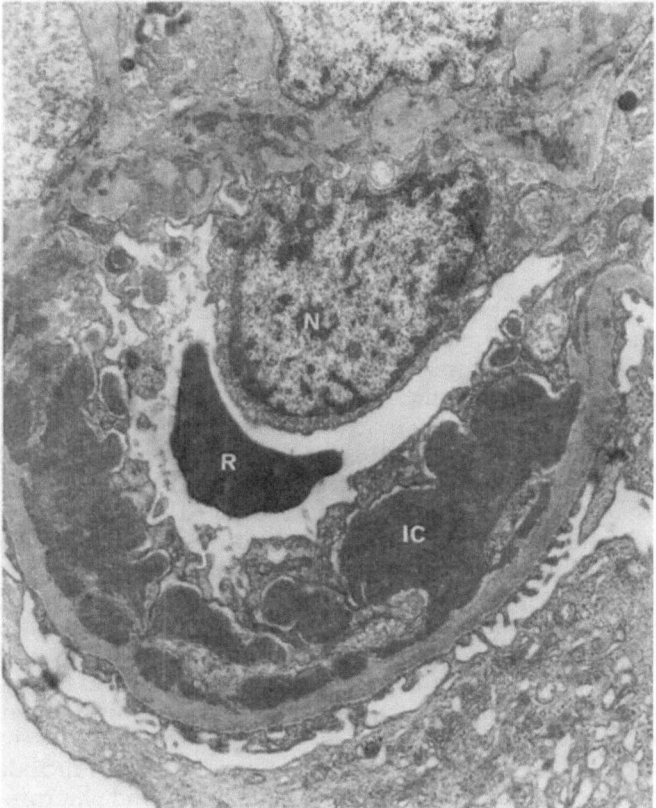

Fig. 7.4. Glomerular capillary. Electron micrograph (× 7800) showing dark deposits of immune complexes on the basement membrane (*IC* = immune complexes, *R* = red cell in lumen, *N* = nucleus of endothelial cell). By courtesy of the late Dr. Colin Tribe.

In bigger vessels such as arterioles and small muscular walled arteries a frank arteritis results from the deposition of immune complexes. The complexes are phagocytosed by polymorphs with the release of lysosomal enzymes and the production of local fibrinoid necrosis. Vaso-active amines and prostaglandins are released causing an increase in vascular permeability and the exudation of serum from the damaged vessels.

In the skin, immunoglobulin, also probably derived from deposited complexes, accumulates at the junction of dermis and epidermis. Its presence may be shown by immunofluorescent staining of biopsy specimens of apparently normal skin – the basis of the "lupus band test".

Pathology

There are few specific features in the microscopic appearances of the pathological lesions of SLE. The most characteristic is the "haematoxylin body", which is what remains of a cell nucleus after phagocytosis has destroyed polymorph or other cells. These bodies are the tissue counterpart of the "LE cell" nucleus seen in the now-abandoned LE cell test. Another characteristic histological finding is the "onion skin" appearance of vessel walls in the spleen resulting from vasculitis.

Drug-Induced SLE

A number of drugs, of which hydralazine and procainamide are the major examples, are capable of inducing a syndrome closely resembling SLE but with certain significant differences. Development of the syndrome is related to the cumulative dosage of the drug. The female preponderance of spontaneous SLE is not found in the drug-induced syndrome, which affects the two sexes roughly equally. Some genetic predisposition is indicated by the increased frequency of the syndrome among slow acetylators, and among carriers of the tissue antigen HLA–DR4. The autoantibodies formed are different: in the drug-induced syndrome antibodies are formed to histone and to ssDNA, but not to dsDNA. They may be found in half or more of individuals exposed to hydralazine or procainamide weeks or months before the clinical syndrome appears, and only a small proportion of those taking the drug, up to 3%, actually manifest the syndrome (Harmon and Portanova 1982).

Clinically, drug-induced SLE is less severe than the spontaneous disease. Cerebral involvement is not seen, and renal lesions are infrequent. There is a non-destructive polyarthritis, often with fever and myalgia, but cutaneous lesions are less common. Pleural and pericardial inflammation and effusions may occur and there are sometimes signs of myocarditis.

Other drugs that are associated with the SLE-like syndrome include anticonvulsants such as phenytoin, also penicillin, sulphonamides and chlorpromazine. The role of the drug may in some cases be that of exacerbating pre-existing disease rather than initiating it. In any case, the syndrome subsides after withdrawal of the drug.

Overlap Syndromes

Some patients present a mixture of manifestations of SLE combined with features of other connective tissue diseases, particularly scleroderma and/or polymyositis – mixed connective tissue disease, or MCTD (Sharp 1974). The "mixed" nature of the disorder may not be apparent at the start, until it has evolved further. Serologically such patients usually do not form dsDNA antibody, but nearly always have antibody to nuclear RNP, which is a characteristic of polymyositis. They may also have antibodies associated with systemic sclerosis (Chap. 9, pp. 198–9). Clinically the disease presents a mixture of features e.g. polyarthritis, Raynaud phenomenon, sclerodactyly and proximal muscle weakness. The more serious cerebral and renal lesions of SLE are uncommon.

As regards the heart, pericarditis may occur, occasionally with a large effusion or tamponade. Examples of myocarditis and heart block are on record, both in adults and in children (Alpert et al. 1983; Emlen 1979; Singsen et al. 1977). Case History 7.1 describes a patient whose illness was precipitated by exposure to sunlight, developing pericarditis and heart block, with recovery.

Case History 7.1

Mixed connective tissue disease
Heart block

Mrs. V.M., Housewife, born 1943

1971	Developed Raynaud phenomenon Arthralgia knees and ankles
1972	Depression, treated with ECT
1973	Arthralgia continued
1978	Swelling of finger joints On holiday had rash from sunlight Fever, chest pain and syncope
June 21	Admitted to hospital Pericarditis, complete heart block (Fig. 7.5) ANF++ (speckled pattern), LE test −ve DNA antibodies absent Given temporary pacemaker, prednisone 80 mg/day
June 30	Pacemaker off, prednisone reduced ECG: 2:1 AV block with Rbbb
July 14	24 hour ECG: mainly 2:1 block and periods of complete block (Fig. 7.6)
July 20	Discharged home in 2:1 block Well on prednisone 10 mg/day
Comment	Serology consistent with MCTD, not SLE. Variable degree of heart block. Acute symptoms probably induced by sunlight

---

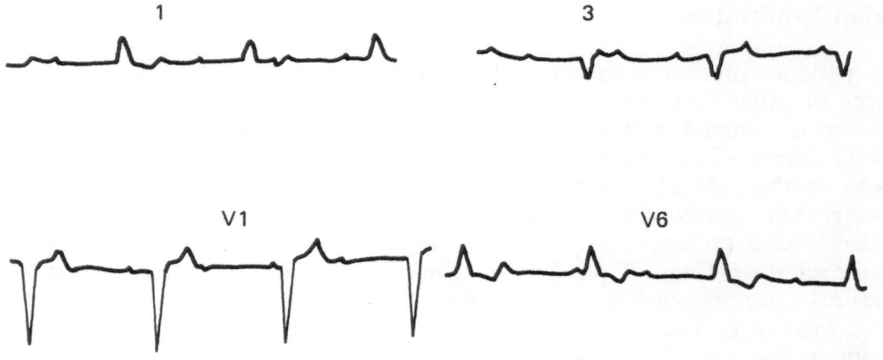

Fig. 7.5. Complete heart block with left bundle branch block in the patient described in Case History 7.1.

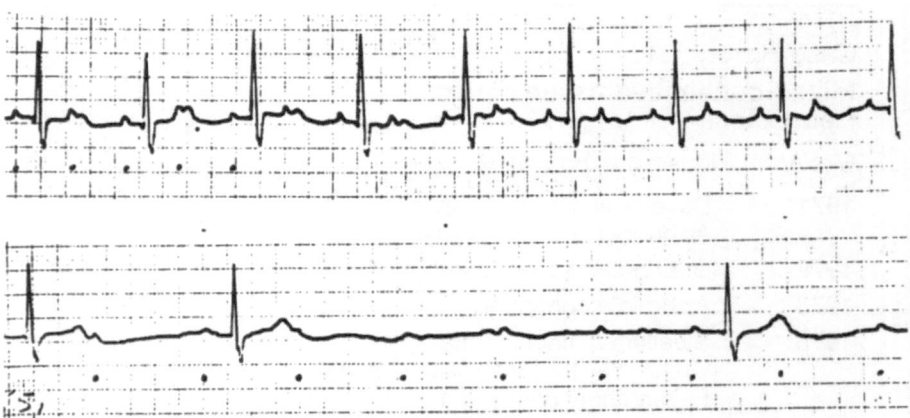

Fig. 7.6. Second degree heart block with 2:1 AV conduction and R bundle branch block (*above*) and a brief period of ventricular asystole (*below*, with P waves marked). From a 24-hour ECG recording made in the patient described in Case History 7.1.

Clinical Features of SLE

General

Being a multi-system disease, SLE has a wide variety of clinical presentations and patterns of evolution. The initial symptoms may be non-specific, with malaise, muscular aching and arthralgia, fever and depression. This stage may then progress to manifestations that are specifically associated with SLE, or it may subside. The course of the disease is unpredictable. In some patients the disease is acute and progressive from the start while in others it is episodic, or it may manifest as a single episode followed by apparent permanent resolution (Grigor et al. 1978).

A gradual progression is described in Case History 7.1, with further episodes at intervals and final remission. A sudden deterioration of SLE is described in Case History 7.2, provoked by sunlight after which the patient's illness ran a stormy course to eventual death.

In an analysis of the manifestations of SLE based on 150 cases, Estes and Christian (1971) noted that about half of their patients presented with musculoskeletal symptoms, about one-fifth with skin lesions and the remainder with a variety of symptoms. Pleurisy and pericarditis were uncommon at the start, being present in 2% or 3% only, but more common later. The frequency of eventual involvement of different systems in their series of patients is shown in Table 7.2.

Table 7.2. Incidence of major clinical manifestations of SLE based on 150 prospectively studied patients. (From Estes and Christian 1971)

Clinical manifestation	Percentage of patients
Musculo-articular	95
Cutaneous	81
Fever	77
Haemotological	
Anaemia	73
Leucopenia	66
Thrombocytopenia	19
Neuropsychiatric	59
Renal	53
Pleural and pulmonary	48
Cardiac	38

Case History 7.2

Systemic lupus erythematosus
Pericardial and pleural effusions
Fatal thrombocytopenia

Mrs. J.M., Housewife, born 1926

1962	Onset of seronegative polyarthritis
1965	Some deteriorations: started prednisone
1966–8	Hospital admissions, hip and knee lesions Rose Waaler and LE tests negative
1969	R hip arthroplasty

1970	ESR 102 mm/hr. Hb 10 g/dl. WBC 3000
May 1971	Exposure to sun on Mediterranean holiday Relapse in arthritis Pleural and pericardial effusions (Fig. 7.7) LE cells + + Anaemia, Coombs test +ve Effusions cleared with prednisone 60 mg/day
Aug 1971	Improved; prednisone 20 mg/day
1972–3	Worsening arthritis, pericarditis, anaemia, leucopenia and thrombocytopenia
1974	Died with uncontrollable thrombocytopenia
Autopsy	Adherent pericardium, partial fusion of two aortic valve cusps Many haemorrhages
Comment	A destructive seronegative polyarthritis, requiring hip surgery. Exposure to sunlight provoked florid SLE. Progressive deterioration and death in spite of all therapeutic efforts

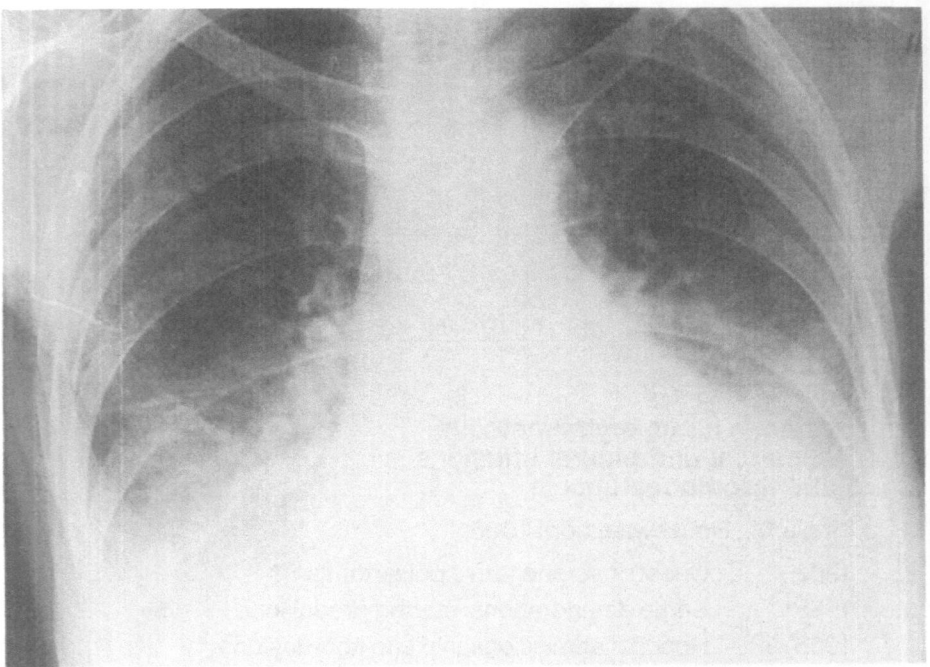

Fig. 7.7. Pleural and pericardial effusions. Chest X-ray film of the patient described in Case History 7.2.

Musculoskeletal Symptoms

Musculoskeletal symptoms include the non-specific myalgia and arthralgia already mentioned, sometimes with tenosynovitis. These symptoms may progress to a frank polyarthritis. Usually this is a non-erosive seronegative arthritis with a relatively good prognosis as regards function, with little deformity. In a few patients the arthritis is identifiable as rheumatoid arthritis i.e. it is seropositive, causes erosion of cartilage, forms nodules and results in considerable joint damage. Rheumatoid arthritis can be the presenting illness, with the addition of the multi-systemic features of SLE later on. In addition, a damaging bony lesion may arise as a result of avascular necrosis e.g. of the femoral head (Case History 7.5).

Renal Symptoms

Nephritis is uncommon as a presenting feature but often develops silently, its onset only being detected if the urine is regularly examined for albumen and casts. Ultimately at least half of SLE patients have some degree of lupus nephritis. Albuminuria is severe enough to produce the nephrotic syndrome in many patients. Renal biopsy is important in assessing the nature of the renal changes (Fig. 7.2) and in planning treatment, which often involves steroid or immunosuppressive drugs. Associated hypertension is common and renal failure may finally be the cause of death (Adu and Cameron 1982; Lee et al. 1977).

Neuropsychiatric Symptoms

Neuropsychiatric symptoms range from depression and migraine to chorea, epilepsy, confusional states and dementia. Definitive proof that such disorders have an organic basis and that this is due to SLE may be difficult to obtain. Changes in the EEG may be demonstrable, but other evidence may require highly specialised investigations such as measurement of cerebral oxygen uptake or imaging by nuclear magnetic resonance. Chorea and some lesions that have a thrombotic basis, such as infarction of brain, or of spinal cord producing myelitis, are now seen to be associated with the presence of anticardiolipin antibody (Asherson et al. 1987; Hughes et al. 1986).

Cutaneous Lesions

The classical malar butterfly erythema is a strong diagnostic pointer but is present in little over a half of SLE patients, and is likely to be transitory. Other skin lesions are alopecia, discoid lupus, urticaria, livedo reticularis and Raynaud's phenomenon.

Haematological Changes

Characteristic blood changes include leucopenia and normochromic anaemia. Haemolytic anaemia and thrombocytopenia may also be part of the clinical picture of SLE, sometimes antedating multisystem SLE by an interval of years. Thrombocytopenia was a terminal feature in Case History 7.2.

Pleural and Pulmonary Symptoms

Pleural and pulmonary symptoms include pleurisy with or without effusion, pneumonia and fibrosing alveolitis (Olsen and Lever 1972). The cytology of the pleural fluid in cases of effusion reflects an inflammatory process; the glucose level in the fluid is not reduced as it usually is in a rheumatoid pleural effusion. Antinuclear antibody may be found in the fluid and a reduction of C3 and C4 complement components. In some instances pleural biopsy has shown perivascular infiltration with lymphocytes and plasma cells with suggestive evidence for the local formation of immune complexes. Recurrent large pleural effusions were a problem in the patient described in Case History 7.3, ultimately requiring the surgical induction of pleural adhesions before the disease came under control.

Slowly progressive shrinkage of the lower lobes of the lungs may be seen on serial X-ray films; this is not explicable on the basis of pulmonary infection or fibrosis, and the cause appears to be a weakening of the diaphragmatic muscle, due to a form of myositis (Turner-Stokes and Turner-Warwick 1982).

Case History 7.3

SLE, Haemolytic anaemia, Thrombocytopenia
Neurological symptoms
Recurrent pleural effusions

Mrs. F.B., Nurse, born 1939

1964	Fever, arthralgia and rash
	Thrombocytopenia
	Haemolytic anaemia LE cells + +
	Responded to prednisone 40 mg/day
1965	Prednisone withdrawn: convulsion
	Prednisone restarted, 15 mg/day
1966	Migraine BP 170/110
	Enlarged liver, spleen and lymph nodes
	Large bilateral pleural effusions
	Pseudo-chylous fluid withdrawn, cholesterol +
	14 aspirations R and 11 L; 1 or 2 litres each
	R thoracotomy after which R effusions ceased
	Migraine continues BP 180/140
	Prednisone dosage 15 to 30 mg/day
1967	Further aspirations L pleural fluid
	L thoracoscopy and introduction of talc
	No further effusions on L
	ECG evidence of pericarditis
	Prednisone reduced to 5 mg/day BP became normal

1973	Minor R hemiparesis and dysphasia, recovered
1979	Well on prednisone 4 mg/day
Comment	Multi-system manifestations. Major problem with pleural effusions, settled after surgical measures. Hypertension apparently related to high steroid dosage and not to renal involvement

Cardiac Features

Involvement of the heart is not a prominent feature of SLE, but of those lesions which do occur pericarditis is the most frequent (Table 7.3). The situation is similar to that in rheumatoid arthritis: the pericardium is not often affected in the initial stages of the disease, but is quite commonly, though silently, involved later on. Signs of pericarditis are commoner at autopsy than clinically. Lesions of the valves, myocardium and coronary vessels may all occur but are relatively rare. Occlusive lesions of major arteries are rare occurrences, but are now seen to be a specific feature of SLE through their association with anticardiolipin antibody. Secondary effects on the heart are a common result of systemic hypertension due to renal disease and also, though rarely, may be the result of pulmonary hypertension.

Table 7.3. Cardiac involvement in SLE

1. *Pericarditis*
    Common clinical finding
    Even commoner pathological finding
2. *Valve lesions*
    Libman–Sacks vegetation on mitral or aortic valve
    Aortic incompetence with fibrinoid necrosis of cusp
    Rarely mitral stenosis
3. *Myocarditis*
    Mainly a pathological finding
    May contribute to heart failure or heart block
4. *Arterial occlusion*
    May affect coronary or other major vessel
5. *Hypertension*
    Systemic hypertension common, secondary to renal disease
    Rarely pulmonary hypertension

Pericarditis

Incidence

Pericarditis is the commonest cardiac manifestation of SLE. Reports of its frequency, as recognised clinically, range from 24% (Lee et al. 1977) and 30% (Dubois and Tuffanelli 1964) to 45% (Harvey et al. 1954), but it is uncommon as a presenting feature of the disease (2% or 3%).

Pericarditis is found more often at autopsy than clinically. Brigden et al. (1960) found signs of present or past pericarditis in 74% of autopsies, but only in 43% of SLE patients: The difference was not so great in Shearn's series (1959), with figures of 44% and 31% respectively. The explanation, as with rheumatoid pericarditis, lies in the mild and often unobtrusive nature of the pericarditis. It is often present without being detected, leaving its residue of adhesions which may be found at autopsy to have obliterated the pericardial cavity.

Pathology

In the active stage of inflammation both surfaces of the pericardium are diffusely thickened and oedematous with a fibrinous exudate and an effusion which is usually small; large effusions are unusual. Histologically, in addition to oedema there are areas of fibrinoid necrosis in which many haematoxylin bodies may be seen; these are the remains of polymorph nuclei. At a later stage, after the effusion has absorbed, light fibrous adhesions form between the two pericardial surfaces. These adhesions are rarely sufficiently dense to impede the heart's action or to cause constriction.

The pericardial fluid is pale yellow and may be lightly blood-stained. There may be up to 20 000 white cells/mm^3 which are mainly polymorphs. The glucose level in the fluid may be reduced, but not so consistently as in rheumatoid pericardial and pleural effusions. The fluid contains antinuclear antibodies and LE cells; the level of complement is reduced and immune complexes may be present, probably formed in situ (Hunder et al. 1974; Michet and Hunder 1984).

Clinical Features

As might be expected, the patient with lupus pericarditis is usually a young or middle-aged woman with SLE in an active phase. However, pericarditis has been noted in the newborn child of a mother with SLE (Doshi et al. 1980) and also in children who may present with juvenile chronic arthritis which evolves subsequently into SLE (Ragsdale et al. 1980).

Pericarditis may develop at any time during the course of SLE while the disease is active. The duration of clinically detectable pericarditis appears usually to be brief, resolving in a matter of days, although it may persist subclinically for weeks with relapses. The commonest symptom is pain, which is either a dull substernal ache or a sharper pain related to respiration or posture, being eased by sitting upright and leaning forward. Pleurisy may also be present in which case pleural symptoms tend to dominate (Case Histories 7.2, 7.3, 7.4).

A friction rub is only heard in a minority of cases, but this depends upon the care with which it is sought and the frequency of examination.

Dyspnoea is only likely if the effusion is a large one, which is unusual. Other factors may contribute to dyspnoea, such as a pleural effusion, anaemia or myocarditis. Occasionally an effusion is large enough to cause tamponade, producing signs of central venous engorgement, hepatomegaly, orthopnoea and pulsus paradoxus (p. 94). Tamponade occurred in only 1 patient in a series of 83 with cardiac involvement (Table 7.4) (Shearn 1969) and in 2 patients in a series of 29, both of whom needed surgical relief (Estes and Christian 1971). A number of individual case reports of tamponade are on record, both in spontaneous SLE (e.g. Carroll and Barrett 1984) and in the drug-induced form (e.g. Stein et al. 1979).

Table 7.4. Pericarditis in SLE: from a study of 83 patients with cardiac involvement; 16 deaths with autopsies (From Shearn 1959)

	Percentage
Clinical evidence of pericarditis in	31
Autopsy evidence of pericarditis (7/16)	44
Pericardial friction rub (16/83)	19
ECG evidence of pericarditis	12
Significant pericardial effusion	7
Tamponade in one patient only	–

Case History 7.4

Systemic lupus erythematosus
Pericarditis and pleural effusions
Minor recurrences and remissions

Mrs. D.C., Housewife, born 1910

1965 Nov	Polyarthralgia for 6 months Transient knee effusions Central chest pain, pericardial friction Bilateral pleural effusions
December	LE cells +++ ESR 110 mm/hr ECG: atrial fibrillation, flattening all T waves Responded to prednisone 30 mg/day
1966 Jan	No signs of pericarditis: sinus rhythm
February	Symptom-free Prednisone 5 mg/day ECG: T waves returning to normal
1967	Recurrence of minor central chest pain Chest X-ray and ECG normal Temporary increase in prednisone Returned to maintenance dose of 5 mg/day
1978 Dec	Transient butterfly rash and arthralgia accompanying chest infection Cleared on penicillin and prednisone 14 mg/day
1979 Feb	Well and symptom-free: prednisone 5 mg/day
Comment	An acute illness in November 1965 with pericarditis, pleurisy and atrial fibrillation. Good response to prednisone, with minor reactivations responding to temporary increase in prednisone

Complications

Constrictive pericarditis is a rare complication in SLE as the fibrous adhesions resulting from pericarditis are usually not particularly dense. A few cases are on record, both in spontaneous SLE (Hejtmancik et al. 1964; Jacobson and Reza 1978; Yurchak et al. 1965) and in a patient with procainamide induced SLE (Sunder and Shah 1975). The evolution from the inflammatory stage of pericarditis is usually slow, but has been observed in a matter of weeks (Starkey and Hahn 1973).

Secondary infection of the pericardium is a possibility in a seriously ill and debilitated patient, or in one whose resistance has been lowered by immunosuppressive drugs. This carries a grave prognosis and may be a terminal event. Staphylococcal pericarditis was described by Knodell and Manders (1974).

Diagnosis

Diagnosis of pericarditis in SLE rests on the same evidence as has been described for rheumatoid pericarditis (p. 95) i.e. the presence of chest pain, dyspnoea and possibly a friction rub and occasionally signs of tamponade. The X-ray film and ECG evidence are as described.

Echocardiography is the most sensitive diagnostic method for revealing even a small effusion or pericardial thickening. Collins et al. (1978) found echocardiographic signs of pericarditis in 35% of a series of SLE patients who had normal chest X-ray films and electrocardiograms. At the same time a study can be made of mitral and aortic valve function (Elkayam et al. 1977).

Treatment

In most cases the pericarditis is sufficiently mild and transitory for specific measures to be unnecessary, beyond the treatment of SLE in general (Hughes 1979). For relief of pain aspirin or non-steroid anti-inflammatory drugs are indicated, and they may assist in the resolution of the pericarditis. If pain persists or if the effusion does not absorb, corticosteroid may be given e.g. prednisone 30 or 40 mg daily, reducing soon after a response is achieved. Antimalarial and immunosuppressive drugs, usually plaquenil and azathioprine, will assist as steroid sparers if not already being given. If pericardial aspiration should be necessary, intrapericardial steroid may be given at the same time e.g. prednisolone acetate 20 mg or triamcinolone hexacetonide 20 mg.

Valve Lesions

General

The classical heart valve lesion in SLE is the low-grade endocarditis with vegetation formation on the mitral valve, originally described by Libman and Sacks (1924) (Fig. 7.8). At the time they saw this as an autonomous lesion, and it was Gross (1940) who recognised it as being part of systemic lupus.

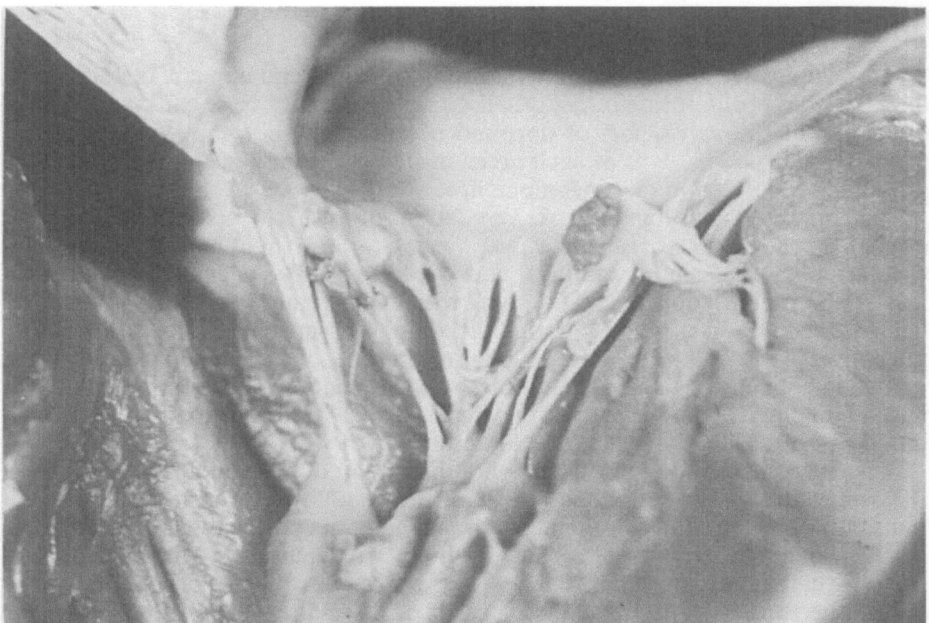

Fig. 7.8. Mitral valve (× 1.6) showing a characteristic small Libman–Sacks vegetation on the posterior cusp.

Other valves, particularly the aortic, may be affected too, and minor pathological changes are often present that cannot be detected clinically. The effect on cardiac function of any of these valve lesions is usually slight, although occasionally an aortic or mitral lesion of importance may arise.

Incidence

Pathological endocardial changes are found in a half or more of hearts examined at autopsy (Dubois 1974; Harvey et al. 1954) but valve lesions are only recognised in life in under a quarter of patients with SLE. Brigden et al. (1960) found abnormalities in the valves of half of the hearts (13 of 27) examined at autopsy, but could only recognise a valve lesion clinically in one-fifth (12 of 60) of the patients seen. They found organic mitral murmurs in 8 and aortic murmurs in 6, 2 patients having both mitral and aortic lesions. Tricuspid and pulmonary valve lesions are rarely, if ever, diagnosed in life, although some pathological changes may be seen in these valves at autopsy.

Bulkley and Roberts (1975) commented that since the introduction of corticosteroid treatment for SLE, Libman–Sacks lesions had become fewer and also smaller than previously. However, they also found an increased incidence in hypertension and coronary atherosclerosis which they attributed to the influence of corticosteroids.

Pathology

The affected valve cusp shows mild fibrous thickening and appears oedematous; there is often proliferation of endothelial cells on the surface of the cusp. Within the tissue of the valve, foci of fibrinoid necrosis may be seen, with scattered haematoxylin bodies. It is at such areas of necrosis that a cusp may perforate, producing fenestration and incompetence.

The characteristic Libman-Sacks vegetation forms on the ventricular aspect of a cusp of the mitral or aortic valve, near the cusp margin (Fig. 7.8). The vegetation consists mainly of fibrin, and three zones have been described within it: a superficial zone of exudation with amorphous protein, fibrin and haematoxylin bodies (Fig. 7.9), a middle zone of organisation with proliferating fibroblasts and capillaries, and an innermost zone of neo-vascularisation with maturing connective tissue. Immunofluorescent staining shows deposits of IgG and complement components in the thickened cusp, and in the walls of small blood vessels (Bidani et al. 1980; Shapiro et al. 1977).

Vegetations are thought to begin with disruption of the endothelial surface of the valve due to the turbulence of blood flow, followed by the deposition of immune complexes and complement. Increased tissue permeability leads to local oedema of the valve tissue and finally there is organisation with fibrosis and neo-vascularisation.

For the most part these pathological changes make little difference to the functioning of the affected valve. But thickening and fibrosis are sometimes sufficient to cause mitral or aortic incompetence, or adhesions may form between the mitral cusps and produce stenosis; however, aortic stenosis has not been recorded. Calcification may be a late sequel in a damaged valve.

Clinical Features

Most mitral and aortic valve lesions in SLE cause few symptoms, but if a significant lesion develops the physical signs are the same as those already described for mitral incompetence, mitral stenosis and aortic incompetence due to rheumatic heart disease (Chap. 2). However, symptoms such as dyspnoea, fatigue, oedema and venous engorgement may arise from other effects of the disease, being added to the symptoms due to the valve lesion. For example, anaemia, renal disease, pleurisy, pericarditis and hypertension may each contribute to the symptomatology.

The stage in the course of SLE at which a valve lesion may develop is very variable. A mitral or an aortic valve lesion may appear in the first year of the disease or not until some years later. In Case History 7.5, severe mitral stenosis developed within 2 years of onset and required surgical valve replacement. The case of Vaughton et al. (1979) was similar. Three patients with aortic incompetence in the early stages of the disease are described by Bernhard et al. (1969). A number of accounts are available of mitral stenosis (Paget et al. 1975; Reilly et al. 1988), of mitral incompetence (Myerowitz et al. 1974), and of mixed stenosis and incompetence (Milne et al. 1981), developing at various stages in the course of the disease.

As with rheumatic heart disease, mitral stenosis may lead to secondary pulmonary hypertension; also, combined mitral and aortic valve disease may occur.

Sudden deterioration in a patient with an aortic valve lesion may be due to perforation of a cusp, producing severe regurgitation and precipitating left ventricular failure and pulmonary oedema; this was the case in one of the three patients described by Shulman and Christian (1969). A mitral lesion, too, may be made suddenly worse by rupture of one of the chordae tendineae or of a papillary muscle (Murray et al. 1975).

Valvular heart disease is one of the possible causes of death in SLE, though an uncommon one. While a number of surgical successes have been achieved, some patients are too ill to face cardiac surgery e.g. with renal failure, or may suffer further pathological developments after initial success.

Case History 7.5

SLE: Mitral stenosis
Mitral valve replacement

Paul R., Electrician, born 1948

1976 March	Febrile illness, arthralgia Mitral stenosis found Apical presystolic and mid-diastolic murmurs LE cell test + DNA binding 24% Serum complement reduced
April	Improved on prednisone 15 mg/day Arthralgia gone
1978 Jan	Becoming dyspnoeic
April	Marked deterioration, urgent dyspnoea Pulmonary embolus and LLL pneumonia *Open heart surgery* Pulmonary hypertension at systemic level Mitral orifice reduced to 5 mm diameter Granulation tissue and thrombus extending from mitral valve on to LV wall (Fig. 7.9) Mitral valve replaced with heterograft
June	Doing well, prednisone 20 mg/day reducing later to 8 mg/day
1979 April	Well but now has bilateral hip lesions
1980	Bilateral hip arthroplasties
1985	Died with staphylococcal septicaemia
Comment	Mitral stenosis an early development in the course of his SLE. Post-operative progress initially good, marred by developing hip lesions and later death from septicaemia

With acknowledgements to Dr. Justin Clark and Dr. M. Cawley

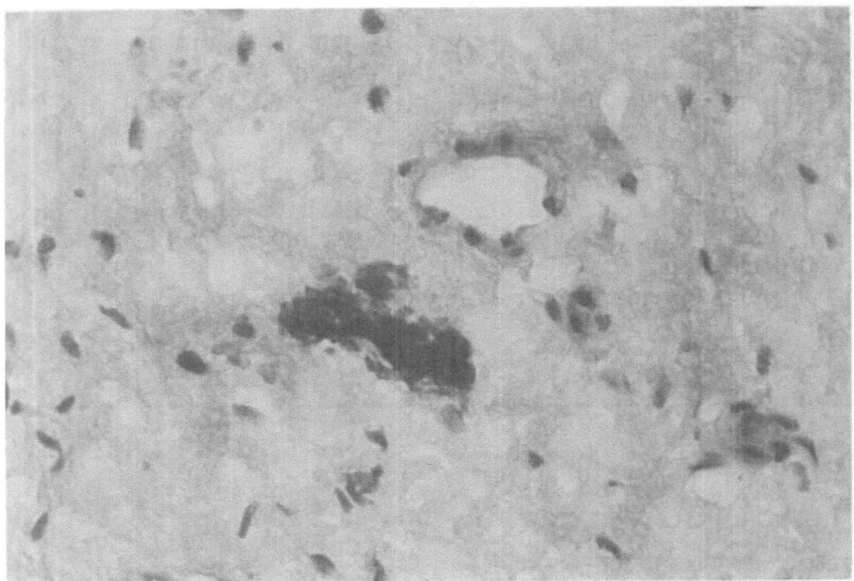

Fig. 7.9. Granulation tissue from mitral valve in the patient described in Case History 7.5. Scattered haematoxylin bodies are seen (× 180). With acknowledgements to Dr. PJ Gallagher.

Diagnosis

Auscultation. A heart murmur in a patient with SLE is not necessarily a sign of a valve lesion, as functional murmurs are common. The significant organic murmurs that do indicate valve lesions are the apical pansystolic murmur of mitral incompetence, the apical mid-diastolic murmur of mitral stenosis with an opening snap, and an aortic diastolic murmur. Other causes of systolic murmurs include "functional" mitral incompetence due to dilatation of the left ventricle secondary to hypertension, coronary disease or myocarditis, the systolic murmur of a prolapsing mitral cusp, and the functional systolic murmur found with a hyperdynamic heart action in the presence of anaemia or fever.

Chest X-ray. Chest X-ray films may not be helpful. The size of the cardiac shadow may be enlarged by a pericardial effusion; genuine cardiomegaly may be due to hypertension, myocarditis or coronary disease, and not necessarily to a valve lesion. There may be calcification at the mitral or aortic valve, but there are a number of other possible causes for this. Fluoroscopy may be of help in identifying mitral or aortic regurgitation.

Electrocardiography. The ECG may be abnormal in various ways and is only likely to contribute indirectly to the diagnosis of a valve lesion. ST and T wave changes may be caused by pericarditis, myocarditis, and left ventricular hypertrophy. Arrhythmias such as atrial fibrillation or flutter may be seen, or conduction defects.

Echocardiography. This technique is valuable for the same reasons that it is in the diagnosis of rheumatic valvular heart disease. It can reveal thickening of mitral or aortic valve cusps, or reduction of mitral closing rate due to valve disease. The size of the mitral aperture can be measured and visualised with 2-D echocardiography. Serial examinations over a period enable the progress of valve pathology to be watched. Collins et al. (1978) reported finding abnormalities at the mitral valve in a quarter of the patients with SLE studied by echocardiography, as well as finding evidence of pericarditis in a third. Maniscalco et al. (1975) found a reduction in the EF slope in 9 of 25 patients, indicating an abnormality of mitral cusp movement, although only 1 patient had signs of mitral cusp thickening. Kahan et al. (1985) drew attention to the advantages of 2-D echocardiography over one-dimensional M mode studies, in helping to differentiate between the vegetation and cusp thickening of SLE and the vegetation of infective endocarditis.

Differential Diagnosis. The valve lesions of SLE may be indistinguishable from those of rheumatic heart disease other than in the general clinical setting. Also, lone aortic incompetence may occur in SLE whereas it is accompanied by an appreciable mitral lesion in rheumatic heart disease. A prolapsing mitral cusp produces an apical and central systolic murmur and a systolic click which is characteristic; echocardiography shows the typical pattern of echo caused by the prolapse. But a prolapsing mitral cusp may be present in a patient with SLE. Infective endocarditis may be difficult to distinguish from a mitral or aortic lesion in SLE, perhaps accompanied by fever. Close clinical observation, repeated blood cultures and echocardiography (preferably 2-D) will help to distinguish between the two.

Treatment

The presence of a progressive valve lesion is an indication for corticosteroid treatment, particularly if the disease generally is active. This is on the grounds that endocardial lesions are modified by corticosteroids, with evidence of healing and stabilisation. In view of the risks of using corticosteroids, both generally and in promoting coronary atherosclerosis and hypertension (Bulkley and Roberts 1975), the policy should be to treat the patient for a period of weeks or months with an effective dose, such as prednisone 30 mg daily, closely following the signs of valvular disease and reducing dosage to a minimum as soon as appropriate. The aim should be ultimately to withdraw corticosteroids altogether.

Long-term anticoagulant treatment e.g. with warfarin, is advisable with valve lesions, particularly mitral stenosis, accompanied by atrial fibrillation. An additional indication is the finding of anticardiolipin antibodies, because of their known link with thrombosis.

Diuretics are needed for relief of systemic or pulmonary oedema. Digitalisation is indicated if there are signs of congestive failure and is best given indefinitely if there is established atrial fibrillation. Potassium levels must be monitored if digitalis and diuretics are given together, as hypokalaemia adds to the risk of digitalis toxicity. If there is any impairment of renal function serum digoxin levels should be monitored too as renal failure reduces the excretion rate of digoxin.

Cardiac Surgery. Surgical valve replacement is sometimes necessary for a mitral or aortic lesion, and a number of successful results are reported in the references cited above (p. 150). The indications for surgery are as given for rheumatic valve disease, essentially being worsening cardiac function with actual or threatened left ventricular or congestive failure not controllable by medical means. The situation is sometimes urgent, if for example there has been sudden valve damage caused by perforation of a cusp, a ruptured mitral chorda or superimposed bacterial infection.

The estimation of the risks of surgery has to take into account other possible adverse effects of systemic lupus such as pericarditis, myocarditis and pleural or renal pathology.

Myocarditis

The diagnosis of lupus myocarditis can rarely be made on clinical grounds alone, although pathological changes in heart muscle are a common finding at autopsy. The clinical signs which might indicate the presence of myocarditis may also have other more obvious causes, such as coronary atherosclerosis, hypertension or a valve lesion so that the effects of myocarditis may be overshadowed by other cardiovascular manifestations of SLE.

Incidence

Pathological changes in the myocardium are seen in approximately half of autopsied cases of SLE (e.g. Harvey et al. 1954; Shearn 1959), although the proportion quoted in other reports varies according to the histological criteria. In patients who have received long-term corticosteroid therapy the severity of myocardial and endocardial changes appears to be reduced, but the probability of coincident hypertension and coronary atherosclerosis is increased (Bulkley and Roberts 1975).

Myocarditis has been recognised clinically in about 8% of systemic lupus patients (Dubois 1974; Estes and Christian 1971). The higher figure of 40% given by Shearn (1959) is based on purely electrocardiographic changes. Echocardiography suggests that the majority of patients with SLE have some myocardial functional abnormality (Chia et al. 1981; Del Rio et al. 1978). However, as Bennett (1984) has pointed out, it is virtually impossible to know whether impaired myocardial function should be attributed to myocarditis, coronary atherosclerosis or arteritis.

Pathology

There are no apparent changes in the myocardium visible to the naked eye. Histologically there is infiltration by plasma cells and lymphocytes in the fibrous septa between the myocardial cells, with oedema and foci of fibrinoid necrosis and occasional haematoxylin bodies. Degenerative changes within myocardial cells, and areas of necrosis due to small vascular occlusions caused by arteritis, may be seen. Occasionally a medium-sized coronary artery may be the site of necrotising arteritis leading to occlusion and myocardial infarction. Myocardial damage resulting from coronary atherosclerosis may also be present, and this is a commoner finding in SLE than is primary myocarditis.

Clinical Features

Classically, myocarditis causes weakening and stretching of the myocardium, dilatation of the heart, low output failure with gallop rhythm and possibly arrhythmias and conduction defects. This full clinical picture is rare in SLE. In those patients in whom myocarditis is suspected, it is usually on the grounds of cardiomegaly, tachycardia and echocardiographic and ECG abnormalities and frank congestive failure is unlikely. Brigden et al. (1960) found no example among 60 patients of congestive failure purely attributable to myocarditis, but considered hypertension was the chief factor in the 22 patients who did have heart failure.

Diagnosis

Diagnosis is based on clinical findings, with X-ray evidence of cardiomegaly and ECG and echocardiographic changes. The ECG may show T wave inversions, atrial fibrillation, ventricular ectopic beats or first degree or bundle branch block. Complete block is discussed below.

Echocardiography is the most sensitive indicator of myocarditis. M mode recording may show dilatation of the left ventricle with a reduced fractional shortening of the ventricular diameter in systole (normally 30% or more). The distinction between myocarditis and myocardial damage from coronary disease cannot be made by M mode recording, but it may be possible to distinguish between the two by 2-D (cross-sectional) visualisation. This may reveal regional defects in ventricular wall motion in the case of coronary disease but not with myocarditis.

Myocarditis may be a feature of mixed connective tissue disease, when it is associated with myositis (Lash et al. 1986). Antibody to RNP is usually present.

Treatment

The finding of myocarditis is an indication for corticosteroid treatment. In view of reports of myocarditis healing after prolonged treatment, a course of 3 to 6 months on prednisone is justified. A suitable dose would be 30 mg daily at first, reducing to a maintenance dose of 10 mg according to progress.

There is a dilemma here, as Bennett (1984) points out, in that corticosteroid may exacerbate coronary atheroma or hypertension, but this therapy is justified nevertheless for the relief of myocarditis or coronary arteritis.

Heart Block

Adult Form

Small vessel vasculitis in SLE may damage nodal or conducting tissue in the heart, producing heart block. Destruction of the sinus node or of the atrioventricular node has been described, with replacement of nodal tissue by granulation tissue or fibrosis (Bharati et al. 1975). Complete heart block results, although this is a rare event in SLE (Bourel et al. 1971; Moffitt 1965) or in mixed connective tissue disease (Emlen 1979). Bundle branch block has also been noted (Hejtmancik et al. 1964), sometimes as a temporary stage in the progression to complete block.

Atrial fibrillation or atrial standstill can occur as a complication of pericarditis due to the inflammatory process spreading into the area of the sinus node, which lies very near the surface of the atrial myocardium (Hover and Koppes 1979; James et al. 1965).

The treatment of complete block is by pacing, which gives good long-term results and a good prognosis, subject to the disease in general remaining under control (Wray and Iveson 1975).

Congenital Form

Congenital heart block in the newborn is now recognised as a possible result of systemic lupus in the mother during pregnancy, even though the disease may not be fully expressed in her (Case History 7.6, Fig. 7.10) (Berube et al. 1978; Chameides et al. 1977).

The improved prognosis for mother and child in pregnancy has encouraged more patients with SLE to proceed to term rather than have the pregnancy terminated, as previously recommended. Some manifestations of systemic lupus may appear in the child, as a result of maternal antibodies crossing the placenta. Some effects are of short duration and recover spontaneously within days or weeks, e.g. lupus rash, pericarditis (Doshi et al. 1980), anaemia, leucopenia or thrombocytopenia, but heart block is probably always permanent (Chameides et al. 1977; Davies 1984; Hess and Spencer-Green 1979).

Surveys of pregnancies in women with SLE have revealed neonatal heart block with might otherwise have gone unrecognised (McCue et al. 1977).

Heart block may be recognised during foetal life, and it is important to distinguish it from the bradycardia of foetal distress (Berube et al. 1978). Some infants tolerate complete heart block well, as the idioventricular rate in the newborn is 60 to 80/minute, and not all will require pacing. In some instances the true nature of the child's bradycardia has not been recognised until much later in life, possibly coinciding with the development of SLE or a related form of autoimmune disease.

Esscher and Scott (1979), reviewing the health of the mothers of babies born with complete heart block, found that one-third of them either had SLE, possibly in an incomplete form, or would develop SLE in subsequent years. Of the 27 cases in their series, foetal heart block was diagnosed antenatally in 24. Nine infants died and at autopsy 7 of these had endomycardial fibrosis.

Similarly, McCune et al. (1987) reviewed 21 families in which 24 children had been born with evidence of systemic lupus: 12 infants had heart block, 10 had cutaneous lupus and 2 had both. Five of the 11 surviving children with heart block now have pacemakers. Of the mothers, half were initially asymptomatic, but 18 of the 21 later developed SLE; of 12 children born in subsequent pregnancies, 3 had signs of neonatal lupus.

Maddison et al. (1983) studied sera from 41 mothers of infants with congenital heart block and found anti Ro (SSA) antibodies in 25 of them (61%): the same antibody was identified in the sera of the children of those mothers, up to the age of 6 months. After that time the antibody disappeared in the children although heart block persisted. The implication is that antibody of maternal origin crossed the placenta and was present in the foetus at the time of development of the cardiac conducting system, inflicting permanent damage, but disappearing from the child some months after birth.

Treatment of neonatal heart block is not always required as many infants tolerate the bradycardia well. But if dyspnoea, distress or syncope follow, pacing becomes necessary. There are important lessons regarding prophylaxis: any pregnancy in a mother with systemic lupus must be monitored carefully for signs of foetal or neonatal heart block, or for other signs of neonatal lupus. And following the diagnosis of heart block in any newborn child, the mother must be screened for signs of systemic lupus or related autoimmune disease, not merely at the time of childbirth but also in later years (Davies 1984).

Case History 7.6

**Congenital complete heart block
Latent maternal SLE**

Mrs. K.B., Housewife, born 1958

1979 June 1	Caesarian section at 38 weeks in first pregnancy for presumed foetal distress with foetal heart rate of 80 Baby had complete heart block (Fig. 7.10) Mother had been well during pregnancy No history suggesting SLE
June 18	Mother developed iliofemoral venous thrombosis, given anticoagulants Plasma viscosity raised, 2.02 Hb 9.0 WBC 6.7 Total globulin raised, 34 g/l ANF +, speckled pattern DNA binding 15%, anti DNA −ve
1980	Baby well but still in complete block Mother well
1985	Mother developed arthralgias and then nephrotic syndrome: renal biopsy showed crescentic glomerulonephritis Reponded to pulsed steroid + azathioprin

1986   Photosensitive dermatitis in mother
            Child remains well, bradycardia still

Comment   Discovery of heart block in child led to recognition of
            incomplete form of SLE in mother, more fully expressed by
            renal lupus 7 years later

With acknowledgements to Professor Peter Maddison

___

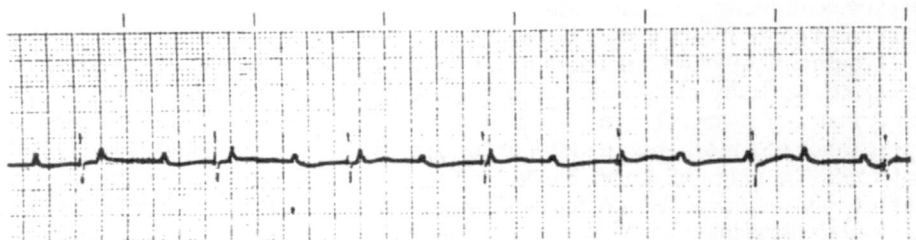

Fig. 7.10. Complete heart block in the newborn child described in Case History 7.6. The atrial rate is 110 and the ventricular rate 60/minute.

Coronary Arteritis

Vasculitis in systemic lupus is the result of the deposition of immune complexes and complement on the endothelium of small vessels, usually of the calibre of arterioles and venules. In the heart this process plays a part in the causation of lesions in the myocardium and, to a less extent, in the endocardium and pericardium.

Medium-sized and larger muscular walled arteries, including the coronary arteries, may sometimes be the site of a more serious necrotising arteritis resembling polyarteritis nodosa. Histologically there is an accumulation of polymorphs in all layers of the arterial wall, with oedema, resulting in narrowing or obliteration of the lumen (Fauci et al. 1978). It has been suggested that this focal arterial damage may be a predisposing factor in the later development of atherosclerosis (Parrillo and Fauci 1980). If so, the observed higher incidence of coronary atherosclerosis in corticosteroid-treated patients with SLE (Bulkley and Roberts 1975; Tsakraklides et al. 1974) may be explainable on the basis that corticosteroid treatment favours healing of coronary arteritis and atherosclerosis develops later at the site of the arteritic lesions.

On clinical grounds coronary arteritis should be suspected when angina or myocardial infarction develop in a patient with SLE, particularly if the patient is young, female and under treatment with corticosteroids. Several examples are on record, even in teenagers and children (Bonfiglio et al. 1972; Homcy et al. 1982; Ishikawa et al. 1978; Jensen and Sigurd 1973; Meller et al. 1975). At the same time, arteritis may manifest in other major arteries, e.g. in the lower limb causing gangrene (Gladstein et al. 1979). Coronary arteritis has also been reported in mixed connective tissue disease (Alpert et al. 1983).

Laboratory findings which support the diagnosis of arteritis include a raised ESR and C-reactive protein, antinuclear antibodies, reduced serum complement, cryoglobulinaemia and positive tests for circulating immune complexes.

Coronary arteriography may reveal the sites of arterial narrowing, which may be numerous (Haider and Roberts 1981). In one report a distinctive pattern was seen, with saccular aneurysms in the coronary vessels as well as obstructive lesions (Heibel et al. 1976).

Antiphospholipid (anticardiolipin) antibodies have been shown to be associated with occlusion of major arteries e.g. of main limb arteries (Asherson et al. 1986a), of the coronary arteries (Asherson et al. 1986b), and even of the aorta (Drew et al. 1987). In these lesions arteritis was absent, but a primary thrombotic tendency was present probably caused by abnormal platelet agglutination. Appropriate therapy in this situation is with anticoagulants or anti-platelet drugs.

Treatment of arteritis is with high dosage corticosteroid, commencing at the level of 60 to 80 mg prednisone daily, reducing in 1–3 weeks to half this level. If there is evidence of persistent or recurrent arteritis, indicating the need for prolonged treatment, a change may be made to an alternate-day regime, combined with immunosuppressive drugs such as azathioprine or cyclophosphamide as steroid sparers. Where thrombosis rather than arteritis is the underlying cause of arterial obstruction anticoagulant treatment is indicated.

Hypertension

Patients with systemic lupus are frequently hypertensive, generally as a result of renal disease, adding the possibility of hypertensive heart disease to the other effects of the disease upon the heart. Brigden et al. (1960) found 26 of their 60 patients to be hypertensive (43%), renal lupus being the cause in 20. Bulkley and Roberts (1975) in their clinical and autopsy study of 36 patients with SLE treated with corticosteroids, reported a higher incidence, 69%, with autopsy confirmation of hypertensive heart disease. They commented that this was almost a five-fold greater incidence of hypertension than was found in pre-steroid days; Klemperer et al. (1941) had found 15% to be hypertensive. The implication is that the widespread use of corticosteroids in the treatment of SLE, often given for long periods and sometimes in high dosage, has contributed to the more frequent association of hypertension with SLE. This has been a contributory factor in the more frequent finding of coronary atherosclerosis.

The presence of hypertension obviously adds to the frequency of heart disease in SLE, and calls for treatment with anti-hypertensive drugs, such as beta blockers, nifedipine, angiotensin-converting enzyme (ACE) inhibitors and diuretics. This may bring further problems of reaction to drugs. Some patients with drug-related SLE are hypertensives who have proved to be sensitive to hydralazine. Russell et al. (1987), reviewing 20 such patients, described improvement in the signs of SLE after withdrawal of hydralazine, but a relapse after the substitution of the ACE inhibitor captopril. It is important, therefore, to find a safe anti-hypertensive regime in view of the dangers of leaving hypertension inadequately treated, including the risk of an adverse effect on renal function and progression to malignant hypertension. The advantages of the management of SLE with minimum recourse to corticosteroids are clear.

Pulmonary Hypertension

Pulmonary hypertension is a rare but significant development in systemic lupus. Occasional case reports have described the finding, in a patient with SLE, of right ventricular hypertrophy, tricuspid incompetence and congestive failure resulting from pulmonary arterial hypertension for which no underlying pulmonary cause could be found. Similarly pulmonary hypertension of an apparently primary nature is an occasional finding in systemic sclerosis, mixed connective tissue disease and rheumatoid arthritis.

The symptoms of severe pulmonary hypertension are of progressive effort dyspnoea, sometimes with angina and syncope on effort, cyanosis and congestive failure. On physical examination there are signs of right ventricular hypertrophy, with a palpable right ventricular "heave" in the xiphisternal area, an accentuated second heart sound in the pulmonary valve area and confirmation of right ventricular hypertrophy by X-ray, ECG and echocardiography. Cardiac catheter studies may show the pulmonary arterial pressure to be at least double its normal value of about 20/10 mmHg, and sometimes to be the equal of systemic arterial pressure. Such findings have been described as unexplained or primary pulmonary hypertension, mainly in girls or young women, occurring in isolation, but sometimes associated with Raynaud's syndrome (Wade and Ball 1957; Walcott et al. 1970).

More recent reports have described similar pulmonary hypertension in association with SLE (Gladman and Sternberg 1985) and the finding of the "lupus anticoagulant" in this setting (Asherson et al. 1983; Asherson and Oakley 1986). The known association of the lupus anticoagulant with anticardiolipin antibody and a thrombotic tendency suggests that pulmonary hypertension may result from vascular thrombosis in small pulmonary vessels raising the pulmonary arterial resistance; multiple small pulmonary embolisation is another possible explanation, though rather less likely.

It therefore seems possible that a number of instances of unexplained or primary pulmonary hypertension may have a basis of autoimmune disease.

Treatment of pulmonary hypertension is notoriously difficult, but some success has been reported with nifedipine.

References

Adu D, Cameron JS (1982) Lupus nephritis. Clin Rheum Dis 8: 153–182

Alpert MA, Goldberg SH, Singsen BH (1983) Cardiovascular manifestations of mixed connective tissue disease in adults. Circulation 68: 1182–1193

Asherson RA, Oakley CM (1986) Pulmonary hypertension and systemic lupus erythematosus (editorial). J Rheumatol 13: 1–5.

Asherson RA, Mackworth-Young CG, Boey ML et al. (1983) Pulmonary hypertension in systemic lupus erythematosus. Br Med J 287: 1024–1025

Asherson RA, Derkson RHWM, Harris EN et al. (1986a) Large vessel occlusions and gangrene in systemic lupus erythematosus and "lupus-like" disease. J Rheumatol 13: 740–747

Asherson RA, Mackay AR, Harris EN (1986b) Myocardial infarction in a young man with systemic lupus erythematosus, deep vein thrombosis and antibodies to phospholipid. Br Heart J 56: 190–193

Asherson RA, Derkson RHWM, Harris EN et al. (1987) Chorea in systemic lupus erythematosus and "lupus-like" disease: association with antiphospholipid antibodies. Semin Arthritis Rheum 16: 253–259

Bakke AC, Kirkland PA, Kitridou RL et al. (1983) T lymphocyte subsets in systemic lupus erythematosus. Arthritis Rheum 26: 745–750

Bennett RB (1984) Myocardial involvement in SLE. In: Ansell BM, Simkin PA (eds) The heart and rheumatic disease. Butterworths, London, pp 39–43

Bernhard GC, Lange RL, Hensley GT (1969) Aortic disease with valvular insufficiency as the principal manifestation of SLE. Ann Intern Med 71: 81–87

Berube S, Lister.G, Toews WH, Creasy RK, Heymann MA (1978) Congenital heart block and maternal systemic lupus erythematosus. Am J Obstet Gynecol 130: 595–596

Bharati S, Fuente DJ, Kallen RJ, Freij Y, Lev M (1975) Conduction system in systemic lupus erythematosus with atrioventricular block. Am J Cardiol 35: 299–304

Bidani AK, Roberts JL, Schwartz MM, Lewis EJ (1980) Immunopathology of cardiac lesions in fatal SLE. Am J Med 69: 849–858

Bonfiglio TA, Botti RE, Hagstrom JWC (1972) Coronary arteritis, occlusion and myocardial infarction due to lupus erythematosus. Am Heart J 83: 153–158

Bourel G, Gouffault J, Boudesseul B (1971) Cardiovascular manifestations of disseminated lupus erythematosus. Coeur Med Intern 10: 535–544

Brigden W, Bywaters EGL, Lessof MH, Ross IP (1960) The heart in systemic lupus erythematosus. Br Heart J 22: 1–16

Bulkley BH, Roberts WC (1975) The heart in SLE and the changes induced in it by corticosteroid therapy. Am J Med 58: 243–264

Carroll N, Barrett JA (1984) Systemic lupus erythematosus presenting with cardiac tamponade. Br Heart J 51: 452–453

Chameides L, Truex RC, Vetter V, Rashkind WJ, Galioto FM, Noonan JA (1977) Association of maternal systemic lupus erythematosus with congenital heart block. N Engl J Med 297: 1204–1206

Chia BL, Mak BKM, Feng PH (1981) Cardiovascular abnormalities in SLE. J Clin Ultrasound 9: 237–242

Collins RL, Turner RA, Nomeir AM et al. (1978) Cardiopulmonary manifestations of SLE. J Rheumatol 5: 299–306

Davies MJ (1984) The conduction system in systemic lupus erythematosus. In: Ansell BM, Simkin PA (eds) The heart and rheumatic disease. Butterworths, London, pp 66–68

Del Rio A, Varquez JJ, Sobrino JA et al. (1978) Myocardial involvement in systemic lupus erythematosus. Chest 74: 414–417

Doshi N, Smith B, Klionsky B (1980) Congenital pericarditis due to maternal SLE. J Pediatr 96: 699–701

Drew P, Asherson RA, Zuk RJ, Goodwin FJ, Hughes JRV (1987) Aortic occlusion in SLE associated with antiphospholipid antibodies. Ann Rheum Dis 46: 612–616

Dubois EL (1974) Systemic lupus erythematosus. Univ S Calif Press, Los Angeles

Dubois EL, Tuffanelli DL (1974) Clinical manifestations of systemic lupus erythematosus: computer analysis of 520 cases. JAMA 190: 104–111

Elkayam U, Weiss S, Laniado S (1977) Pericardial effusion and mitral valve involvement in SLE: echocardiographic study. Ann Rheum Dis 36: 349–353

Emlen W (1979) Complete heart block in mixed connective tissue disease. Arthritis Rheum 22: 679–680

Esscher E, Scott JS (1979) Congenital heart block and maternal SLE. Br Med J 1: 1235–1238

Estes D, Christian CL (1971) The natural history of systemic lupus erythematosus by prospective analysis. Medicine (Baltimore) 50: 85–95

Fauci AS, Haynes BF, Katz P (1978) The spectrum of vasculitis. Ann Intern Med 89: 660–676

Fessel WJ (1974) Systemic lupus erythematosus in the community. Arch Intern Med 134: 1027–1035

Gladman DD, Sternberg L (1985) Pulmonary hypertension in SLE. J Rheumatol 12: 365–367

Gladstein GS, Rynes RI, Parhami N, Bartholomew LE (1979) Gangrene of a foot secondary to SLE with large vessel vasculitis. J Rheumatol 6: 549–553

Grigor RR, Edmonds J, Lewkonia R, Bresnihan B, Hughes GRV (1978) Systemic lupus erythematosus: a prospective analysis. Ann Rheum Dis 37: 121–128

Gross L (1940) The cardiac lesions in Libman–Sacks disease with a consideration of its relationship to acute diffuse lupus erythematosus. Am J Pathol 16: 375–407

Haider YS, Roberts WC (1981) Coronary arterial disease in systemic lupus erythematosus. Am J Med 70: 775–781

Harmon CE, Portonova JP (1982) Drug-induced lupus: clinical and serological studies. Clin Rheum Dis 8: 121–135

Harvey AM, Shulman LE, Tumulty A, Conley CL, Schoenrich EH (1954) Systemic lupus erythematosus: review of the literature and clinical analysis of 318 cases. Medicine (Baltimore) 33: 291–437

Heibel RH, O'Toole JD, Curtiss EL et al. (1976) Coronary arteritis in systemic lupus erythematosus. Chest 69: 700–703

Hejtmancik MR, Wright JC, Quint R, Jennings FL (1964) The cardiovascular manifestations of SLE. Am Heart J 68: 119–130

Hess EV, Spencer-Green G (1979) Congenital heart block and connective tissue disease. Ann Intern Med 91: 645–646

Hochberg MC (1987a) Prevalence of systemic lupus erythematosus in England and Wales, 1981–2. Ann Rheum Dis 46: 664–666

Hochberg MC (1987b) Mortality from systemic lupus erythematosus in England and Wales, 1974–83. Br J Rheumatol 26: 437–441

Homcy CJ, Liberthson RR, Fallon JT, Gross S, Mills LM (1982) Ischaemic heart disease in the young: report of 6 cases. Am J Cardiol 49: 478–484

Hover AR, Koppes GM (1979) Atrial standstill and complete heart block in SLE. Chest 76: 230–231

Howard PF, Hochberg MC, Bias WB, Arnett FC, McLean RH (1986) Relationship between C4 null genes, HLA-D region antigens and genetic susceptibility to SLE in Caucasian and black Americans. Am J Med 81: 187–193

Hughes GRV (1979) Systemic lupus erythematosus: treatment and prognosis. Br Med J 2: 1019–1022

Hughes GRV, Harris NN, Gharavi AE (1986) The anticardiolipin syndrome (editorial). J Rheumatol 13: 486–489

Hunder GG, Mullen BJ, McDuffie FC (1974) Complement in pericardial fluid of lupus erythematosus. Ann Intern Med 80: 453–458

Ishikawa S, Segar WE, Gilbert EF, Burkholder PM, Levy JM, Visekul C (1978) Myocardial infarct in a child with SLE. Am J Dis Childh 132: 696–699

Jacobson EJ, Reza MJ (1978) Constrictive pericarditis in SLE. Demonstration of immunoglobulin in the pericardium. Arthritis Rheum 21: 972–974

James TN, Rupe CE, Monto RW (1965) Pathology of the cardiac conduction system in SLE. Ann Intern Med 63: 402–410

Jensen G, Sigurd B (1973) Systemic lupus erythematosus and myocardial infarct. Chest 64: 653–654

Kahan A, Amor B, Vernejoul F de, Saporta L (1985) Libman–Sacks endocarditis: the diagnostic importance of 2 dimensional echocardiography. Br J Rheumatol 24: 187–190

Klemperer P, Pollack AD, Baehr G (1941) The pathology of disseminated lupus erythematosus. Arch Path 32: 569–631

Knodell RG, Manders SJ (1974) Staphylococcal pericarditis in a patient with SLE. Chest 65: 103–105

Lachmann PJ (1987) Complement – friend or foe? Heberden Oration 1986. Br J Rheumatol 26: 409–415

Lash A, Wittman AL, Quismorio FP (1986) Myocarditis in mixed connective tissue disease. Clinical and pathological study of 3 cases and review of literature. Semin Arthritis Rheum 15: 288–296

Lee P, Urowitz ME, Bookman AAM et al. (1977) Systemic lupus erythematosus. Q J Med 46: 1–32

Libman E, Sacks B (1924) A hitherto undescribed form of valvular and mural endocarditis. Arch Intern Med 33: 701–715

Maddison PJ, Provost TT, Reichlin M (1981) Serological findings in patients with "ANA negative" SLE. Medicine (Baltimore) 60: 87–94

Maddison PJ, Skinner RP, Esscher E, Taylor PV, Scott O, Scott JS (1983) Serological studies in congenital heart block. Ann Rheum Dis 42: 218–219

Maniscalco BS, Felner JM, McCans JL, Chiapella JA (1975) Echocardiographic abnormalities in SLE. Circulation 52: 211

McCue CM, Mantakas ME, Tingelstad JB et al. (1977) Congenital heart block in newborns of mothers with connective tissue disease. Circulation 56: 82–90

McCune AB, Weston WL, Lee LA (1987) Maternal and foetal outcome in neonatal lupus erythematosus. Ann Intern Med 106: 518–523

Meller J, Conde CA, Deppisch LM, Denoso E, Dack S (1975) Myocardial infarction due to coronary atherosclerosis in three young adults with SLE. Am J Cardiol 35: 309–314

Michet CJ, Hunder GG (1984) Pericarditis in systemic lupus erythematosus. In: Ansell BM, Simkin PA (eds) The heart and rheumatic disease. Butterworths, London, pp 11–13

Milne JR, Doyle DV, Banim SE, Huskisson EC (1981) Systemic lupus erythematosus as a cause of severe mixed mitral valve disease. J Rheumatol 8: 516–518

Moffitt GR Jr (1965) Complete atrio-ventricular dissociation with Stokes Adams attacks due to disseminated lupus erythematosus: report of a case. Ann Intern Med 63: 508–511

Morgan SH, Hughes GRV (1984) Connective tissue disorders: systemic lupus erythematosus. Medicine International 2: 397–402

Murray FT, Fuleihan DS, Cornwall CS, Pinals RS (1975) Acute mitral regurgitation from ruptured chordae tendineae in SLE. J Rheumatol 2: 454–459

Myerowitz PD, Michaelis LL, McIntosh CL (1974) Mitral valve replacement for mitral regurgitation due to Libman–Sacks endocarditis. J Thor Cardiovasc Surg 67: 869–874

Olsen EGJ, Lever JV (1972) Pulmonary changes in systemic lupus erythematosus. Br J Dis Chest 66: 71–77

Paget SA, Bulkley BH, Grauer LE, Seningen S (1975) Mitral valve disease of SLE. A cause of severe congestive heart failure reversed by valve replacement. Am J Med 59: 134–139

Parrillo JE, Fauci AS (1980) Necrotising vasculitis, coronary angiitis and the cardiologist. Am Heart J 99: 547–554

Ragsdale C, Petty RE, Cassidy JT, Sullivan DB (1980) The clinical progression of apparent juvenile rheumatoid arthritis to systemic lupus erythematosus. J Rheumatol 7: 50–55

Reilly PA, Maddison PJ, Thomas RD, Poole-Wilson PA (1988) Mitral stenosis in SLE: successful management by mitral valve replacement. Europ J Cardiothorac Surg; in the press

Russell GI, Bing RF, Jones JAG, Thurston H, Swales JD (1987) Hydralazine sensitivity: clinical features, autoantibody changes and HLA-DR4 phenotype. Q J Med 65: 845–852

Rynes RI (1982) Inherited complement deficiency states and SLE. Clin Rheum Dis 8: 29–47

Shapiro RF, Gamble CN, Wiesner KB et al. (1977) Immunpathogenesis of Libman–Sacks endocarditis. Ann Rheum Dis 36: 508–516

Sharp GC (1974) Mixed connective tissue disease. Bull Rheum Dis 25: 828–831

Shearn MA (1959) The heart in systemic lupus erythematosus. Am Heart J 58: 452–466

Shulman HJ, Christian CL (1969) Aortic insufficiency in SLE. Arthritis Rheum 12: 138–145

Singsen BH, Bernstein BH, Kornreich HK, King KK, Hanson V, Tan EM (1977) Mixed connective tissue disease in childhood. J Pediatr 90: 893–900

Starkey RH, Hahn BH (1973) Rapid development of constrictive pericarditis in a patient with SLE. Chest 63: 448–450

Stein HB, Dodek A, Lawson L, Rae A (1979) Procaine induced LE. Report of a case with large pericardial effusion and fluid analysis. J Rheumatol 6: 543–548

Sunder SK, Shah A (1975) Constrictive pericarditis in procainamide-induced lupus erythematosus syndrome. Am J Cardiol 36: 960–962

Tan EM, Cohen HS, Fries JF et al. (1982) The 1982 revised criteria for the classification of SLE. Arthritis Rheum 25: 1271–1276

Tsakraklides VG, Blieden LC, Edwards JE (1974) Coronary atherosclerosis and myocardial infarction associated with SLE. Am Heart J 87: 637–641

Turner-Stokes L, Turner-Warwick M (1982) Intrathoracic manifestations of SLE. Clin Rheum Dis 8: 229–242

Vaughton KC, Walker DR, Sturridge MF (1979) Mitral valve replacement for mitral stenosis caused by Libman–Sacks endocarditis. Br Heart J 41: 730–733

Wade G, Ball J (1957) Unexplained pulmonary hypertension. Q J Med 26: 83–119
Walcott G, Burchell HB, Brown AL (1970) Primary pulmonary hypertension. Am J Med 39: 70–79
Wood PHN (1977) The incidence of rheumatoid arthritis and SLE in Great Britain. In: The
    challenge of arthritis and rheumatism. British League Against Rheumatism, London
Wray R, Iveson M (1975) Complete heart block and SLE. Br Heart J 37: 982–983
Yurchak PM, Levine SA, Gorlin R (1965) Constrictive pericarditis complicating disseminated lupus
    erythematosus. Circulation 31: 113–118

Chapter 8

Ankylosing Spondylitis and Reiter's Disease

Introduction

Although very different in their clinical presentation and course, ankylosing spondylitis and Reiter's disease have a number of significant features in common. The most important of these are sacro-iliitis, a high incidence of the histocompatibility antigen HLA–B27, and their effects on the heart.

In the early stages of each a few patients may have a mild and transient pericarditis or may be found to have first degree heart block. These are symptomless events, subsiding without complication and usually passing unnoticed.

More seriously, after some years, a small proportion of patients develop an aortitis with aortic valve incompetence, or a degree of heart block, or both together. Identical lesions may occur in either ankylosing spondylitis or Reiter's disease, mainly in patients who have more severe and continuously active forms of the disease. In the case of ankylosing spondylitis the patient is likely to have peripheral joint disease as well as spondylitis. In the case of Reiter's disease the patient will have sacro-iliitis as well as peripheral arthritis and possibly spondylitis too. In either case the patient with an aortic lesion or with heart block will be male and will be a carrier of the histocompatibility antigen HLA–B27.

Seronegative Spondylarthropathy and HLA–B27

Seronegative Spondylarthropathy

Ankylosing spondylitis and Reiter's disease are the two main members of a group related disorders originally identified by Moll et al. (1974) as having a number of features in common. They named the group "seronegative spondylarthritides", although the term "spondylarthropathies" is also used. Besides ankylosing spondylitis and Reiter's disease the other members of the group are psoriatic arthropathy, the arthritis of inflammatory bowel disease (ulcerative colitis and Crohn's disease), Whipple's disease and Behçet's syndrome. Spondylitis is not an invariable component in all of these disorders, and when it does occur there are minor differences in its clinical and radiological features in different settings in the group (McEwen et al. 1971). Sacro-iliitis is a more consistent finding in the group than spondylitis.

The elements linking these disorders are: the absence of rheumatoid factor and of rheumatoid nodules, sacro-iliitis with or without spondylitis, peripheral arthritis and familial aggregation. In some members of the group there may be uveitis, lesions of the skin or of the genito-urinary tract. Identical forms of cardiac involvement may be found in ankylosing spondylitis and Reiter's disease and very occasionally have been known to accompany the spondylitis of psoriasis or inflammatory bowel disease (Masi 1979; Moll 1983).

HLA–B27

The discovery of the association between ankylosing spondylitis and the histocompatibility antigen HLA–B27 led to the realisation that this antigen was the biological link between the members of this group of diseases (Brewerton et al. 1973). The antigen is present with different frequencies in different members of the group, as shown in Table 8.1; it is carried on the cell surface of all nucleated cells.

Table 8.1. HLA–B27 in the spondylarthropathies. (From Nicholls (1979) and Calin (1984))

	HLA–B27 frequency (%)	Relative risk[a]
Ankylosing spondylitis	95	×90
Reiter's disease	78	×36
Juvenile chronic arthritis	26	×4.5
Psoriatic arthritis (spondylitic)	40	×9
Psoriatic arthritis (peripheral)	15	×2.5
Colitis and Crohn's arthritis	60	
Salmonella arthritis	67	×18
Yersinia arthritis	80	×18

[a] This column shows the relative risk of acquiring the disease in individuals carrying the B27 antigen compared with those without it.

The clinical feature with which B27 is most often associated is sacro-iliitis, for which it is a marker; to a less extent it is a marker for spondylitis and uveitis. The inherited presence of the antigen increases an individual's risk of developing one or other of the conditions for which it is a marker, and the estimated risk factor is shown in Table 8.1. Other genetic determinants evidently also influence the development of ankylosing spondylitis, for family studies have shown a greater incidence of spondylitis in the relatives of B27-positive spondylitic patients than in the relatives of B27-positive individuals who do not have spondylitis (Calin et al. 1983).

The association between HLA–B27 and the spondylarthropathies crosses all ethnic and geographic boundaries. In some races the natural frequency of the B27 antigen is low (e.g. in African blacks and Australian aborigines) and among them spondylitis is rare. In other races, such as some American Indians, B27 is carried more frequently and spondylitis is found with correspondingly greater frequency. Between 10% and 20% of those carrying the antigen have some evidence of sacro-iliitis, in both sexes, although symptomatically it is less apparent in women (Calin 1983).

Being a marker for sacro-iliitis and spondylitis, B27 is therefore associated with the heart lesions found with spondylitis. Can the antigen act as an independent marker predisposing to forms of spondylitic heart disease in the absence of spondylitis? Bergfeldt and his associates believe that it can. They cite examples of B27-positive patients with heart block and aortitis in the presence of only partially expressed clinical features of spondylitis or Reiter's disease (1984 a, b). They have also shown that patients with heart block may sometimes have unrecognised B27-positive spondylitis (Bergfeldt et al. 1982a, b).

However, surveys of patients with "lone" aortic incompetence do not suggest that they have unrecognised spondylitis, nor do they have a higher incidence than normal of the antigen B27 (Calin et al. 1976; Hollingworth et al. 1979). Nevertheless, aortic incompetence has been found in some patients who are B27 positive before radiological evidence of sacro-iliitis had become apparent, both in adults (Bulkley and Roberts 1973) and in teenage boys (Kean et al. 1980; Stewart et al. 1978).

Reactive Arthritis

Another significant association of the B27 antigen is with the predisposition to arthritis following enteritis caused by Shigella, Salmonella and Yersinia organisms. Individuals carrying the B27 antigen tend to develop "reactive" arthritis more often and more severely after these infections than those who are B27-negative. The arthritis may take the form of a limited polyarthritis or of Reiter's disease with eye and skin involvement and sometimes spondylitis. Shortly after the acute infection there may be signs of a mild carditis, with transient pericarditis or first-degree block; the later, more serious, lesions of aortitis, aortic incompetence or complete block have not so far been reported after Yersinia although they have been found, with spondylitis, as late sequelae to Shigella and Salmonella infections. (Laitinen et al. 1977; Leirosalo et al. 1982).

Ankylosing Spondylitis

Description

Ankylosing spondylitis is a disease in which a low-grade inflammatory process, usually beginning in the sacro-iliac joints, gradually spreads up the spine producing stiffness, rigidity and eventual ankylosis in the sacro-iliac, interspinal and costo-spinal joints. Its onset is most often in young male adults or adolescents aged between 15 and 30 years. In about one-third there is arthritis in peripheral joints as well as the spine, mainly affecting hips, knees and shoulders.

Peripheral arthritis usually follows some years after spinal disease has begun but sometimes, especially in younger patients, a peripheral joint, or the cervical spine, may be the first to be affected.

The progress of ankylosing spondylitis is unpredictable. It may be insidiously progressive and practically symptomless or it may advance with periods of considerable inflammatory activity, causing systemic and local symptoms. It may appear to arrest at any stage. Characteristic symptoms are low backache and stiffness, worst in the morning, and nocturnal back pain; however, restriction in spinal movement and in chest expansion may develop without the patient being aware of these changes.

Non-articular connective tissue lesions include painful plantar fasciitis, inflammation of tendinous and ligamentous attachments (enthesiopathy) and of costochondral junctions. Other extra-articular lesions are uveitis, often recurrent, in about 25%, aortitis with aortic valve incompetence and/or heart block in up to 10%, apical pulmonary fibrosis, and secondary amyloid disease as a late complication of severe prolonged spondylitis.

The New York criteria for the diagnosis of probable and definite ankylosing spondylitis are based on clinical and radiological findings as set out in Table 8.2.

Table 8.2.   New York diagnostic criteria for ankylosing spondylitis. (From Bennett and Wood 1968)

Minimal requirements
Clinical examination of back and chest including chest expansion and AP radiographs for all males over 15 years and females over 45 years

Clinical criteria
1. Limitation of motion of lumbar spine in all 3 planes, anterior, lateral, extension
2. History of presence of pain at dorsolumbar junction or in lumbar spine
3. Limitation of chest expansion to 1 inch or less at level of 4th intercostal space

Grading of radiographs
Sacro-iliac joint on either side to be graded separately.
0 = normal
1 = suspicious changes
2 = minimal abnormality
3 = unequivocal abnormality
4 = severe abnormality or total ankylosis

Definite ankylosing spondylitis
grade 3–4 bilateral sacro-iliitis with any one clinical criterion
or grade 3–4 unilateral sacro-iliitis with clinical criterion 1
or grade 2 bilateral sacro-iliitis with clinical criterion 1 or clinical criteria 2 and 3

Probable ankylosing spondylitis
grade 3–4 bilateral sacro-iliitis without any clinical criteria

Prevalence

A clinical survey in England in 1963 estimated the prevalence of spondylitis as 4 per 1000 men and 0.5 per 1000 women, giving a male:female ratio of about 9:1 (Lawrence 1963). Rather lower estimates were given by corresponding American surveys, the mean figures being 1.5 per 1000 men and 0.15 per 1000 women (Calin and Fries 1975). In blacks and orientals the prevalence is very much lower while in some American Indians it is higher, being related to the prevalence of the HLA–B27 antigen in different racial groups.

A reassessment of the true prevalence of ankylosing spondylitis, in forms that are not always clinically apparent, has followed the careful epidemiological studies of the carriers of the HLA–B27 antigen. As approximately 8% of Caucasians carry the antigen, if about 10% of them have minor stigmata of spondylitis (as these studies imply), the true incidence of ankylosing spondylitis in the general population of Caucasian origin is likely to approach 1%. Many of these, especially women, will have evidence of sacro-iliitis so mild as to be overlooked, or too mild to meet the New York diagnostic criteria (Cohen et al. 1976; Van der Linden et al. 1983).

Pathology

The characteristic pathological lesion is the enthesiopathy, or inflammation at the sites of tendinous or ligamentous attachment to bone. This is found in the earliest stages of the pelvic and spinal lesions at sacro-iliac, intervertebral and spinocostal articulations. It is also found at extra-articular sites, notably at the attachment of tendons and ligaments to the iliac crests and the ischial tuberosities, also in the soles of the feet causing plantar fasciitis. At these sites the histological appearance is one of infiltration by lymphocytes and plasma cells with local erosion of cortical bone. The end-result is a vigorous production of fibrous tissue and ultimately calcification and ossification at the site of the enthesiopathy, forming bony spurs or bridges between neighbouring bones (Ball 1980). A similar cellular reaction may occur in the aortic wall leading to destruction of elastic tissue with replacement fibrosis but no calcification.

In the inflamed joint synovium the histological appearance is very like that seen in rheumatoid arthritis, and antiglobulins have been identified in the synovium, but not rheumatoid factor. There is some evidence for the production of immune complexes locally, but not on the scale seen in rheumatoid arthritis and SLE; immune complexes are not released into the general circulation and vasculitis is not seen. However, in the blood, activated lymphocytes can be identified while the disease is in an active phase (Eghtedari et al. 1976).

Causation

The reasons for this pathological reaction and the precise role of the HLA–B27 antigen are still not understood. The nature of the inflammatory reaction points to a prolonged immunologically-based response. Analogy with the known bacterial initiation of Reiter's disease and other forms of reactive arthritis suggests a triggering of the inflammation by an antigen of bacterial origin.

A leading hypothesis is that a causative organism, by carrying an antigen closely related in molecular structure to that of the B27 antigen, may in some way give rise to a chronic inflammatory process manifesting mainly at entheses and synovia. One proposed mechanism would be a parallel to the role of the streptococcus in causing rheumatic heart disease (Ebringer 1983). Suspicion centring on Klebsiella organisms in the intestine in this role has not been substantiated (Brewerton 1983). Nevertheless, the central position of the B27 antigen in the aetiology of the spondylarthropathies, and our now detailed knowledge of its molecular structure, strongly encourage a search for an, as yet, unidentified causative organism (McGuigan et al. 1985; Archer and Winrow 1987).

Cardiovascular Lesions

The most important cardiovascular lesions found with ankylosing spondylitis are aortitis, associated with aortic valve incompetence, and heart block (see pp. 173–182 and pp. 182–188). There are also less serious effects on the pericardium and myocardium.

Pericardium. Pericarditis is an infrequent finding, reported in about 1% of spondylitics (Bernstein and Broch 1949; Graham and Smythe 1958; Wilkinson and Bywaters 1958). As it is symptomless and transient it is only likely to be found by chance, recognised either by the presence of a friction rub or by ECG changes. It is found during a phase of inflammatory activity in the spondylitis, at any stage in the disease, including the early stages though not as often as it is found in the early stages of Reiter's disease. It is without clinical significance, but is responsible for the pericardial adhesions that may be found at autopsy (Davidson et al. 1963).

Myocardium. Inflammatory changes in the myocardium are usually slight and confined to the area immediately adjoining the central fibrous body and the AV node. However, clinical signs suggestive of cardiomyopathy were described by Takkunen et al. (1970) causing cardiac enlargement and pulmonary venous engorgement in a number of spondylitics, although this observation was not supported by pathological evidence. This, and the report of an increased mortality rate among spondylitics (Radford et al. 1977), have suggested that the myocardium may be affected more than has been realised.

In support of this, a functional abnormality in the myocardium has been shown by echocardiography. Brewerton et al. (1987) reported a measurable delay in the early phase of diastolic movement in the left ventricle in 16 of the 30 spondylitic men studied. This was not associated with dilatation of the left atrium or ventricle. It was attributed to a diffuse increase in myocardial interstitial connective tissue, including reticulin, which they noted on histological examination of the myocardium in autopsied cases.

Also, Ribeiro et al. (1984) have reported echocardiographic evidence of a poorly contracting left ventricle in 5 of 28 patients with spondylitis, not associated with aortic valve disease or heart block.

Radio nuclide studies have confirmed a functional abnormality affecting left ventricular wall movement in diastole. Gould et al. (1988) found that the peak filling rate was lower in spondylitic subjects than in normal controls, although the spondylitic subjects had no overt heart disease. The abnormality of left ventricular wall motion, both at rest and on exercise, suggested a decreased compliance in ventricular muscle.

Reiter's Disease

Description

The classical triad of Reiter's disease consists of urethritis, arthritis and conjunctivitis, following two to three weeks after either bacillary dysentery or urethritis. Its name commemorates the description by Hans Reiter in 1916 of a patient in the German army who had contracted the disease after an attack of dysentery. In the French literature it is referred to as the Fiessinger–LeRoy syndrome in recognition of their description, also in 1916, of the disease during an epidemic of dysentery in the French army. However, a clear account of the disease was given by Sir Benjamin Brodie in 1818, associated with urethritis, including an account of typical recurrences (Good 1974).

The triad of symptoms is not always complete as either the conjunctivitis or, less often, the urethritis may not occur, or may be slight and therefore pass unobserved. Urethritis is part of the triad in those cases that follow dysentery. In women, who only make up about 10% of reported cases, the genito-urinary manifestation may be cervicitis rather than urethritis, and this too may go unreported or unrecognised as part of the syndrome.

The arthritis is acute and is not likely to be overlooked. It was present in 96% of the series of 410 patients described by Csonka (1979). It mainly affects a number of joints of the lower part of the body – the knees, ankles, feet, hips or sacro-iliacs, usually in an asymmetrical fashion.

Additional lesions often seen are muco-cutaneous ulcerations (balanitis or stomal ulcers), plantar fasciitis, calcanean spur formation, Achilles tendinitis and keratoderma blenorrhagica, a rash closely resembling pustular psoriasis (Willkens et al. 1982).

In due course the arthritis subsides but may take weeks or months to do so. In subsequent years the syndrome may recur a number of times, each recurrence mimicking the clinical pattern of the original attack. Recurrences may follow sexual exposure but often are apparently spontaneous, without precipitating cause. After 5 years about 80% of patients show signs of active disease. Permanent joint damage may result, and considerable disability was reported in 30% of a series of 131 cases by Fox et al. (1979), particularly resulting from symptoms in the feet and ankles.

In some 20% sacro-iliitis and ascending spinal disease lead to the characteristic appearance of ankylosing spondylitis; some of the earlier descriptions of ankylosing spondylitis were in fact the result of Reiter's disease. However, the spinal lesions differ in some respect from those of classical "idiopathic" ankylosing spondylitis. Following Reiter's disease the spinal changes seen radiologically are less extensive and consist often of asymmetrically placed syndesmophytes forming bony bridges between neighbouring pairs of vertebrae (Cliff 1971; McEwen et al. 1971).

Prevalence

In Europe and North America Reiter's disease is generally the result of sexually acquired urethritis and in venereal disease clinics in Britain it accounts for 1% to 2% of the cases seen. The sex ratio of 10 male to one female patient probably underestimates the occurrence in women for the reasons given above. Elsewhere, e.g. in Africa and Asia, dysentery is the commoner cause, and anywhere in the world, in time of war, epidemic dysentery may be responsible.

The biggest epidemic occurrence of Reiter's disease was the result of an epidemic of Flexner dysentery in Finnish troops in 1944. Over 300 cases were reported by Paronen (1948) among an estimated 150 000 cases of dysentery, i.e. 0.2%. A follow-up of 100 of these cases 20 years later showed that 80 of them still had arthritic symptoms, of whom 32 had spondylitis and 30 peripheral arthritis; 2 cases had aortic incompetence (Sairanen et al. 1969). Of the patients tested, 78% were B27-positive (Sairanen and Tiilikainen 1975).

Another well-documented epidemic occurred in a US naval ship when 9 men developed Reiter's disease out of 602 who contracted Shigella dysentery, i.e. 1.5% (Noer 1965).

Pathology

Reiter's disease is a form of reactive arthritis which may be initiated by a number of infections in the bowel (Shigella, Salmonella, Yersinia, Campylobacter) or in the urogenital tract (Mycoplasma, Chlamydia). In some cases no organism can be incriminated and an onset following trauma has been suggested. Although the HLA–B27 antigen has an important role, this is still far from clear, and about 20% of cases arise in B27-negative subjects.

In the affected joints the inflamed synovium has much the same histological appearance as in rheumatoid arthritis, with no particular distinguishing features. There is little evidence of immune complex formation or complement consumption, and rheumatoid factor is absent. In more actively inflamed joints there is a tense effusion. The fluid may have a cell count up to $50\,000/mm^3$, mainly of polymorphs, and in less acutely inflamed joints T lymphocytes are prominent. No organisms are found in the joint, but Keat et al. (1987) have reported finding elemental bodies in the synovium and fluid that were identified by monoclonal antibody reaction as being derived from *Chlamydia trachomatis*. This may well be proof of a causative role for *Chlamydia* (Editorial (*Lancet*) 1985).

Enthesiopathy is a significant pathological feature, just as it is in ankylosing spondylitis. It is well-marked in the ligamentous attachments around the sacro-iliac and interspinal joints.

The Heart

The most important cardiovascular lesions are aortitis, aortic incompetence and heart block; they are identical with the corresponding lesions in ankylosing spondylitis, and are described below. Less serious involvement of the pericardium and myocardium also occurs.

Pericardium. Pericarditis has been observed in 1%–2% of patients in the acute stages of Reiter's disease. Csonka and Oates (1957) reported it in 2 of 128 patients and Paronen (1948) in 7 of 308 patients in the Finnish epidemic. It may cause central chest pain or discomfort but is probably too mild always to be complained of by patients suffering an acute arthritis. Recurrences of pericarditis have been noted coinciding with recurrences of Reiter's disease (Csonka et al. 1961) but there are no sequelae.

Myocardium. There are many reports of heart block in the acute stages of the disease; it is usually a transient first degree block, with a probable incidence of 4% or 5% (Good 1974; Paronen 1948). In a few patients this degree of heart block was still present on follow-up some years later, and in one had progressed to complete block.

Although the appearance of first degree heart block is frequently attributed to myocarditis, as in rheumatic fever, there is little evidence for any pathological changes in the myocardium beyond the immediate vicinity of the AV node and conducting bundle. There are a few reports of a more serious form of myocarditis, such as that of Blétry et al. (1979). They described a patient who developed cardiomegaly with congestive and left ventricular failure 20 years after the onset of Reiter's disease, not attributable to an aortic valve lesion. He also had a florid psoriasiform rash, and ultimately responded dramatically to methotrexate. This case appears to be the parallel of the cardiomyopathy reported by Takkunen in ankylosing spondylitis.

The Aortic Lesion

Historical

The striking spinal rigidity of ankylosing spondylitis has been recognised for at least 200 years, but it was not until the late nineteenth century that clear clinical descriptions appeared from Strumpell, Bechterew and Marie, whose names are still linked eponymously with the disease. Mallory (1936) was the first to report the lesions of the aorta and aortic valve, but at that time spondylitis was seen as a variant of rheumatoid arthritis and the valve lesion was attributed to coincidental rheumatic heart disease.

It was Bauer, Clark and Kulka who first realised that the aortic and aortic-valve lesions were a specific feature of spondylitis, which was then becoming accepted as a disease separate from rheumatoid arthritis (Bauer et al. 1951; Clark et al. 1957).

Other early reports confirming the occasional development of aortitis and aortic incompetence in patients with ankylosing spondylitis came from Schilder et al. (1956), Ansell et al. (1958), Graham and Smythe (1958), Crow (1960), and Davidson et al. (1963), among others. The additional presence of heart block was noted by these authors.

The development of the same heart lesions as a late sequel to Reiter's disease was appreciated by Graham and Smythe, and was also reported by Sobin and Hagstrom (1962), Siguier et al. (1970) and Paulus et al. (1972) and was reviewed in detail by Good (1974).

The identity of the heart lesions of ankylosing spondylitis and of Reiter's disease was thus recognised before the discovery of their common disease marker, the HLA–B27 antigen.

Description

The clinical picture that emerges from these many publications is of the appearance of aortic incompetence in a male patient with a past history of ankylosing spondylitis usually of 10 years' duration or more, which is sometimes the result of Reiter's disease. The aortic valve lesion, at first symptomless, slowly progresses causing cardiac enlargement, dyspnoea and sometimes angina, ultimately producing congestive heart failure. This may be the cause of death, but associated heart block, in the days before pacing became available, sometimes caused death during a Stokes–Adams attack. At autopsy the essential pathological changes are in the wall of the proximal aorta, in the aortic valve and sometimes in the mitral, and there may be damage to the AV node and conducting tissue.

Case History 8.1 illustrates such a course, with characteristic pathological changes at autopsy.

Case History 8.1

Reiter's disease
Ankylosing spondylitis
Aortic incompetence
Death in heart failure

Mr. E.W., Business representative, born 1907

1944	Dysentery, conjunctivitis, urethritis Discharged from Army with "post-dysenteric arthritis"
1956	Ankylosing spondylitis diagnosed Treated with radiotherapy
1960	Corticosteroid treatment Duodenal ulcer, haematemesis Found to have aortic incompetence BP 130/40 Cardiac enlargement, LV+
1962	Developed attacks of LV failure Died in congestive failure
Autopsy	Proximal aortitis; aortic valve cusps thickened and contracted. LV hypertrophy Regurgitant endocardial jet lesion See Figs. 8.1, 8.2, 8.3, 8.4
Comment	Spondylitis recognised 12 years after post-dysenteric Reiter's disease. Death 2 years after discovery of aortic valve lesion

---

Pathology

Aortitis is in most cases confined to the first few centimetres of the ascending aorta. Macroscopically, the intima is thickened, with longitudinal creases or scars wrinkling its surface as is seen in syphilitic aortitis. The adventitia is also thickened and fibrous and the aortic diameter may be slightly widened, though not to the extent of aneurysm formation. The aortic valve cusps are thickened and slightly contracted and their free margins too are thickened or rolled. Some fibrous adhesions may form between the cusps, but only at the commissures, and there is no stenosis (Fig. 8.1). The coronary orifices remain patent. Thickening of the endocardium below the valve may spread downwards to involve the mitral valve, mainly its aortic cusp, and this too may be somewhat thickened and contracted so that the valve is incompetent. A localised fibrous thickening or ridge at the base of the mitral cusp is often seen (Bulkley and Roberts 1973).

Histologically, there is hyaline thickening of the aortic intima, and in the media, disruption of the elastic fibres with collagenous replacement (Figs. 8.2, 8.5). The adventitia too is thickened as a result of the laying down of collagen associated with a low grade inflammatory process: foci of lymphocytic infiltration may be seen (Fig. 8.3) and the vasa vasorum in the adventitia may show endarteritis obliterans (Fig. 8.4).

Similar low-grade inflammatory changes, i.e. with foci of round cell infiltration and laying down of collagen, may be traced downwards from the base

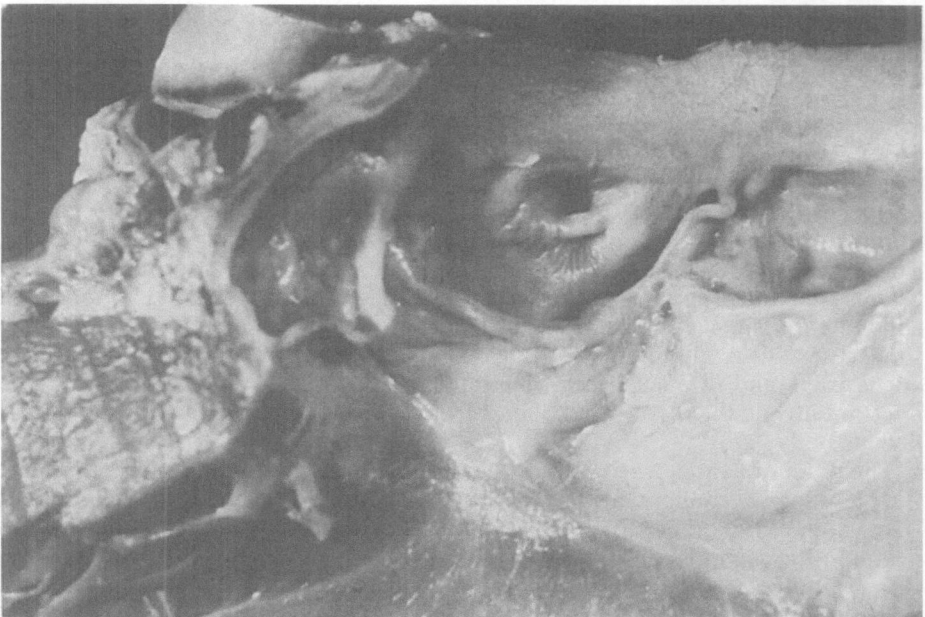

Fig. 8.1. Aortic valve from the autopsy on the patient in Case History 8.1. The valve cusps are thickened and shortened with rolled margins. There is some adhesion formation at the commissures and an endocardial jet lesion below the valve. (From Cosh and Lever 1984, by permission of Messrs Butterworths.)

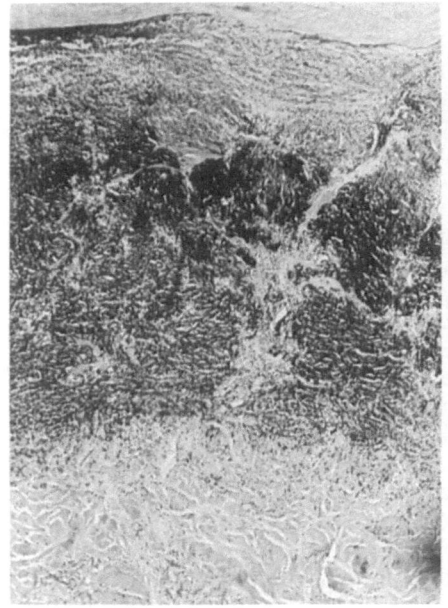 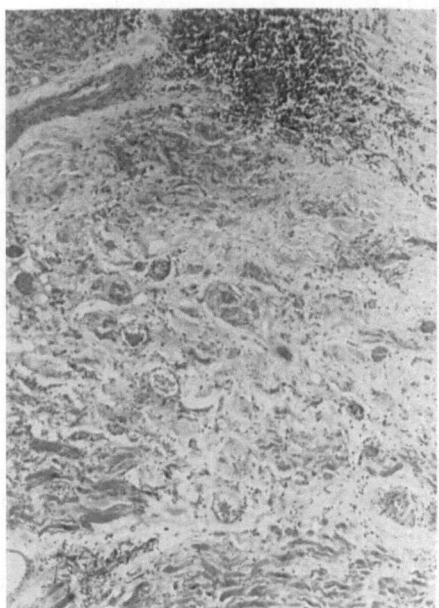

Fig. 8.2.   **Fig. 8.3.**

Fig. 8.2. Aortic wall from Case History 8.1; the elastic fibres in the media are grossly disrupted. The intima is above and the adventitia below. (Van Gieson × 60). (From Cosh and Lever 1984, by permission of Messrs Butterworths.)

Fig. 8.3. Aortic adventitia from Case History 8.1, showing focal lymphocytic infiltration and increased vascularity (H and E × 60).

of the aortic valve cusps (where there may be a localised increase in vascularity) to the aortic valve ring and into the central fibrous body of the heart (Fig. 8.6). This is the "fibrous skeleton" of the heart, anchoring the roots of the great vessels and the upper part of the septum. It is here that the AV node and conducting tissue can be damaged or destroyed by the inflammatory process; in some cases this is where the pathological process begins, with involvement of the aortic valve and the aorta following later, if at all. The inflammatory reaction does not invade the myocardium apart from the immediate vicinity of the central fibrous body.

The extent of the aortitis is variable. At one extreme the aorta is spared and the pathological changes are confined to the central fibrous body and conducting tissue and, at the other, aortitis may extend throughout the arch and descending aorta: in the second case of Ansell et al. (1958) the aorta was involved as far as the origin of the renal arteries. In some atypical cases there has been an aortic arch syndrome in which one or more of the major branches of the aorta have been partially or totally obstructed at their origins (Hull et al. 1984; Toone et al. 1959).

Light pericardial adhesions may be found at autopsy or, occasionally, there is an active serofibrinous pericarditis.

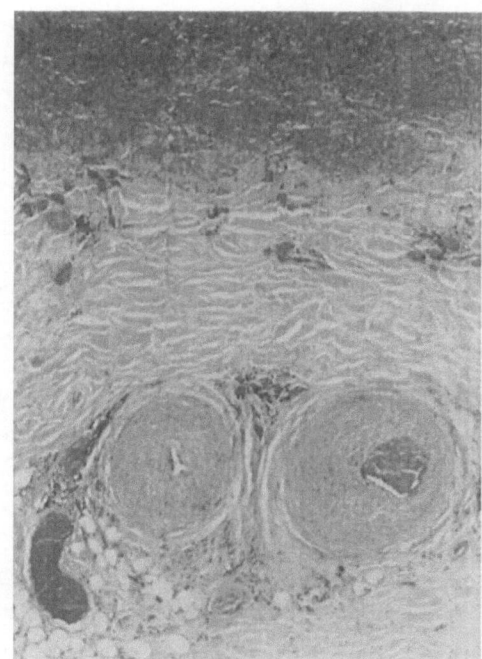

Fig. 8.4. Aortic adventitia from Case History 8.1 showing marked endarteritis obliterans of the vasa vasorum (H and E × 60). (From Cosh and Lever 1984, by permission of Messrs Butterworths.)

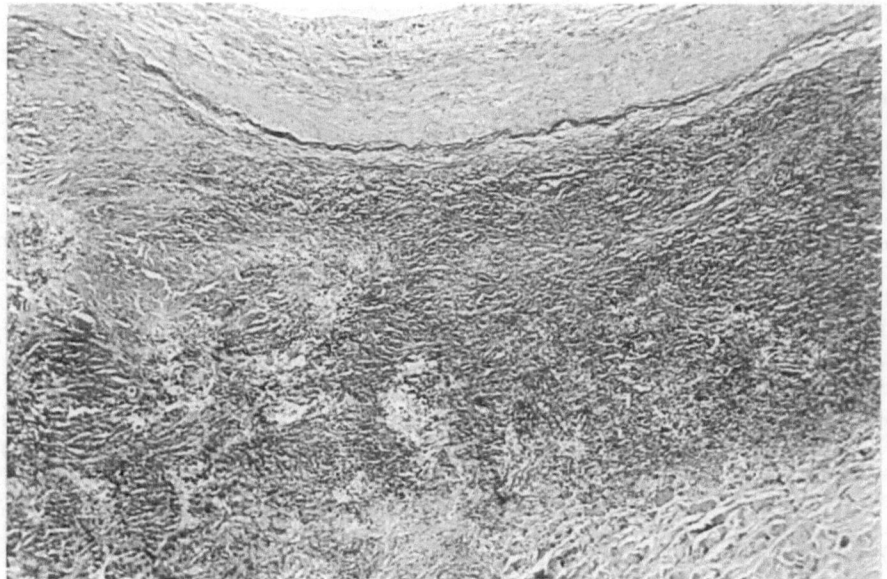

Fig. 8.5. Section of aortic wall from a patient with spondylitic aortitis. The elastic fibres of the media are fragmented and there is scanty round cells infiltration of the media (H and E × 60). (From Cosh and Lever 1984, by permission of Messrs Butterworths.)

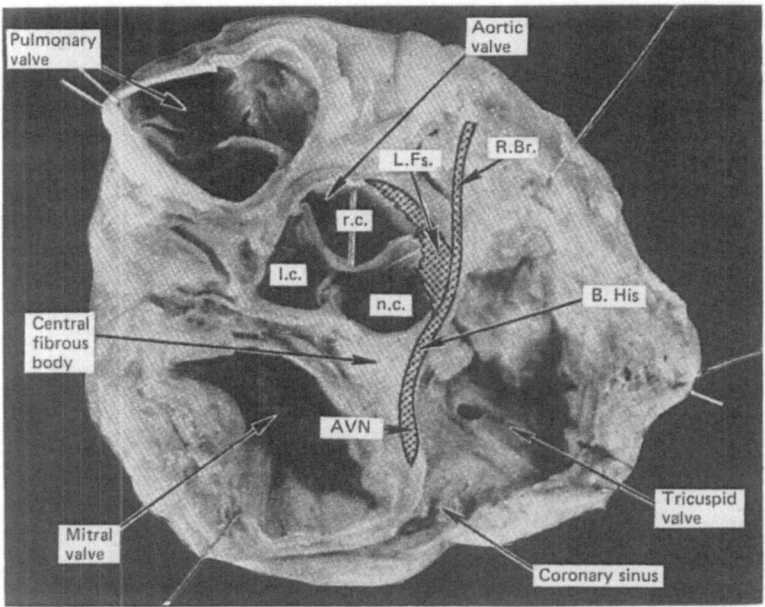

Fig. 8.6. The heart seen from above with the atria and great vessels removed to show the close relationship between the aortic root and the central fibrous body with the AV node and the bundle of His (B. His). L Fs = left fascicles; R.Br = right bundle branch. The three aortic cusps are: r.c. right coronary cusp: l.c. left coronary cusp: n.c. non coronary cusp. (From Hudson 1967 with the permission of the author and the Editor and Publishers of the British Heart Journal and Messrs Butterworths.)

Prevalence

The prevalence of aortic lesions among spondylitic patients is variously reported as between 1% (Ansell et al. 1958) and 10% (Kinsella et al. 1974). The figure is higher with a longer duration and a more severe form of spondylitis. Graham and Smythe (1958) found an overall figure of 5% in their series of over 500 spondylitics, but analysis showed that it was only 1% among the younger men with uncomplicated spondylitis whereas aortic lesions were found in 18% of older men with longer histories and more serious disease, i.e. including peripheral arthritis and iritis.

At the Mayo Clinic Davidson and colleagues (1963) found 24 cases of valve disease among 1000 spondylitics i.e. 2.4%; of these, 11 cases involved the aortic valve alone, but it is likely that some of the remainder had rheumatic heart disease. Of the 25 autopsies that they reported 6 had valve lesions: two were of the aortic valve alone, one of the mitral valve alone and in three both valves were affected.

Henssge et al. (1970) found 3 cases of lone aortic incompetence among 100 spondylitic patients. A review of 128 spondylitics in Bath revealed 3 patients with aortic incompetence (2.3%), 5 with forms of heart block and 2 with arrhythmias. The 3 patients with aortic incompetence had had ankylosing spondylitis for 11 years or more (Table 8.3).

Table 8.3. Cardiac abnormalities among 128 spondylitics seen at the Royal National Hospital for Rheumatic Diseases, Bath (with acknowledgement to Professor N Gerber)

Sex	Length of history of spondylitis (years)	Aortic incompetence	Heart block (degree)	Heart rhythm
M	41	0	First	Normal
F	37	0	First	Normal
M	26	+	0	Atrial fibrillation
M	22	0	First	Normal
M	16	+	First	Normal
M	11	+	Lbbb	Normal
M	9	0	0	Atrial flutter

Aortic incompetence in 3 (2%–3%)
First degree heart block in 4 (3%)

The evidence of spondylitis among patients with aortic incompetence selected for surgery reveals the association rather more often. Schilder et al. (1956) found 5 spondylitics among 100 referred with aortic incompetence. Qaiyumi et al. (1985) found 7 among 100, 4 with idiopathic ankylosing spondylitis and 3 following Reiter's disease; 6 of the 7 had heart block in addition.

Among black races ankylosing spondylitis itself is rare owing to the lower frequency of the B27 antigen among them. Two cases of aortic incompetence in B27-positive black men were reported by Eversmeyer et al. (1978) but the overall prevalence of spondylitic heart disease in blacks is unknown.

With the present recognition of many milder forms of spondylitis the true prevalence of spondylitic heart disease is likely to be lower than the 2% to 5% quoted here, and probably nearer to the 1% noted among Graham and Smythe's milder cases.

Clinical Features

Aortic incompetence often presents with the finding of an aortic diastolic murmur on routine examination of a spondylitic patient who is free from cardiac symptoms. The discovery comes generally between 10 and 20 years after the onset of spondylitis or the first attack of Reiter's disease. The ECG may show first degree heart block or bundle branch block, but the heart is not enlarged and is in sinus rhythm. In the 5 cases reported by Paulus et al. (1972) the average interval between the onset of Reiter's disease and the finding of the valve lesions was 15 years.

The symptom-free period may then continue for up to 6 years, as in the 8 patients of Bulkley and Roberts (1973) before cardiac symptoms appear: effort dyspnoea, angina and ultimately episodes of left ventricular failure or congestive failure. By this time, the cardiac rhythm may have changed to atrial fibrillation or the degree of heart block may have advanced to complete block.

Alternatively, among spondylitic patients whose progress is not being monitored, the valve lesion may only be discovered because cardiac symptoms have arisen, and the situation may already be serious.

Exceptionally, in children or adolescents, the aortic lesions may develop in advance of the signs of sacro-iliitis or spondylitis. Deterioration can then be rapid and the need for cardiac surgery may become urgent. Stewart et al. (1978) report such a case in a young man aged 18 years in whom both the aortic and mitral valves were replaced successfully; the diagnosis of B27-positive spondyl-arthropathy only became clear 5 years later. Demoulin et al. (1983) describe a similar situation with a young man aged 19 years whose valve lesion deteriorated rapidly; he was known to have had spondylitis for 10 years. Other young patients with less urgent aortic lesions were reported by Hubscher et al. (1984) and Kean et al. (1980).

Diagnosis. The diagnosis of an aortic valve lesion presents few difficulties, and the physical findings are as described for rheumatic heart disease in Chap. 2. There may be a spondylitic mitral valve lesion as well, and this must be differentiated from a functional mitral incompetence caused by left ventricular dilatation; the mid-diastolic mitral murmur of Austin Flint may also be present if aortic regurgitation is considerable, and this does not indicate organic mitral stenosis. Catheter studies or angiocardiography may be necessary to assess the state of the mitral valve if surgery is being considered.

Echocardiography. This technique is valuable in estimating ventricular dimension and function (Brewerton et al. 1987), or the state of the aortic and mitral valve cusps and the dimension of the aorta. The normal aortic diameter is not more than 3.7 cm just above the aortic valve (Feigenbaum 1980). Guiney et al. (1987) have found this measurement helpful in distinguishing between aortic incompetence due to dilatation of the aorta and valve ring, and incompetence due to aortic cusp lesions. They found that spondylitic aortic lesions came in the former class, with detectable widening of the proximal aorta.

Evidence for widening of the proximal aorta in advance of the development of valvular incompetence has been sought by 2-D echocardiography, but has not been found except in one out of 35 spondylitics (Tucker et al. 1982). However, they and LaBresh et al. (1985) were able to detect the subaortic fibrous "bump" described by Roberts et al. (1974) in 6 out of 35 and in 11 out of 36 spondylitic patients respectively; this is evidence of a pathological change at a pre-clinical stage.

Complications. Heart block: this frequently accompanies an aortic valve lesion, and complete block will probably require pacing. *Arrhythmias*: atrial fibrillation or flutter are common developments with a deteriorating valve lesion, and ventricular arrhythmias may complicate left ventricular hypertrophy or ischaemia. *Infective endocarditis*: may arise even before a valve lesion becomes clinically recognisable. Case History 4.2 describes a spondylitic patient with infection on the mitral valve, which had previously been considered normal. After cure of the infection surgical replacement of the damaged mitral valve was successfully carried out. *Amyloid disease*: a late complication of severe spondylitis or Reiter's disease rather than of valve disease; its main effect is on the kidneys, producing heavy albumenuria, nephrotic syndrome and renal failure (Miller et al. 1979).

Treatment

If aortic incompetence is recognised in the pre-symptomatic stage the only necessary action is periodic surveillance, watching for any signs of deterioration in the valve lesion or for evidence of heart block. When dyspnoea or decompensation develop, as is probable in the course of time, a diuretic is indicated and probably digitalis if there is atrial fibrillation and a rapid heart rate. At the same time the patient may need continuing attention to his spondylitis or arthritis, with postural and mobilising exercises and probably analgesic or anti-inflammatory drugs.

Problems of drug interaction may arise; for example, indomethacin may induce fluid retention, antagonising the effect of a diuretic, while thiazide diuretics tend to lower the blood level of indomethacin, reducing its effectiveness. Either a change of drug or an increased dose may be needed.

If any grade of heart block is present digitalis should be avoided as its vagal effect may add to the degree of block. In the treatment of angina, in the presence of even first degree heart block, beta blockers or verapamil should be avoided for a similar reason; nifedipine is a safer drug in these circumstances.

Surgery. Deterioration in aortic or mitral valve function calls for the consideration of surgical valve replacement. Assessment prior to surgery may require not only cardioangiography but also coronary angiography if coronary disease is a possibility. Renal function too must be assessed.

In the absence of contra-indications, a good result to aortic or mitral valve replacement may be anticipated. Many successes are on record, dating from the reports of aortic valve surgery by Malette et al. (1969) and Spangler et al. (1970) and of combined aortic and mitral valve surgery by Roberts et al. (1974) and Stewart et al. (1978). It is an advantage if the valve prosthesis used does not require subsequent long-term anticoagulant treatment, which would inevitably raise problems of drug interaction in a patient with spondylitis or arthritis. The rigidity of the spine and thorax in a spondylitic patient call for extra post-operative care but do not add significantly to the difficulty of the operation.

Case History 8.2 describes a patient with aortic incompetence due to Reiter's disease who had a good result to aortic valve replacement.

Case History 8.2

**Reiter's disease
Aortic incompetence
Aortic valve replacement
First degree heart block**

Mr. B., Builder, born 1921

1951	Urethritis, conjunctivitis and polyarthritis
1955	Recurrence of arthritis
1960	Recurrence of arthritis
	Aortic diastolic murmur heard

1967   Free aortic regurgitation
            Dyspnoea and angina
            Cardiac enlargement LV+
            BP 185/65 PR interval 0.24 sec

1968   *Aortic valve replacement*

1972   Prosthesis working well: symptom-free
            Still LV hypertrophy and PR 0.24 sec

Comment   Aortic incompetence developing 9 years after first attack of
            Reiter's disease. Aortic valve replacement after a further 8
            years. First degree block persists

            The ECG strip in Fig. 8.7 shows temporary AV dissociation in
            this patient with the ventricular rate slightly faster than the
            atrial rate

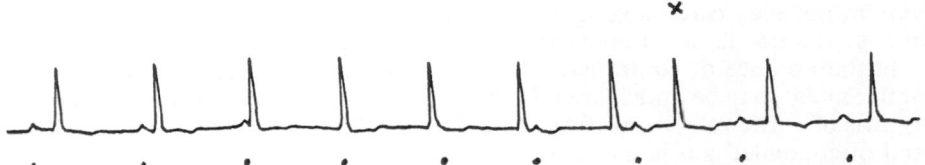

Fig. 8.7.   A–V dissociation in the ECG from the patient in Case History 8.2. The ventricular rate is
75 and the atrial rate 60. One beat, marked, is slightly premature, in response to the previous atrial
contraction.

Heart Block

Description

In Reiter's disease the appearance of temporary first degree heart block in 4% or
5% of patients in the acute initial attack has been noted by a number of authors
(see p. 173). As a rule, conduction returns to normal, but first degree block may
recur in subsequent relapses of the disease. It is found rather more frequently in
the later stages, 10 years or more after the onset. It may then still be first degree
block, or it may have advanced to second degree or complete block. There
seems to be no regular progression and it is not clear whether those patients with
heart block in the later stages are the same individuals who manifested it

originally. As first and second degree block are symptomless their occurrence is naturally only noted irregularly if and when the ECG is recorded.

In ankylosing spondylitis first degree block is found infrequently in the early stages but first degree or complete block may occur after 10 years or more much as with Reiter's disease. In both conditions heart block may be associated with aortitis and aortic incompetence although either of these complications can occur without the other.

Case History 8.3 describes a patient with ankylosing spondylitis, aortic incompetence and left bundle branch block; his ECG and chest X-ray films are shown in Figs. 8.8 and 8.9.

Case History 8.3
Ankylosing spondylitis
Aortic incompetence
L bundle branch block
Aortic valve replacement and coronary artery bypass

Mr. G.B., Warehouseman, born 1933

1952	Bilateral heel pain, plantar fasciitis
1959	Onset of low back pain and stiffness
1969	Established ankylosing spondylitis Arthritis knees and ankles Normal heart ESR 67
1971	Soft aortic diastolic murmur heard No cardiac symptoms BP 150/70 ECG: L bundle branch block
1977	Mild dyspnoea and angina on effort Aortic diastolic murmur louder BP 140/70 ECG unchanged: Lbbb (Fig. 8.8) Cardiac enlargement, LV+ (Fig. 8.9)
1979	Cardiac catheter and assessment Surgery not yet necessary
1981	Symptoms increasing Angina worse *Aortic valve replacement and coronary artery bypass*
1987	Cardiac condition good; ECG now normal In-patient spondylitis rehabilitation programme
Comment	Symptomless aortic incompetence found after 12 years spondylitis. Very gradual deterioration and surgical valve replacement 10 years after murmur found

---

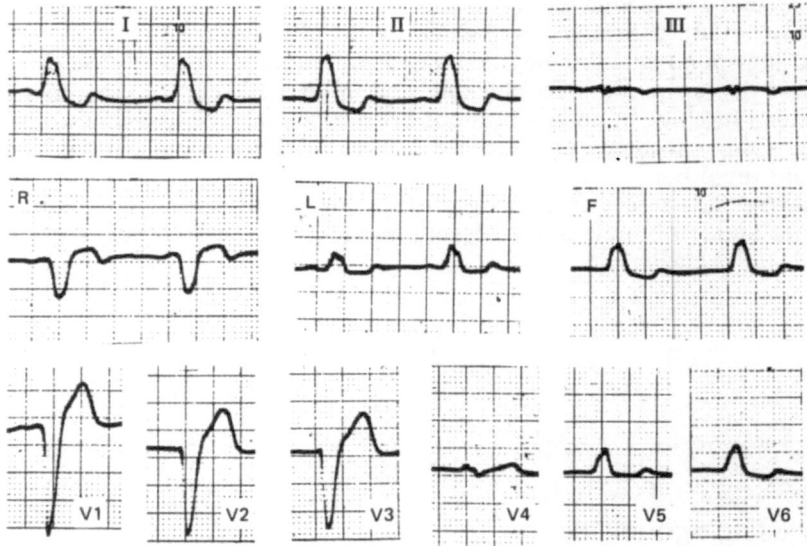

Fig. 8.8.   Left bundle branch block in an ECG from the patient in Case History 8.3. His ECG later returned to normal.

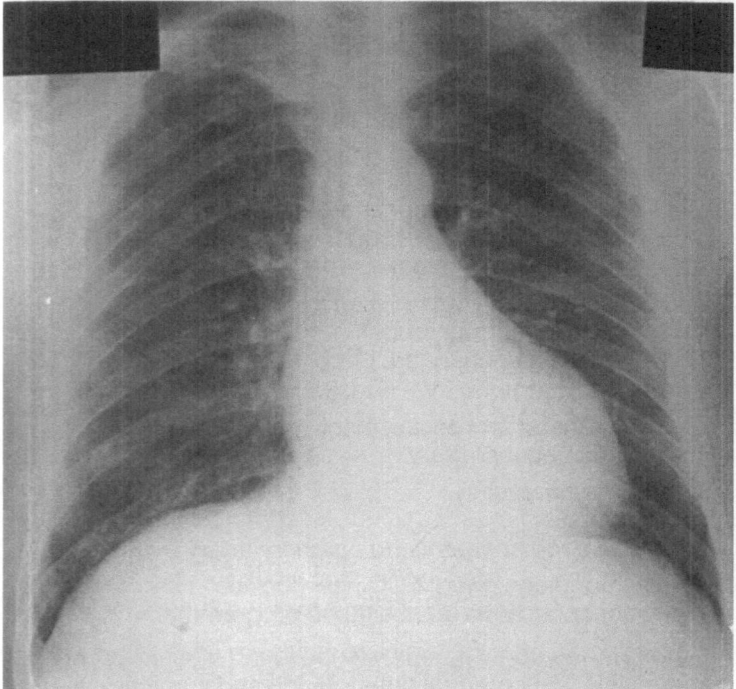

Fig. 8.9.   Chest X-ray film from the patient in Case History 8.3, showing cardiomegaly and left ventricular hypertrophy.

Pathology

This was well described in the report of Weed et al. (1966). They described two male patients with ankylosing spondylitis of some 20 years' duration with aortic incompetence. One patient had complete heart block which was successfully paced. The other had various atrial arrhythmias and later heart block and died. At autopsy the findings were characteristic of many later reports by other authors. "A fibrous tissue sleeve nearly surrounded the aortic root and blended into the aortic valve ring and into the membranous septum . . . Microscopically . . . the tissue was relatively acellular but numerous focal areas of infiltration by chronic inflammatory cells (mainly lymphocytes) were associated with dilated capillaries. Arterioles in the region of fibrosis often had strikingly thickened walls and narrowed lumens . . . Step sections showed continuity of the process from the base of the aortic valve to the apex of the muscular septum . . . The penetrating portion of the AV bundle was almost completely replaced by fibrous tissue." Similar pathological findings were reported by Sobin and Hagstrom (1962).

Figure 8.10, taken from Weed's paper, and Figs. 8.6 and 8.11 illustrate the close proximity of the AV node and the conducting bundle to the central fibrous body and the aortic root.

Davies (1984) also illustrates the pathological changes that may involve the AV node and the conducting bundle or its branches, showing the marked endarteritis of the artery to the node in which the lumen is very largely obstructed by the extreme intimal thickening.

The intensity and the progression of this inflammatory process evidently fluctuate, so accounting for the often transient nature of the failure of conduction. Even after complete block appears to have become permanent and a cardiac pacemaker has been provided spontaneous recovery of conduction may follow (Kinsella et al. 1974; Bergfeldt et al. 1982a).

Prevalence

In the many published reports on the subject, the prevalence of heart block in ankylosing spondylitis or Reiter's disease is variously estimated as between 1% and 15% and an average figure is the 8% given by Weed et al. (1966). The frequency of heart block clearly depends in part on the duration of the spondylarthropathy. In the biggest series, that of Graham and Smythe (1958), the figure was 1% in younger men who had relatively mild disease, and 15% in older men with more severe and long-standing spondylitis – figures very similar to their corresponding observations on aortic incompetence in spondylitis (p. 179).

Among patients with aortic incompetence referred for cardiac surgery heart block may be found as well as previously unsuspected spondylitis or Reiter's disease. Thus Qaiyumi et al. (1985) among 100 such patients found 3 with complete block associated with unrecognised spondylitis and 3 (one with complete and two with first degree block) associated with an unsuspected history of Reiter's disease.

Similarly, the study of patients who have been given pacemakers for complete heart block has shown that many of them had evidence of undiagnosed

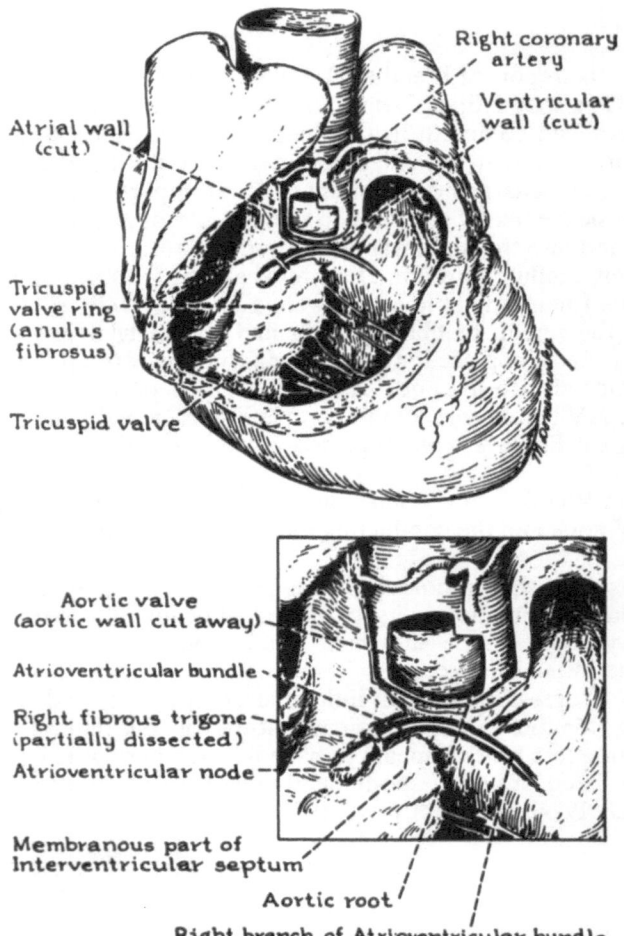

Right coronary
artery

Ventricular
wall (cut)

Atrial wall
(cut)

Tricuspid
valve ring
(anulus
fibrosus)

Tricuspid valve

Aortic valve
(aortic wall cut away)

Atrioventricular bundle

Right fibrous trigone
(partially dissected)

Atrioventricular node

Membranous part of
Interventricular septum

Aortic root

Right branch of Atrioventricular bundle

Fig. 8.10. Root of aorta with part of the aortic wall cut away to show the proximity of the bundle of His to the aortic root. (From Weed et al. (1966) *Archives of Internal Medicine* 117: 804; with permission of the author and of the Editor and Publishers of the Archives of Internal Medicine.)

spondylarthropathy. Bergfeldt et al. (1982b) found 19 with radiological evidence of sacro-iliitis among 223 men with pacemakers (8.5%); 15 of them fulfilled the criteria for ankylosing spondylitis (6.7%). The same authors, reviewing 68 patients with a 25-year history of spondylitis and who had had frequent ECG recordings performed, found some degree of block in 22; this was often temporary, but it gives the highest known prevalence figure of 33%. Six of them had complete heart block from which one patient made a spontaneous recovery (Bergfeldt et al. 1982a).

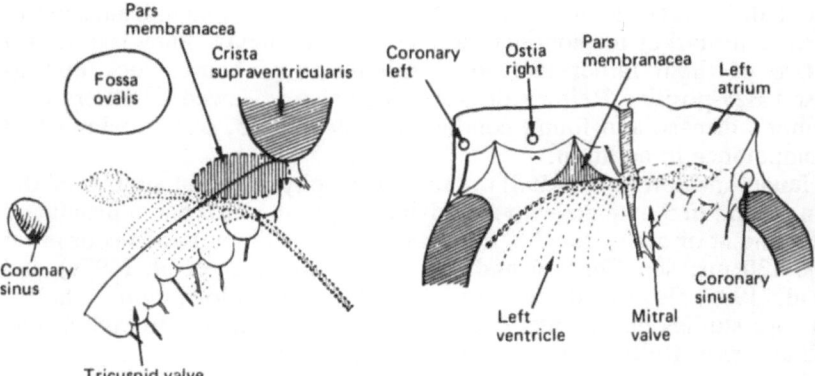

Fig. 8.11. Anatomical relationships of the AV node and bundle of His, showing proximity to the tricuspid valve (left) and to the mitral valve, aortic root and septum (right). (From Hudson 1957 with permission of the author and the Editor and Publishers of the British Heart Journal, and Messrs Butterworth.)

Clinical Features

As first and second degree block are symptomless, symptoms only appear if AV dissociation becomes complete. The patient may merely suffer dyspnoea, fatigue or faintness on exertion owing to the bradycardia; in others there may be syncope induced by effort, or a full-blown Stokes–Adams attack with syncope due to failure of the idioventricular rhythm. Such attacks can be fatal. Palliative treatment with slow release isoprenaline is of help in the short term, but the only lasting solution is an implanted pacemaker (see p. 125).

Electrophysiology

Investigations of the physiological nature of the failure of conduction in spondylarthropathy have been reported by a number of authors. Bergfeldt et al. (1984b) made electrophysiological studies on 12 patients, who were B27-positive, with complete heart block, permanent or temporary, attributed to spondylitis in 8 of them. In 10 of the 12 patients the site of the delay was shown to be at or above the AV node ("suprahisian"), below the main bundle in one ("infrahisian"), while one patient was normal at the time of study. In 3 the sinus node function was impaired and in 6 there was fascicular or bundle branch block also.

Having demonstrated conduction defects in some B27-positive patients who had only incomplete forms of spondylarthropathy, Bergfeldt and his colleagues concluded that the B27 antigen is, in its own right, a marker which genetically predisposes a patient to disorders of conduction, predominantly at the AV node, although the conduction system may be widely affected.

Ruppert et al. (1982) came to a similar conclusion about the significance of the B27 antigen as a marker for conduction defects in the heart. They reported 3 patients, two of them father and son, with forms of heart block due to unrecognised B27-positive Reiter's disease. They also reviewed 19 others with known Reiter's disease and found conduction defects in 5, one of whom had aortic incompetence in addition.

Nitter-Hauge and Otterstad (1981) made electrophysiological studies of the conduction system in 5 patients with spondylarthropathy. All 5 had a prolonged conduction time at or above the AV node with an A–H time of 160 ms or more (normal 60–130 ms: see Chap. 6 and Fig. 6.15). Mazieres et al. (1979) and Rossen et al. (1975) also found "suprahisian" delay with prolongation of the A–H time in case studies of patients with heart block associated with ankylosing spondylitis and with Reiter's disease respectively.

Other Spondylarthropathies

Psoriatic Arthropathy

Psoriatic arthropathy manifests in various forms, among which groups or subsets having similar patterns of joint involvement can be identified. About 20% have radiological evidence of sacro-iliitis and some signs of spondylitis. As shown in Table 8.1, B27-positivity is found more often in the spondylitic forms than in the peripheral forms of psoriatic joint disease (40% compared with 15%).

A more detailed analysis of the histocompatibility antigens in 158 patients with psoriatic arthropathy was made by Gladman et al. (1986). They found the B27 antigen in 25% of all forms of psoriatic joint disease, compared with 7% of psoriatic patients without joint disease, and 8% of normal controls. In 54 psoriatic patients with spinal involvement B27 was present in 37%. They also noted an increased frequency of HLA–DR4 in patients with a rheumatoid-like form of psoriatic arthritis, 53%, compared with 30% in controls.

Heart disease in psoriatic spondylarthropathy is rare; an example of aortic incompetence is quoted by Muna et al. (1980).

Inflammatory Bowel Disease

Patients with ulcerative colitis or Crohn's disease may develop either a peripheral form of polyarthritis or a spinal form. The latter form may legitimately be classed among the spondylarthropathies, carrying the B27 antigen in 50% or 60% of cases with a risk of cardiac involvement as in ankylosing spondylitis.

Behçet's Syndrome

This is a doubtful member of the group of spondylarthropathies. Arthritis is not prominent among its various symptoms. However, three patients with Behçet's syndrome and spondylitis were reported by Dubost et al. (1985), two of whom were B27-positive. Cardiac involvement in Behçet's syndrome, when it occurs, takes different forms from those found in the spondylarthropathies (see Chap. 10).

References

Ansell BM, Bywaters EGL, Doniach I (1958) The aortic lesion of ankylosing spondylitis. Br Heart J 20: 507–515

Archer JR, Winrow VR (1987) HLA–B27 and the course of arthritis: does molecular biology help? Ann Rheum Dis 46: 713–715

Ball J (1980) Pathology and pathogenesis. In: Moll JMH (ed) Ankylosing spondylitis. Churchill Livingstone, Edinburgh, pp 96–112

Bauer W, Clarke WS, Kulka JP (1951) Aortitis and aortic endocarditis; an unrecognised manifestation of rheumatoid arthritis. Ann Rheum Dis 10: 470–471

Bennett PH, Wood PHN (eds) (1968) Population studies of the rheumatic diseases. Excerpta Medica Foundation, Amsterdam, pp 456–457

Bergfeldt L, Edhag O, Vallin H (1982a) Cardiac conduction disturbances, an underestimated manifestation in ankylosing spondylitis. Acta Med Scand 212: 217–223

Bergfeldt L, Edhag O, Vedin L, Vallin H (1982b) Ankylosing spondylitis: an important cause of severe disturbances of the cardiac conducting system. Prevalence among 223 pacemaker treated men. Am J Med 73: 187–191

Bergfeldt L, Edhag O, Rajs J (1984a) HLA–B27 associated heart disease. Am J Med 77: 961–967

Bergfeldt L, Vallin H, Edhag O (1984b) Complete heart block in HLA–B27 associated disease. Electrophysiological and clinical characteristics. Br Heart J 51: 184–188

Bernstein L, Broch OJ (1949) Cardiac complications in spondylarthritis ankylopoietica. Acta Med Scand 135: 185–194

Blétry O, De Prost Y, Scheuble C, Frank R, Godeau P (1979) Syndrome de Fiessinger–Leroy – Reiter avec cardiomyopathie non-obstructive. Arch Mal Coeur 72: 799–805

Brewerton DA (1983) A search for infective agents in spondylitis and uveitis. Br J Rheumatol 22 (suppl 2): 91–92

Brewerton DA, Caffrey M, Hart FD, James DCO, Nicholls A, Sturrock RD (1973) Ankylosing spondylitis and HLA–27. Lancet I: 94–907

Brewerton DA, Gibson DG, Goodard DH et al. (1987) The myocardium in ankylosing spondylitis. A clinical, echocardiographic and histopathological study. Lancet I: 995–998

Bulkley BH, Roberts WC (1973) Ankylosing spondylitis and aortic regurgitation. Circulation 48: 1014–1027

Calin A (1983) Spondylarthropathy in Caucasians and non-Caucasians. J Rheumatol 10 (suppl 10); 16–18

Calin A (1984) Seronegative arthritis. Medicine International 2 (22): 912–917

Calin A, Fries JF (1975) Striking prevalence of ankylosing spondylitis in "healthy" W27 positive males and females: a controlled study. N Engl J Med 293: 835–839

Calin A, Fries JF, Stinson JE, Payne R (1976) Normal frequency of HLA–B27 in aortic insufficiency. N Engl J Med 294: 397

Calin A, Marder A, Becks E, Burns T (1983) Genetic differences between B27 positive patients with ankylosing spondylitis and B27 positive healthy controls. Arthritis Rheum 26: 470–474

Clark WS, Kulka JP, Bauer W (1957) Rheumatoid aortitis with aortic regurgitation, an unusual manifestation of rheumatoid arthritis (including spondylitis). Am J Med 22: 580–592

Cliff JM (1971) Spinal bony bridging and carditis in Reiter's disease. Ann Rheum Dis 30: 171–179

Cohen LM, Mittal KK, Schmid FR, Rogers LF, Cohen KL (1976) Increased risk of spondylitis stigmata in apparently healthy HLA–W27 men. Ann Intern Med 84: 1–7

Cosh JA, Lever JV (1984) The aortic valve. In Ansell BM, Simkin PA (eds) The heart and rheumatic disease. Butterworths, London, pp. 83–119

Crow RS (1960) Aortic incompetence in ankylosing spondylitis. Br Med J 2: 271–273

Csonka GW (1979) Clinical aspects of Reiter's syndrome. Ann Rheum Dis; 38 (suppl) 4–7 and 24–28

Csonka GW, Oates JK (1957) Pericarditis and electrocardiographic changes in Reiter's syndrome.
    Br Med J 1: 866–869
Csonka GW, Litchfield JW, Oates JK, Willcox, RR (1961) Cardiac lesions in Reiter's disease. Br
    Med J I: 243–247
Davidson P, Baggenstoss AH, Slocumb CH, Daugherty GW (1963) Cardiac and aortic lesions in
    rheumatoid spondylitis. Mayo Clin Proc 36: 427–435
Davies MJ (1984) Disorders of the conduction system. In: Ansell BM, Simkin PA (eds) The heart
    and rheumatic disease. Butterworths, London, pp 69–73
Demoulin JC, Lespagnard J, Bertholet M, Soumagne D (1983) Acute fulminant aortic regurgitation
    in ankylosing spondylitis. Am Heart J 105: 859–861
Dubost JJ, Sauvezie B, Galtier B et al. (1985) Behçet's syndrome and ankylosing spondylitis. Rev
    Rhum Mal Osteoartic 52: 457–461
Ebringer A (1983) The cross-tolerance hypothesis, HLA–B27 and ankylosing spondylitis. Br J
    Rheumatol 22 (suppl 2): 53–66
Editorial, Lancet (1985) Is Reiter's syndrome caused by chlamydia? Lancet I: 317
Eghtedari AA, Davis P, Bacon PA (1976) Immunological reactivity in ankylosing spondylitis. Ann
    Rheum Dis 35: 155–157
Eversmeyer WH, Rosenstock D, Biundo JJ (1978) Aortic insufficiency with mild ankylosing spondy-
    litis in black men. JAMA 240: 2652–2653
Feigenbaum H (1980) Echocardiography. In: Braunwald E (ed) Heart disease. Saunders, London pp
    96–146
Fox R, Calin A, Gerber RC, Gibson D (1979) The chronicity of symptoms and disability in Reiter's
    syndrome. An analysis of 131 consecutive patients. Ann Intern Med 91: 190–193
Gladman DD, Anhorn KAB, Schachter RK, Mervart AH (1986) HLA antigens in psoriatic arthritis.
    J Rheumatol 13: 586–592
Good AE (1974) Reiter's disease; a review with special attention to cardiovascular and neurogenic
    sequelae. Semin Arthritis Rheum 3: 253–286
Gould BA, Turner J, Keeling DH, Hickling P, Marshall AJ (1988) Myocardial dysfunction in
    ankylosing spondylitics. Br Heart J 59: 129
Graham DC, Smythe HA (1958) The carditis and aortitis of ankylosing spondylitis. Bull Rheum Dis
    9: 171–175
Guiney TE, Davies MJ, Parker DJ, Leech GJ, Leatham A (1987) The aetiology and course of
    isolated severe aortic regurgitation: a clinical, pathological and echocardiographic study. Br
    Heart J 58: 358–368
Henssge R, Boehme A, Muller A (1970) Herzbeteiligung bei der Spondylitis ankylopoietica. Dtsch
    Gesundheitwes 25: 391–393
Hollingworth P, Hall PJ, Knight SC, Newman R (1979) Lone aortic regurgitation, sacro-iliitis and
    HLA–B27: case history and frequency of association. Br Heart J 42: 229–230
Hubscher O, Graci y Susini J (1984) Aortic insufficiency in Reiter's disease of juvenile onset. J
    Rheumatol 11: 94–95
Hudson REB (1967) Surgical pathology of the conducting system of the heart. Br Heart J 29: 646–
    670
Hull RG, Asherson RA, Rennie JAN (1984) Ankylosing spondylitis and an aortic arch syndrome.
    Br Heart J 51: 663–665
Kean WF, Anastassiades TP, Ford PM (1980) Aortic incompetence in HLA–B27 positive juvenile
    arthritis. Ann Rheum Dis 39: 294–295
Keat A, Thomas B, Dixey J, Osborn M, Sonnex C, Taylor-Robinson D (1987) Chlamydia trachoma-
    tis and reactive arthritis: the missing link. Lancet I: 72–74
Kinsella TD, Johnson LG, Sutherland RI (1974) Cardiovascular manifestations of ankylosing
    spondylitis. Canad Med Assoc J 111: 1309–1311
LaBresh KA, Lally EV, Sharma SC, Ho G (1985) Two dimensional echocardiographic detection of
    preclinical aortic root abnormalities in rheumatoid variant diseases. Am J Med 78: 908–912
Laitinen O, Leirosalo M, Skylv G (1977) Relation between HLA–B27 and clinical features in
    patients with yersinia arthritis. Arthritis Rheum 20: 1121–1124
Lawrence JS (1963) The prevalence of arthritis. Br J Clin Pract 17: 699–705
Leirosalo M, Skylv G, Kousa M et al. (1982) Follow up study on patients with Reiter's disease and
    reactive arthritis with special reference to HLA–B27. Arthritis Rheum 25: 249–259
Malette WG, Eiseman B, Danielson GK, Mazzoleni A, Rams JJ (1969) Rheumatoid spondylitis and
    aortic insufficiency. J Thorac Cardiovasc Surg 57: 471–474
Mallory TB (1936) Case records of the Massachusetts General Hospital. N Engl J Med 214: 690–698
Masi AT (1979) Epidemiology of B27 associated diseases. Ann Rheum Dis 38 (suppl): 131–134

Mazieres B, Constans R, Donzeau JP, Sacau P, Dardenne P, Arlet J (1979) Etude electrophysiologique de deux cas de bloc auriculo-ventriculaire secondaire a une spondylarthrite ankylosante. Rev Rhum Mal Osteoartic 46: 137–140

McEwen C, Ditata D, Lingg C, Porini A, Good A, Rankin T (1971) Ankylosing spondylitis and spondylitis accompanying ulcerative colitis, regional enteritis, psoriasis and Reiter's disease. Arthritis Rheum 14: 291–318

McGuigan LE, Geczy AF, Edmonds JP (1985) The immunopathology of ankylosing spondylitis – a review. Semin Arthritis Rheum 15: 81–105

Miller LD, Brown EC, Arnett FC (1979) Amyloidosis in Reiter's syndrome. J Rheumatol 6: 225–231

Moll JMH (1983) Seronegative arthropathies (Editorial). J R Soc Med 76: 445–448

Moll JMH, Haslock I, Macrae IF, Wright V (1974) Associations between ankylosing spondylitis, psoriatic arthritis, Reiter's disease, the intestinal arthropathies and Behcet's syndrome. Medicine (Baltimore) 53: 343–364

Muna WF, Roller DH, Craft J et al. (1980) Psoriatic arthritis and aortic regurgitation. JAMA 244: 363–365

Nicholls A (1979) HLA antigens and rheumatic disease. Medicine, 3rd series: 690–692

Nitter-Hauge S, Otterstad JE (1981) Characteristics of atrioventricular conduction disturbances in ankylosing spondylitis. Acta Med Scand 210: 197–200

Noer HR (1966) An "experimental" epidemic of Reiter's syndrome. JAMA 197: 117–122

Paronen I (1948) Reiter's disease; a study of 344 cases observed in Finland. Acta Med Scand; 131 (suppl 212): 1–114

Paulus HE, Pearson CM, Pitts W (1972) Aortic insufficiency in 5 patients with Reiter's syndrome. Am J Med 53: 464–472

Qaiyumi S, Hassan ZU, Toone E (1985) Seronegative spondylarthropathies in lone aortic insufficiency. Arch Intern Med 145: 822–824

Radford EP, Doll R, Smith PG (1977) Mortality among patients with ankylosing spondylitis not given X-ray therapy. N Engl J Med 297: 572–576

Ribeiro P, Morley KD, Shapiro LM, Garnett RAF, Hughes GRV (1984) Left ventricular function in patients with ankylosing spondylitis and Reiter's disease. Eur Heart J 5: 419–422

Roberts WC, Hollingworth JF, Bulkley BH et al. (1974) Combined mitral and aortic regurgitation in ankylosing spondylitis. Am J Med 56: 237–243

Rossen RM, Goodman DJ, Harrison DC (1975) Atrio-ventricular conduction disturbances in Reiter's syndrome. Am J Med 58: 280–284

Ruppert G, Lindsay J, Barth WF (1982) Cardiac conduction abnormalities in Reiter's syndrome. Am J Med 73: 335–340

Sairanen E, Tiilikainen A (1975) HL–A27 in Reiter's disease following shigellosis. Scand J Rheumatol 4 (suppl 8): abstract 30/11

Sairanen E, Paronen I, Mahonen H (1969) Reiter's syndrome: a follow up study. Acta Med Scand 185: 57–63

Schilder DP, Harvey WP, Hufnagel CA (1956) Rheumatoid spondylitis and aortic insufficiency. N Engl J Med 255: 11–17

Siguier F, Godeau P, Herreman G et al. (1970) Insuffisance aortique, spondylarthrite ankylosante et syndrome de Fiessinger-Leroy-Reiter. Coeur Med Interne 9: 457–465

Sobin LH, Hagstrom JWC (1962) Lesions of cardiac conduction tissue in rheumatoid aortitis. JAMA 180: 1–5

Spangler RD, McAllister BD, McGoon DC (1970) Aortic valve replacement in patients with severe aortic valve incompetence associated with rheumatoid spondylitis. Am J Cardiol 26: 130–134

Stewart SR, Robbins DL, Castles JJ (1978) Acute fulminant aortic and mitral insufficiency in ankylosing spondylitis. N Engl J Med 299: 1448–1449

Takkunen J, Vuopala U, Isomaki H (1970) Cardiomyopathy in ankylosing spondylitis. I. Medical history and results of clinical examination in a series of 55 patients. Ann Clin Res 2: 106–112

Toone EC, Pierce EL, Hennigar GR (1959) Aortitis and aortic regurgitation associated with rheumatoid spondylitis. Am J Med 26: 255–263

Tucker CR, Fowles RE, Calin A, Popp RL (1982) Aortitis in ankylosing spondylitis: early detection of aortic root abnormalities with two dimensional echocardiography. Am J Cardiol 49: 680–686

Van der Linden S, Valkenburg H, Cats A (1983) The risk of developing ankylosing spondylitis in HLA–B27 positive individuals: a family and population study. Br J Rheumatol 22 (suppl 2): 18–19

Weed CL, Kulander BG, Mazzarella JA, Decker JL (1966) Heart block in ankylosing spondylitis. Arch Intern Med 117: 800–817
Wilkinson M, Bywaters EGL (1958) Clinical features and course of ankylosing spondylitis. Ann Rheum Dis 17: 209–228
Willkens RF, Arnett FC, Bitter T et al. (1982) Reiter's syndrome. Evaluation of preliminary criteria for definite disease. Bull Rheum Dis 32: 31–34

Chapter 9

Systemic Sclerosis

Introduction

Systemic sclerosis is a multi-system disease in which "the cutaneous features dominate the patient's appearance, but visceral involvement determines the patient's survival" (Campbell and Leroy 1975). The most serious visceral lesions are those affecting the kidneys, lungs, heart and gastro-intestinal tract.

Scleroderma

Scleroderma, the cutaneous aspect of systemic sclerosis, most often affects the fingers, hands, face and neck, frequently with a prolonged prodromal phase in which the patient is subject to Raynaud's phenomenon. The onset of scleroderma is an insidious affair, caused by slowly progressive obliteration of small vessels. It develops usually in middle or later adult life, affecting women more than men in a ratio of about 3:1. Chronic tissue ischaemia leads to minor local swelling and stiffness at first, with excessive laying down of collagen in the dermis and subcutaneous tissue. This diffuse fibrosis causes an unnatural firmness and loss of elasticity in the skin, leading to restriction of finger movements and reduced mobility of facial expression. Finally there is atrophy and shrinkage of subcutaneous tissue, which is most obvious in the hands, face and neck.

Associated changes in the skin include calcinosis (the Thibierge–Weissenbach syndrome) in the form of densely calcified nodules or plaques in the hands or limbs (Fig. 9.1) and telangiectases, mainly on the face. These develop through the dilatation of some capillaries resulting from the obliteration of others. Atrophy and ischaemia of the finger tips lead to trophic sores and necrotic ulcers, while radiographs may reveal shrinkage of the terminal phalanx due to bony absorption.

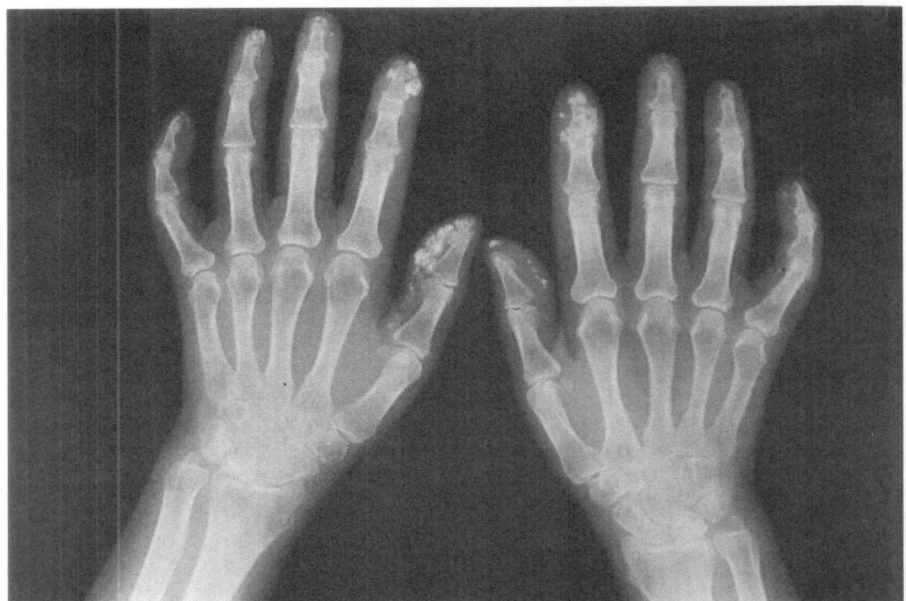

Fig. 9.1. Calcinosis in the hands of a patient with systemic sclerosis. This radiograph shows the deposits of calcium in the pulp of the thumbs and finger tips.

Visceral Lesions

Visceral lesions develop in half or more of patients with scleroderma and, like the skin lesions, result from slowly progressive obstructive changes in small vessels. Occasionally the visceral lesions develop first but generally they follow the skin changes after an unpredictable interval of months or years (Table 9.1).

Table 9.1. Visceral involvement in 261 patients with systemic sclerosis (Campbell and Leroy 1975)

	Percentage of patients affected
Scleroderma in skin	90
Raynaud's phenomenon	78
Oesophagus	52
Lungs	43
Heart	40
Kidney	35
Anaemia	27
Articular	25
Hypertension	21
Muscle	20
Intestine	15
Pericardium	11

Gastro-intestinal Tract. The oesophagus is often affected by changes similar to those taking place in the skin. Oesophageal contractility and peristalsis are impaired resulting in dysphagia and stasis of oesophageal contents. In the small intestine atrophic changes in the mucosa and muscle coat cause loss of motility with stasis, secondary bacterial infection, malabsorption and steatorrhoea.

Lungs. There is slowly progressive pulmonary fibrosis with deterioration in respiratory function, namely reduction in vital capacity and in carbon monoxide diffusing capacity. These changes precede the radiological appearance of pulmonary fibrosis (Schneider et al. 1982; Steen et al. 1985). Measurement of carbon monoxide diffusion capacity has been found to be an aid to prognosis: reduction below 40% of the predicted normal is associated with a significantly lower 5-year survival rate (Peters-Golden et al. 1984).

In addition there may be progressive thickening of the walls of pulmonary arterioles, narrowing their lumen and increasing pulmonary vascular resistance, causing pulmonary hypertension (Trell and Lindstrom 1971). No close parallel has been found between the pulmonary vascular changes and pulmonary fibrosis (Young and Mark 1978) but an association with impaired respiratory function has been noted (Ungerer et al. 1983).

Kidney. "Scleroderma kidney" is the most serious of the visceral lesions of systemic sclerosis. Ischaemic changes in the kidney and reduction in glomerular perfusion cause progressive renal failure and hypertension. Malignant hypertension with rapidly advancing renal failure, "scleroderma renal crisis", carries a high mortality rate (Rodnan et al. 1957; Traub et al. 1983).

The Heart. Pericarditis is the commonest cardiac lesion. It is usually not serious and may go unobserved. The classical "scleroderma heart" is a form of diffuse fibrosis developing in an irregular fashion throughout the myocardium, and may lead to congestive failure. Arrhythmias of all kinds are frequent and occasionally there is heart block. The heart is also affected secondarily as a result of systemic or pulmonary hypertension should these develop.

The CREST Syndrome

The CREST syndrome is a milder and more slowly evolving variant of systemic sclerosis, so named because of the combination of Calcinosis, Raynaud's phenomenon, Esophageal dysfunction, Sclerodactyly and Telangiectasia. It has fewer visceral lesions and renal and cardiac involvement are uncommon; it has a better prognosis than the majority of cases of systemic sclerosis. It is associated with the anti-centromere antibody (p. 198) and also with pulmonary hypertension (Salerni et al. 1977; Ungerer et al. 1983).

Mixed Connective Tissue Disease

Mixed connective tissue disease (MCTD) is an "overlap syndrome" in which features of more than one rheumatic disease appear together (Dubois et al. 1971; Sharp 1974, 1975). In MCTD scleroderma, sometimes with its characteristic visceral lesions of oesophagus or lungs, is combined with polymyositis or with some of the features of systemic lupus erythematosus, such as arthralgia, rash, lymphadenopathy or fever (p. 140). In the heart MCTD causes pericarditis in about 25% of cases and some evidence of myocarditis, but not the extensive myocardial changes of systemic sclerosis or the valve lesions of SLE (Alpert et al. 1983; Singsen et al. 1977). Complete heart block has been reported (Emlen 1979). MCTD has a low incidence of renal involvement and consequently a relatively favourable prognosis.

Prevalence and Course

Systemic sclerosis is uncommon. In Britain it has been estimated that there is one case of systemic sclerosis for every 500 of rheumatoid arthritis (Wood 1977). In the USA its incidence has been calculated as 2 or 3 new cases per million population per annum (Medsger and Masi 1979).

Scleroderma alone, without any visceral involvement, runs a very chronic course lasting many years; the patient's condition may appear to stabilise, with arrest of the progression of scleroderma. However, the development of visceral lesions is unpredictable, and when they do arise the prognosis worsens (Medsger et al. 1971). In one review, deterioration and death was associated with four features in particular: pulmonary involvement, impaired renal function, ECG evidence of cardiac involvement, and the presence of scleroderma in the skin of the trunk (Bennett et al. 1971).

Diagnosis

The clinical recognition of scleroderma is not difficult when the skin involvement has become established. The combination of dermal thickening, and restriction of movement in the fingers and in the face, especially around the mouth, is unmistakable. A history of Raynaud's phenomenon is strongly suggestive, especially if the onset was in the third or fourth decade, whereas uncomplicated Raynaud's phenomenon begins in childhood or adolescence. The finding of flecks of calcification in the digits on radiographs of the hands is confirmatory. An impressive, though non-specific physical sign is the finding of low-pitched friction bruits on auscultation over tendon sheaths in the hand and wrists when the fingers are flexed and extended. The symptom of dysphagia is usually the first sign that visceral involvement has started.

Serological tests may support the diagnosis but cannot be relied on in the early stages, when antinuclear antibodies may not always be present. In mixed connective tissue disease they will be absent, but antibodies to nRNP will be present, often in high titre and, clinically, there will be suggestive features of myositis and/or SLE.

Preliminary diagnostic criteria were outlined by the ARA subcommittee in 1980. The sole major criterion is the presence of sclerodermatous skin changes proximal to the metacarpophalangeal joints in the hands or the metatarsophalangeal joints in the feet and legs. Alternatively the diagnosis may be made on the presence of two of the three minor criteria. These are: sclerodactyly, digital pitting scars on the finger tips or loss of substance in the distal finger pad, or bilateral basal pulmonary fibrosis.

Pathology

In the early stages of scleroderma there are signs of a low-grade inflammatory process in the skin, connective tissue, tendon sheaths and joint synovia. Perivascular infiltration with mononuclear cells is seen on biopsy, and this is followed by intimal proliferation in small arteries such as the digital arteries (Fig. 9.2). Collagen is laid down extensively (Herbert et al. 1974; Jayson 1984) and this process of fibrosis appears to be the result of progressive ischaemic changes which ultimately may lead to tissue atrophy or areas of necrosis. The evolution of these processes is extremely slow and may progress at different rates at different sites. The essential primary change is in the microvasculature, both in the skin and in affected viscera (Campbell and Leroy 1975; Norton and Nardo 1970).

The same process of progressive obliteration of the lumen is seen in small arteries, of 1 mm diameter and less, in the skin (Rodnan et al. 1980), the lungs (Fig. 9.3) (Trell and Lindstrom 1971; Young and Mark 1978), the myocardium (James 1974) and the kidneys (Rodnan et al. 1957). Intimal thickening and medial hyperplasia reduce the lumen until it is much narrowed or finally obstructed, the final step sometimes being a platelet thrombus. Larger arteries show similar changes, though not often to the point of obstruction; in part, these may be the result of hypertension either in the systemic or the pulmonary circulation.

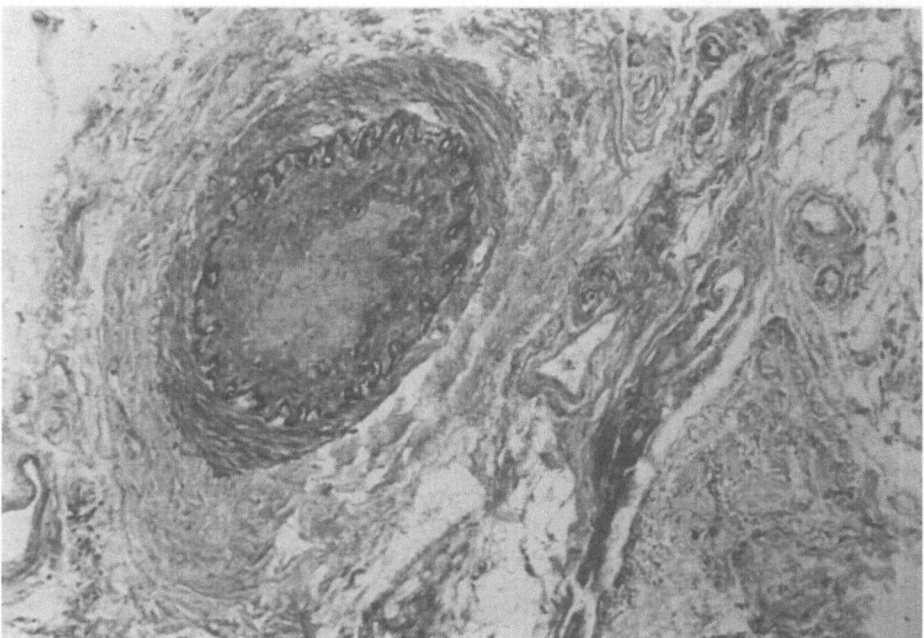

Fig. 9.2. Digital artery in systemic sclerosis. Photomicrograph of a digital artery in a patient with scleroderma showing thickening of the intima and obliteration of the lumen by thrombus (H and E × 200).

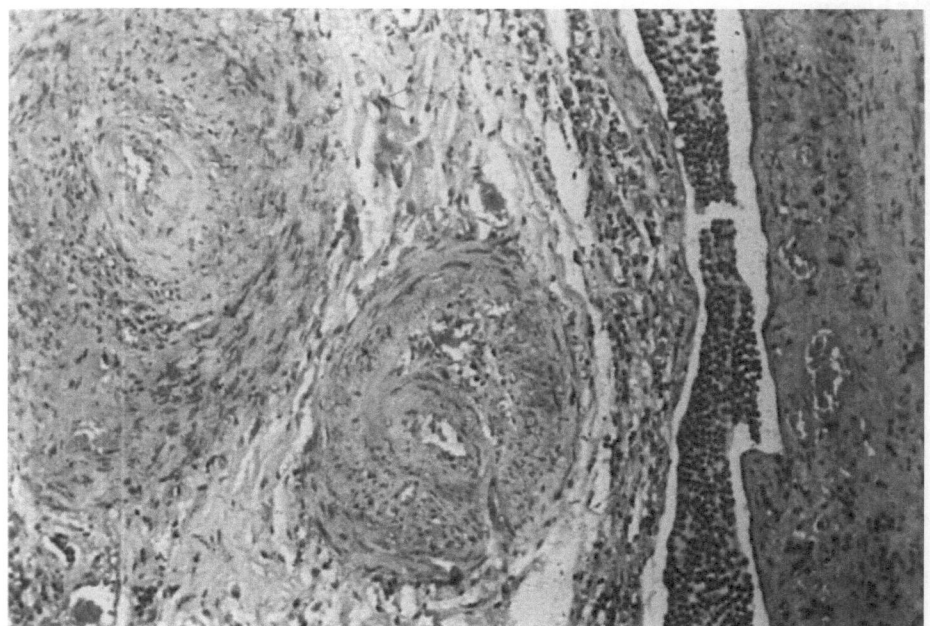

Fig. 9.3. Pulmonary artery in systemic sclerosis. Photomicrograph of a small pulmonary artery in a patient with pulmonary hypertension showing marked thickening of the intima and narrowing of the lumen (H and E × 200).

Capillary abnormalities may be seen and studied by nailfold microscopy. This can be of diagnostic value in distinguishing, in the early stages, between simple Raynaud's phenomenon and scleroderma (Harper et al. 1982; Lefford and Edwards 1986; Maricq et al. 1976). In scleroderma there is dilatation and distortion of some capillary loops with obliteration of others producing avascular areas; in Raynaud's phenomenon the capillary loops are normal.

Immunology

Many observations point to an immunological basis for systemic sclerosis, although its fundamental cause is unknown. Antinuclear antibodies were found in some 40% of sera from patients with systemic scerlosis, using the indirect immunofluorescent technique with an organ substrate such as mouse kidney. But when tissue cultured cells are used as substrate antibodies are found in 95% of sera (Aitcheson and Tan 1982; Catoggio et al. 1983; Tan et al. 1980). Different patterns of nuclear and nucleolar staining may be distinguished. One specific pattern is of staining localised to the centromere region of chromosomes visible in dividing cell nuclei. This anti-centromere antibody is present in 50% or more of sera from patients with the CREST syndrome (Catoggio et al. 1983; Fritzler et al. 1980; McCarty et al. 1983; Miller et al. 1987).

A number of antibodies to extractable nuclear antigens have been identified by precipitation techniques in about half of patients with systemic sclerosis. These include antibodies to the antigen Scl 70, present in some 20% of sera and associated with pulmonary lesions (Catoggio et al. 1983).

Circulating immune complexes are present in the sera of some patients, rather more often in MCTD than in patients with diffuse systemic sclerosis and are associated to some extent with pulmonary and cardiac involvement (Cunningham et al. 1980; Pisko et al. 1979). Both immune complexes and inflammatory cells have been recovered from the lower respiratory tract by broncho-alveolar lavage, undertaken during bronchoscopy. The fact that immune complexes were present in far greater concentration in the lavage fluid than in the serum suggested that they were either being segregated from the blood, or else generated in the lower respiratory tract of affected patients (Silver et al. 1986).

Mixed connective tissue disease characteristically has a high level of antibodies to the extractable nuclear antigen nRNA, in the absence of other antinuclear antibodies (Aitcheson and Tan 1982).

The HLA tissue antigens have no clear-cut role in systemic sclerosis comparable to their role in ankylosing spondylitis or rheumatoid arthritis. There are reports of an increased frequency of HLA–DR5: Gladman and colleagues (1981) found this antigen present in 53% of patients compared with 18% of controls, and the DR5-positive patients had a higher score of skin involvement, though not of visceral lesions. Other reports have confirmed this observation, and to a less extent have shown an increased frequency also of DR1 (Alarcon et al. 1985; Black et al. 1984).

Direct evidence for an immunological basis for arteriopathy was reported by Evans et al. (1987). In an autopsy study of a patient who had had severe and rapidly progressive systemic sclerosis, immunoglobulin was identified in the media of the renal and other arteries. After extraction it was shown to be capable of binding to the muscle and elastic fibres in the coats of small arteries.

The Heart in Systemic Sclerosis

The main cardiac abnormalities seen at autopsy in systemic sclerosis, and the frequency with which they are found, are shown in Table 9.2. These figures are based on the combined reports of McWhorter and Leroy (1974) and Sackner et al. (1966).

Table 9.2. Frequency of cardiac abnormalities in systemic sclerosis, based on 59 autopsies (From McWhorter and Leroy (1974) and Sackner et al. (1966)

	Present at autopsy	Frequency (%)
Cardiomegaly	38/59	64
Pericarditis	33/59	56
Myocardial fibrosis	20/59	34
LV hypertrophy only	21/57	37
RV hypertrophy only	16/57	28
Bilateral ventricular hypertrophy	13/57	23

Pericardium

Pericarditis is a common development in systemic sclerosis but often passes unobserved (Botstein and Leroy 1981; Michet and Hunder 1984; Nasser et al. 1968). In autopsy studies between a half and two-thirds of subjects show evidence of pericarditis, previous or current (D'Angelo et al. 1969; McWhorter and Leroy 1974; Oram and Stokes 1961; Sackner et al. 1966). There may be old pericardial adhesions or an active fibrinous pericarditis which is usually chronic, but is sometimes acute, with or without an effusion.

Pericarditis is recognised clinically in up to 16% of patients with systemic sclerosis on the basis of chest pain, pericardial friction, fever, or ECG and X-ray findings (Botstein and Leroy 1981). Occasionally an effusion is found which is large enough to produce tamponade, when aspiration is required (Uhl and Koppes 1979). Such patients have a poor prognosis on account of associated myocardial or visceral involvement. Constrictive pericarditis is virtually unknown as a sequel.

In some cases pericarditis arises as a result of the complications of systemic sclerosis, e.g. accompanying pleural or pulmonary lesions, or as a result of uraemia. In others it is symptomless and may be unrecognised unless identified on investigation, particularly by echocardiography (Gottdiener et al. 1979). Smith et al. (1979) found echocardiographic evidence of pericardial effusion in 22 of 59 patients (37%) although pericarditis was only clinically apparent in 7 of them.

The pericardial fluid in systemic sclerosis has no distinctive features. There is a moderate pleocytosis, a normal glucose level and the protein content is low. Antinuclear antibody may be detected in the fluid but complement is not reduced, implying that there is no immunological activity in the pericardium. The fluid is thus more characteristic of a transudate than an exudate (Gladman et al. 1976).

Pericarditis is a feature of the CREST syndrome and also of MCTD, though not with the frequency that is noted in diffuse systemic sclerosis. Reports on pericarditis both in adults (Alpert et al. 1983; Oetgen et al. 1983; Sharp 1974) and in children (Singsen et al. 1977) indicate that between a quarter and a third develop pericarditis with MCTD.

Case History 9.1 describes a patient with long-standing systemic sclerosis who died in congestive failure due to myocardial fibrosis; at autopsy she was found to have unsuspected fibrinous pericarditis.

Case History 9.1

Systemic sclerosis
Calcinosis
Cardiomegaly and arrhythmia
Congestive heart failure

Mrs. D.M., Housewife, born 1911

1939   Stiffness and swelling L index finger
              Developed during pregnancy

1942	Scleroderma spread to hands, forearms and face Trunk and lower limbs never involved
1961	Flexion contractures all fingers Heavy calcinosis in hands (Fig. 9.4)
1965	Cardiomegaly ECG: Lbbb Various remedies tried and failed Prednisone 5 mg daily: no apparent benefit
1972	Mild congestive failure Atrial tachycardia AV block 3:1 (Fig. 9.5) Cardioversion twice tried and failed
1976	Dysphagia; oesophagus dilated, aperistaltic
1977	Pressure sores on palms from flexion contractures of fingers
1978	Died in congestive failure Pleural effusions: no signs of pericarditis
Autopsy	Heart much enlarged, 860 g (Fig. 9.6) Parietal pericardium thickened, fibrinous exudate Ventricular walls hypertrophied, areas of softening RV wall 8 mm thick. Coronary arteries normal LV wall thinned at apex, laminated thrombus
Histology	Extensive and irregular fibrosis in myocardium (Fig. 9.7)
Comment	Typically slow evolution of the disease. Cardiac involvement was recognised 26 years after onset of systemic sclerosis and death followed 13 years later

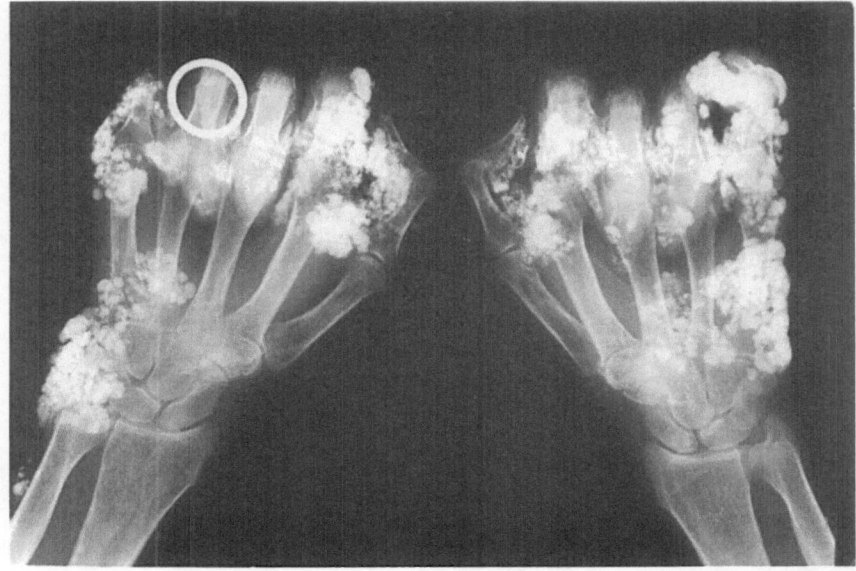

Fig. 9.4. Calcinosis in hands. X-ray film of the hands of the patient described in Case History 9.1.

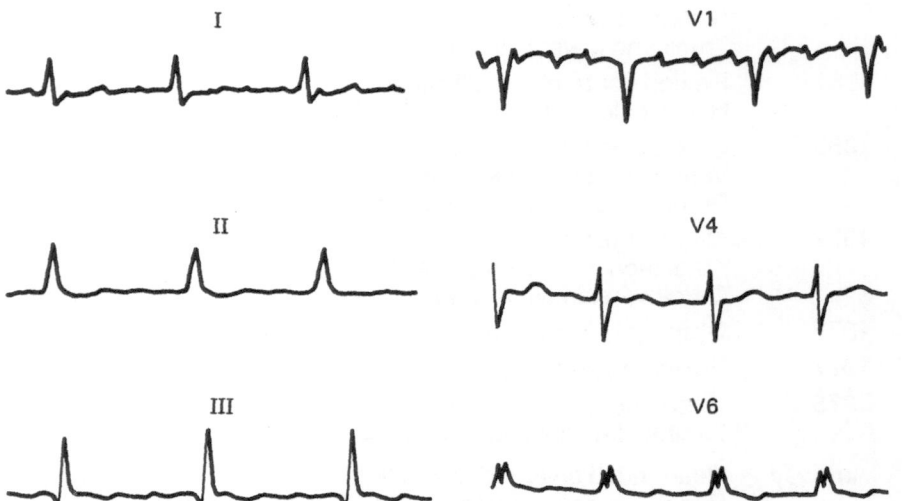

Fig. 9.5. Atrial tachycardia in the patient in Case History 9.1. ECG shows an atrial rate of about 240, with 3:1 AV block. There is also left bundle branch block.

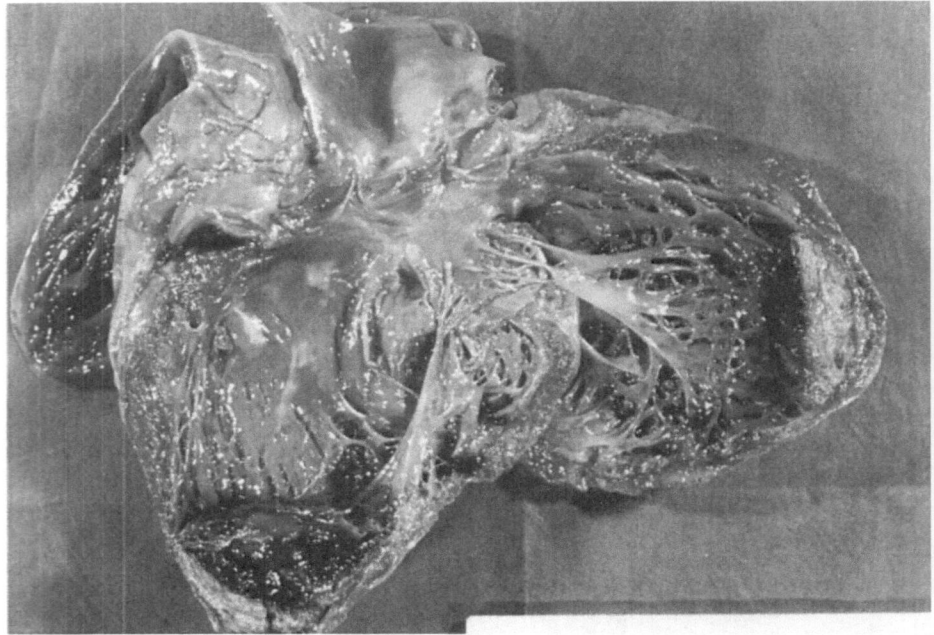

Fig. 9.6. The heart at autopsy on Case History 9.1. The left ventricle is dilated with laminated thrombus at the apex.

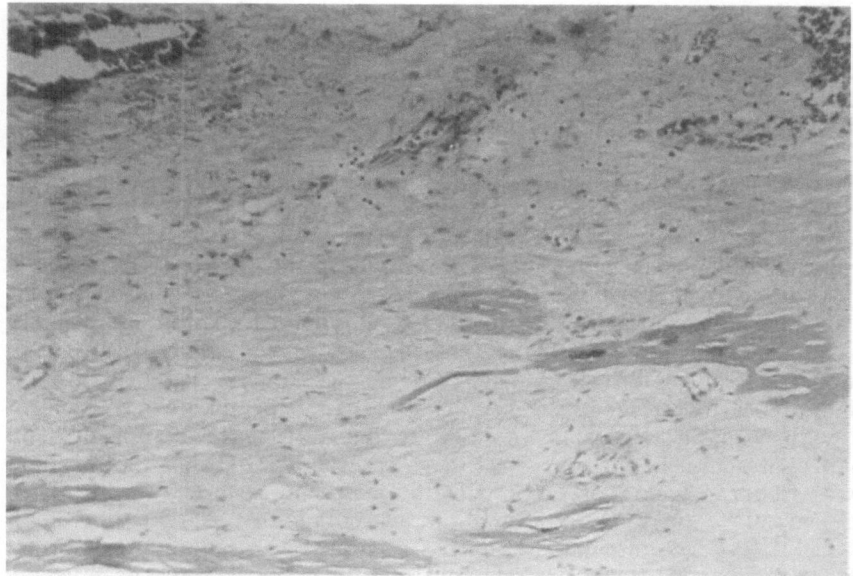

Fig. 9.7. Myocardium from the heart shown in the previous figure, showing diffuse fibrosis with few surviving myocardial fibres. The coronary arteries were of normal calibre and their lumen was unobstructed (H and E × 180).

Myocardium

The characteristic cardiac lesion in systemic sclerosis is the widespread myocardial fibrosis – "scleroderma heart" – which is, in effect, a form of cardiomyopathy. Its essential cause, in common with the cutaneous and other visceral lesions, is ischaemia at a microvascular level.

The fibrosis is irregularly distributed throughout the myocardium of the atria and ventricles, affecting the right ventricle as much as the left. In their description of scleroderma heart Oram and Stokes (1961) drew attention to the fact that the fibrosis and scarring in the myocardium are distributed in a fashion that is quite irregular and bears no relation to the distribution of the main coronary arteries, which are unaffected. In some areas there is dense fibrotic scarring while in others only a diffuse pallor is visible to the naked eye. Between the affected areas the myocardium appears normal.

The earliest histological change is of myocardial cell necrosis, which is followed by a focal inflammatory response leading finally to replacement fibrosis on an extensive scale (Figs. 9.6 and 9.7).

The observations of Oram and Stokes were followed by further accounts by Sackner et al. (1966), Nasser et al. (1968) and D'Angelo et al. (1969) and it became clear that in the myocardium, as elsewhere, "scleroderma is essentially a vascular disease and the primary site of injury is at the microvascular level" (Norton and Nardo 1970).

Microvascular changes in the myocardium were reported by James (1974) in an account of 8 patients with myocardial fibrosis and lesions of the conducting system, 6 of whom had died suddenly of cardiac arrhythmia or arrest. Widespread changes were found in small arteries and arterioles, whose lumen was reduced by endothelial proliferation, intimal fibrosis and medial hyperplasia; in places there was total vascular obstruction by platelet thrombi. The extent of the surrounding myocardial fibrosis seemed out of proportion to the vascular lesions.

Another study of the myocardium in systemic sclerosis, based on 52 autopsied cases, half of whom had fibrotic areas, described the appearance of "contraction band necrosis" in the more severely affected hearts (Bulkley 1979). This pattern of densely staining eosinophilic bands within necrotic myocardial cells is a feature resulting from periods of myocardial ischaemia. It is suggested that episodes of intense arterial spasm, likened to Raynaud's phenomenon in the myocardium, may have been sufficient to induce myocardial cellular necrosis, in due course followed by fibrosis.

Angina, myocardial infarction and sudden death have been known to occur in patients with systemic sclerosis in whom the coronary arteries were normal. The finding of contraction band necrosis in these cases suggested that the terminal event was underperfusion of the myocardium due to severe arterial spasm (Bulkley et al. 1978). In confirmation of circulatory obstruction at a microvascular level, cardioangiography has demonstrated reduced myocardial perfusion with delayed "runoff" in systemic sclerosis in the presence of normally patent main coronary vessels (Gupta et al. 1975).

Calcification may follow in areas of myocardial fibrosis but is unusual. Possibly the poor prognosis does not allow time for this to happen. However, calcification in the myocardium was a striking feature in Case History 9.2, being seen in a wide circle around the mitral valve ring and also in the aortic valve cusps (Fig. 9.8). This patient also had extensive subcutaneous calcinosis in the legs (Fig. 9.9).

In mixed connective tissue disease the myocardium is affected less. Foci of lymphocytic infiltration and limited fibrosis have been reported (Singsen et al. 1977; Whitlow et al. 1980) and luminal narrowing in small arteries due to intimal hyperplasia (Alpert et al. 1983).

Case History 9.2

Systemic sclerosis Gout
Cardiac and pulmonary lesions
Calcification at mitral and aortic valves

Mrs. J.H., Housewife, born 1914

1945	Developed Raynaud's phenomenon
1969	Scleroderma started in fingers Later spread to legs, face, neck
1971	Gout in L hallux: given allopurinol Calcinosis in skin of legs; recurrent ulcers Oesophageal motility reduced
1975	Trials of probenecid and penicillamine failed

1976	Calcinosis disabling: "legs armour plated" (Fig. 9.9)
	Cardiomegaly, dyspnoea BP 180/80
	Mitral and aortic systolic murmurs
	Respiratory tests: impaired gas transfer
	Renal function slightly impaired
	X-ray: calcification in mitral valve ring (Fig. 9.8)
	ECG: LV hypertrophy and ischaemia
1977	Echo: reduced mitral valve excursion; heavy echoes from aortic cusps – ? calcification
1978	Pleural effusions, pneumonia. Gangrene L hallux
	ECG: Lbbb and atrial fibrillation (Fig. 9.10)
	Died in congestive heart failure
Autopsy	Heart much enlarged: wt. 650 g
	Normal pericardium, LV hypertrophy
	Calcification at aortic cusps and in mitral valve ring.
Comment	Cardiac and pulmonary involvement were the causes of her death, but the major clinical problem for 7 years was the disabling leg ulceration with calcinosis

With acknowledgements to Dr. Allan Dixon and Dr. David Yates

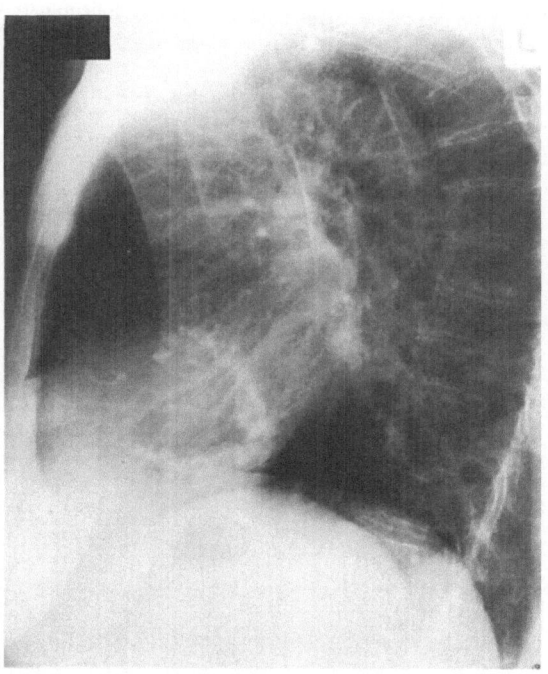

Fig. 9.8. Chest X-ray (left lateral) from the patient in Case History 9.2 showing widespread calcification in the mitral valve ring.

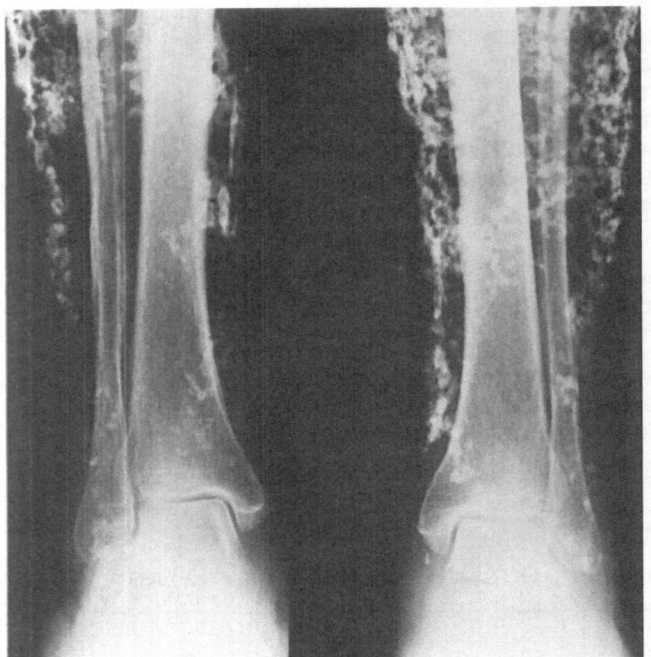

Fig. 9.9. X-ray of legs of the patient in Case History 9.2 showing widespread subcutaneous calcinosis.

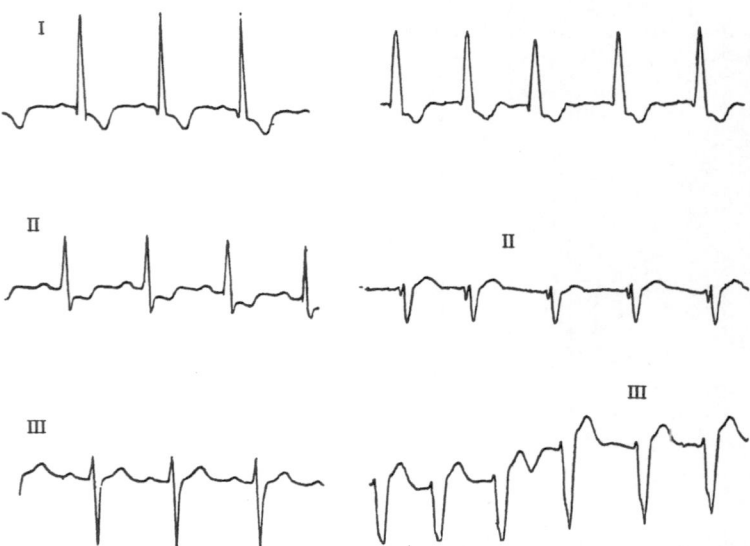

Fig. 9.10. Electrocardiogram from the patient in Case History 9.2, showing (*left*) left ventricular hypertrophy and sinus rhythm in 1976 and (*right*) left bundle branch block and atrial fibrillation in 1978.

Echocardiography. Echocardiography can reveal abnormalities in ventricular dimensions and myocardial function that may otherwise go unrecognised. Left ventricular wall thickening, asymmetrical ventricular hypertrophy and reduced left ventricular compliance have been found in a significant proportion of patients (Ferri et al. 1985; Gottdiener et al. 1979). Some correlation has been shown between right ventricular wall thickness and pulmonary arterial pressure, which is a useful guide to the severity of pulmonary hypertension (Smith et al. 1979).

Radionuclide Scintigraphy. Scintigraphy with thallium-201 has also been used in the assessment of myocardial involvement in systemic sclerosis. Follansbee and colleagues (1984) carried out thallium scans at rest and during exercise on 26 patients with systemic sclerosis. Although only 6 had clinical evidence of cardiac involvement, 20 had abnormal scans, indicating areas of deficient myocardial perfusion. In most cases these were fixed abnormalities, but some defects were revealed only on exercise and recovered on rest, yet the latter were not associated with any arterial abnormality on coronary arteriography. This clearly signifies myocardial vascular insufficiency at the level of small vessels.

Moreover, Alexander et al. (1986) showed that transient reduction in perfusion in a number of segments of ventricular myocardium could be induced by a cold stimulus in 10 of 13 patients in whom there were no signs of myocardial defect. This supports the concept of a form of Raynaud phenomenon affecting the myocardium in response to cold.

Ellis et al. (1986) found a similar myocardial response to cold in 9 of 16 patients, and were able to show that nifedipine reduced the effect of cold, at least for a time. Similar studies by Kahan et al. (1986a, b) confirmed the protective action of nifedipine and dipyridamol against the effect of cold on the myocardium.

Valve Lesions

Valve lesions primarily due to systemic sclerosis are rare. If a valve lesion is found in a patient with systemic sclerosis, the probability is that it is present by coincidence and has a different pathological cause such as rheumatic heart disease or, in an older patient, degenerative disease such as aortic atherosclerosis. Alternatively, it may be a secondary result of systemic sclerosis. Severe hypertension may have caused aortic incompetence, or left ventricular dilatation may have led to functional mitral incompetence. Similarly, severe pulmonary hypertension is sometimes a cause of pulmonary valve incompetence.

There are a few reports of valve lesions which could be attributed to no other cause than systemic sclerosis. Yunus and colleagues (1984) described two such cases, in women with aortic incompetence. The echocardiographic surveys of Gottdiener et al. (1979) and Smith et al. (1979) in patients with systemic sclerosis revealed instances of mitral valve prolapse, but this may well have been a coincidental finding.

Electrocardiographic Abnormalities

A variety of ECG abnormalities are found in systemic sclerosis; they are
common and often are the first, and sometimes the only, sign of cardiac
involvement. They may be present even before the skin lesions appear.

The most frequent findings are changes in rhythm and in conduction; ST and T
wave changes are also seen, or low voltage ventricular complexes, probably the
result of myocardial damage. Table 9.3 lists the ECG changes reported by Oram
and Stokes (1961); more than one type of abnormality may be seen in an
individual patient at different times.

Table 9.3. Electrocardiographic changes in 49 cases of systemic sclerosis. (From Oram and Stokes
1961)

Arrhythmia	24	Ectopic beats: ventricular	11
		atrial	6
		multifocal	3
		Atrial fibrillation	2
		Atrial flutter	1
		Ventricular fibrillation	1
Conduction defect	25	First degree block	10
		Short PR	2
		R bbb	8
		L bbb	3
		Complete heart block	2
ST and T changes	17	T wave inversion	5
		T wave resembling infarct	3
		T wave flat or low	5
		ST depression	4
Hypertrophy	14	Right ventricle	5
		Left ventricle	4
		Atrial	5

48 patients had one or more abnormality

The frequency of ECG abnormalities in different reports ranges from 57%
(Clements et al. 1981) to 70% or more (Cozzi et al. 1983; Roberts et al. 1981).
The incidence of abnormalities obviously depends upon the frequency of ECG
recordings. As might be expected, 24-hour Holter monitoring yields a high
incidence of abnormality; Ferri et al. (1985) noted some form of abnormality in
every one of 52 patients monitored, compared with only 22 revealed by
conventional electrocardiography.

Arrhythmias. Ventricular and atrial ectopic beats are common. Occasionally
atrial fibrillation or flutter are seen or atrial paroxysmal tachycardia. Ventricular
tachycardia has also been described as a presenting feature of systemic sclerosis
(Singh et al. 1974).

In the patient described in Case History 9.1 a sustained atrial tachycardia was
present throughout the last 6 years of her life, usually with 3:1 AV conduction
block (Fig. 9.5). Sinus rhythm was temporarily restored by cardioversion but the

arrhythmia recurred. The patient in Case History 9.2 had terminal atrial fibrillation with left bundle branch block (Fig. 9.10).

Conduction Defects. First degree block is relatively common and so is bundle branch block or hemiblock (Table 9.3) (Davies 1984). Complete heart block is not often seen, but has been noted by Oram and Stokes (1961) and by Summerfield (1975). Lev et al. (1966) also report a case in which a careful study of the conducting tissue was made at autopsy. Complete block mostly presents as such, as in the patient described in Case History 9.3, although it has been known to evolve progressively over a period (Barr et al. 1970). Complete block has also been reported in MCTD (Emlen 1979).

At autopsy the pathological changes in the myocardium may be found to have involved the SA or AV nodes or the Purkinje system. The nodal or Purkinje tissue may be atrophic, or replaced by fibrous tissue; in some cases the arteries supplying the nodes may have their lumen partially or totally obstructed by thickening of the intima or media (James 1974; Lev et al. 1966).

In a study of the conduction system in 35 autopsied cases Ridolfi and colleagues (1976) found fibrotic replacement of the SA node in a third, not necessarily associated with a lesion of the nodal artery or with local myocardial fibrosis. Overlying pericarditis in the close vicinity of the SA node may have contributed to the lesion in some cases. They found the AV node less often affected than the SA node. Correspondence between the pathological lesions of the nodes or the Purkinje system and the ECG recorded before death was not close. In some cases bundle branch block had been present but no corresponding pathological changes could be identified subsequently.

Case History 9.3

Systemic sclerosis
Complete heart block
Oesophageal and intestinal lesions
Death from intestinal obstruction

Mr. C.E., Bus conductor, born 1921

1965	Developed Raynaud's phenomenon
1967	Scleroderma started in hands, later face
1970	Kerato-conjunctivitis sicca: loss of sight of left eye
1971	Cervical sympathectomy for digital ulceration
1972	Facial telangiectases Dysphagia: reduced oesophageal motility Disordered bowel function
1974	Complete heart block, syncope Given pacemaker
1975	Weight loss marked: steatorrhoea Improved on metronidazole

1975 Dec   Developed subacute small bowel obstruction
1976 Jan   Found to have mesenteric torsion
                   Died after laparotomy

Comment   No autopsy study of heart. No cardiac trouble after
                   pacemaker implanted. The major complications were gastro-
                   intestinal

With acknowledgements to Professor Jayson and Professor Read

Left Ventricular Hypertrophy

Left ventricular hypertrophy in systemic sclerosis arises as a response to hypertension caused by renal involvement. Sometimes the progression of the renal disease is so rapid that there is insufficient time for left ventricular hypertrophy to develop before the patient succumbs to renal failure (Rodnan et al. 1957).

At autopsy left ventricular hypertrophy is present in half or more, either alone or in combination with right ventricular hypertrophy (Table 9.2). ECG evidence of left ventricular hypertrophy is seen less often, in about 10% of autopsies. Asymmetrical septal hypertrophy was noted on echocardiographic study of patients with MCTD by Oetgen et al. (1983).

Pulmonary Hypertension

Pulmonary hypertension develops as a result of obliterative changes in the pulmonary vascular bed, which increases the pulmonary vascular resistance. The pulmonary arterial pressure may rise to systemic levels or even higher (Trell and Lindstrom 1971; Wade 1984; Young and Mark 1978). At such pressure levels the main pulmonary arteries become dilated and atheroma may develop in their walls. Some degree of pulmonary hypertension, i.e. a mean pulmonary artery pressure above 22 mm/Hg, was found in 33 of 49 (67%) patients with systemic sclerosis investigated by cardiac catheterisation (Ungerer et al. 1983).

At autopsy right ventricular hypertrophy was found in about 40% of patients, either alone or in combination with left ventricular hypertrophy (Table 9.2) whereas ECG evidence was only seen in about 10%. There is a time lag between the development of pulmonary hypertension and the appearance of hypertrophy in the right ventricle, and ECG changes follow later still. Where pulmonary hypertension progresses rapidly, heart failure and death may supervene before right ventricular hypertrophy and its ECG changes have had time to develop (Trell and Lindstrom 1971).

Pulmonary hypertension may be found in the CREST syndrome; it was severe in 10 of 120 cases reported by Salerni et al. (1971) and was responsible for death in 4 of these. It is an uncommon finding in MCTD (Jones et al. 1978).

Treatment

Scleroderma

Of the many recommended treatments for scleroderma few have more than a local and temporary effect. Simple physical remedies include advice on preserving central body heat, protecting the extremities from cold, avoidance of smoking, and local applications of skin-softening water-miscible cream, to be gently rubbed in with mobilisation of affected skin and tissues.

Some remedies have been proposed in the hope that they might relieve both the dermal and visceral lesions. These include corticosteroids and penicillamine. Corticosteroid may be of use for relief of local inflammation such as synovitis or tenosynovitis, but systemically is likely to do more harm than good. Penicillamine is thought to diminish the laying down of fresh collagen in affected tissues, and sometimes is considered to have relieved myocardial fibrosis (Muers and Stokes 1976).

Severe peripheral ischaemia with threatened tissue necrosis has been relieved at least temporarily by intravenous prostaglandin E_1 infusion, preferably maintained over a period of days (Martin et al. 1981). A dextran infusion has similarly been beneficial in relieving cardiac ischaemia with crescendo angina in a patient with systemic sclerosis.

The calcium antagonist nifedipine, through its direct relaxing effect on arterial smooth muscle is used in the treatment and prevention of Raynaud's phenomenon as well as for hypertension and angina. It has been found to reduce the frequency of attacks of vasospasm in systemic sclerosis also (Hawkins et al. 1986), and was well tolerated in a dose of 10 mg four times daily.

Cardiovascular Lesions

Hypertension

The control of hypertension is vital when it is due to scleroderma kidney, particularly if it is entering the malignant phase or if renal function is impaired. Vigorous treatment with conventional anti-hypertensive drugs such as methyl dopa, hydralazine and diuretics is capable of reversing renal failure, but it is often unsuccessful so that renal dialysis may become necessary (Lam et al. 1978). Among commonly used drugs beta blockers are better avoided owing to their liability to worsen Raynaud's phenomenon, or to exacerbate heart block.

The angiotensin converting enzyme (ACE) inhibitor captopril is well suited for the treatment of renal hypertension which is mediated by angiotensin. Good reports of its use came from Atkinson and Robertson (1979), Lopez-Ovejero et al. (1979), and Thurm and Alexander (1984). But to be effective captopril must be given while renal function is still reasonably good (Whitman et al. 1982). A satisfactory dose is 25 mg three times daily, working up to a maximum of 150 mg three times daily (Thurm and Alexander 1984). Another ACE inhibitor, enalapril, may be used similarly; either drug may be given in combination with other anti-hypertensive agents such as hydralazine, nifedipine, methyldopa or a diuretic.

Pulmonary Hypertension. This has proved almost uniformly unresponsive to treatment, and if severe carries a bad prognosis. However, diazoxide has been found effective in reversing primary pulmonary hypertension (Chan et al. 1987; Hall and Petch 1987) and may well therefore be effective in treating the pulmonary hypertension associated with systemic sclerosis. Nifedipine also may be effective.

Arrhythmias. These, too, are likely to be resistant to treatment. With the exception of beta blockers, conventional drugs may be used, viz: verapamil for atrial arrhythmias, and disopyramide, mexiletine, or phenytoin for ventricular arrhythmias. For paroxysmal ventricular tachycardia, intravenous procainamide or mexiletine may be used, but if the situation is urgent cardioversion is indicated.

Congestive Failure. Congestive or left ventricular failure should be treated conventionally with a diuretic, given intravenously in an emergency. Digoxin may be used in addition, particularly if there is atrial fibrillation with a rapid heart rate, but digoxin should be used with caution in renal failure or in the presence of any form of heart block.

Heart Block. No treatment is necessary with lower grades of block, but a patient with complete heart block should be paced.

References

Aitcheson CT, Tan EM (1982) Antinuclear antibodies. In: Panayi GS (ed) Scientific basis of rheumatology. Churchill Livingstone, Edinburgh, pp 107–111

Alarcon GS, Phillips RM, Wasner CK, Acton RT, Barger BO (1985) DR antigens in systemic sclerosis: lack of clinical correlations. Tissue Antigens 26: 156–158

Alexander EL, Firestein GS, Weiss JL et al. (1986) Reversible cold-induced abnormalities in myocardial perfusion and function in systemic sclerosis. Ann Intern Med 105: 661–668

Alpert MA, Goldberg SH, Singsen BH et al. (1983) Cardiovascular manifestations of mixed connective tissue disease in adults. Circulation 68: 1182–1193

ARA Subcommittee for Scleroderma Criteria (1980) Preliminary criteria for the classification of systemic sclerosis (scleroderma). Arthritis Rheum 23: 581–590

Atkinson AB, Robertson JIS (1979) Captopril in the treatment of clinical hypertension and cardiac failure. Lancet II: 836–839

Barr IM, Abramov A, Dreyfuss F, Yahini JH, Neufeld AN (1970) Progressive heart block in a case of scleroderma. Israel J Med Sci 6: 373–379

Bennett R, Bluestone R, Holt PJL, Bywaters EGL (1971) Survival in scleroderma. Ann Rheum Dis 30: 581–588

Black CM, Welsh KI, Maddison PJ, Jayson MIV, Bernstein RM (1984) HLA antigens, autoantibodies and clinical subsets in scleroderma. Br J Rheumatol 23: 267–271

Botstein GR, Leroy EC (1981) Primary heart disease in systemic sclerosis (scleroderma). Advances in clinical and pathological features, pathogenesis and new therapeutic approaches. Am Heart J 102: 913–919

Bulkley BH (1979) Progressive systemic sclerosis: cardiac involvement. Clin Rheum Dis 5: 131–149

Bulkley BH, Klacsmann PG, Hutchings GM (1978) Angina pectoris, myocardial infarction and sudden death with normal coronary arteries: a clinico-pathological study of 9 patients with progressive systemic sclerosis. Am Heart J 95: 563–569

Campbell PM, Leroy EC (1975) Pathogenesis of systemic sclerosis: a vascular hypothesis. Semin Arthritis Rheum 4: 351–368

Catoggio LJ, Bernstein RM, Black CM, Hughes GRV, Maddison PJ (1983) Serological markers in progressive systemic sclerosis: clinical correlations. Ann Rheum Dis 42: 23–27

Chan NS, McLay J, Kenmure ACF (1987) Reversibility of primary pulmonary hypertension during 6 years treatment with oral diazoxide. Br Heart J 57: 207–209

Clements PJ, Furst DE, Cabeen W, Tashkin D, Paulus HE, Roberts N (1981) The relationship of arrhythmias and conduction disturbances to other manifestations of cardiopulmonary disease in progressive systemic sclerosis (PSS). Am J Med 71: 38–46

Cozzi F, Tessier R, Glorioso S, Peserico A, Todesco S (1983) Electrocardiogram in P.S.S. Analysis of 73 cases. Acta Cardiol 38: 27–34

Cunningham PH, Andrews BS, Davis JS (1980) Immune complexes in progressive systemic sclerosis and mixed connective tissue disease. J Rheumatol 7: 301–308

D'Angelo WA, Fries JF, Masi AT, Shulman LE (1969) Pathologic observations in systemic sclerosis (scleroderma). A study of 58 autopsy cases and 58 matched controls. Am J Med 46: 428–440

Davies MJ (1984) Disorders of the conduction system. In: Ansell BM, Simkin PA (eds) The heart and rheumatic disease. Butterworths, London, pp 68–69

Dubois EL, Chandor S, Friou GJ, Bischel M (1971) Progressive systemic sclerosis and localised scleroderma (morphoea) with positive LE cell test and unusual systemic manifestations compatible with systemic lupus erythematosus. Medicine (Baltimore) 50: 199–222

Ellis WW, Baer AB, Robertson RM, Pincus T, Kronenberg MW (1986) Left ventricular dysfunction induced by cold exposure in patients with systemic sclerosis. Am J Med 80: 385–392

Emlen W (1979) Complete heart block in mixed connective tissue disease. Arthritis Rheum 22: 679–680

Evans DJ, Walport M, Cashman SJ (1987) Progressive systemic sclerosis: autoimmune arteriopathy. Lancet I: 480–482

Ferri C, Bernini L, Bongiorni MG et al. (1985) Non-invasive evaluation of cardiac dysrhythmias and their relationship with multisystemic symptoms in PSS patients. Arthritis Rheum 28: 1259–1266

Follansbee WP, Curtiss EI, Medsger TA et al. (1984) Physiologic abnormalities of cardiac function in progressive systemic sclerosis with diffuse scleroderma. N Engl J Med 310: 142–148

Fritzler MJ, Kinsella TD, Garbutt E (1980) The CREST syndrome: a distinct serological entity with anticentromere antibodies. Am J Med 69: 520–526

Gladman DD, Gordon DA, Urowitz MB, Levy HL (1976) Pericardial fluid analysis in scleroderma (systemic sclerosis). Am J Med 60: 1064–1068

Gladman DD, Keystone EC, Baron M, Lee P, Cane D, Mervert H (1981) Increased frequency of HLA–DR5 in scleroderma. Arthritis Rheum 24: 854–856

Gottdiener JS, Moutsopoulos HM, Decker JL (1979) Echocardiographic identification of cardiac abormalities in scleroderma and related disorders. Am J Med 66: 391–398

Gupta MP, Zoneraich S, Zeitlin W, Zoneraich O, D'Angelo W (1975) Scleroderma heart disease with slow flow velocity in coronary arteries. Chest 67: 116–119

Hall DR, Petch MC (1987) Reversibility of primary pulmonary hypertension during 6 years of treatment with diazoxide. Br Heart J 58: 420

Harper FE, Maricq HR, Turner RE, Lidman RW, Leroy EC (1982) A prospective study of Raynaud phenomenon and early connective tissue disease. Am J Med 72: 883–888

Hawkins SJ, Black CM, Hall ND, McGregor A, Ring EFJ, Maddison PJ (1986) Clinical and laboratory effects of nifedipine in Raynaud phenomenon. Rheumatol Int 6: 85–88

Herbert CM, Lindberg KA, Jayson MIV, Bailey AJ (1974) Biosynthesis and maturation of the skin collagen in scleroderma and effect of D-penicillamine. Lancet I: 187–192

James TN (1974) De Subitaneis Mortibus. VIII. Coronary arteries and conduction system in scleroderma heart disease. Circulation 50: 844–856

Jayson MIV (1984) Systemic sclerosis: a collagen or a microvascular disease? (Editorial). Br Med J; i: 1855–1857

Jones MB, Osterholm RK, Wilson RB, Martin FH, Commers RJ, Bachmeyer JD (1978) Fatal pulmonary hypertension and resolving immune complex glomerulonephritis in mixed connective tissue disease. Am J Med 65: 855–863

Kahan A, Devaux JY, Amor B et al. (1986a) Pharmacodynamic effects of dipyridamol on Thallium 201 myocardial perfusion in progressive systemic sclerosis with diffuse scleroderma. Ann Rheum Dis 45: 718–725

Kahan A, Devaux JY, Amor B et al. (1986b) Nifedipine and Thallium 201 myocardial perfusion in progressive systemic sclerosis. N Engl J Med 314: 1397–1402

Lam M, Ricanati ES, Khan MA, Kuschner I (1978) Reversal of severe renal failure in systemic sclerosis. Ann Intern Med 89: 642–643

Lefford F, Edwards JCW (1986) Nailfold capillary microscopy in connective tissue disease: a quantitative morphological analysis. Ann Rheum Dis 45: 741–749

Lev M, Landowne M, Matchar JC, Wagner JA (1966) Systemic scleroderma with complete heart block. Am Heart J 72: 13–24

Lopez-Ovejero JA, Saal SD, D'Angelo WA, Cheigh JS, Stenzel KH, Laragh JH (1979) Reversal of vascular and renal crises of scleroderma by oral angiotensin converting enzyme blockade. N Engl J Med 300: 1417–1419

Maricq HR, Spencer-Green G, Leroy EC (1976) Skin capillary abnormalities as indicators of organ involvement in scleroderma (systemic sclerosis), Raynaud's syndrome and dermatomyositis. Am J Med 61: 862–870

Martin MFR, Dowd PM, Ring EFJ, Cook ED, Dieppe PS, Kirby JDT (1981) Prostaglandin E1 infusions for vascular insufficiency in progressive systemic sclerosis. Ann Rheum Dis 40: 350–354

McCarty GA, Rice JR, Bembe ML, Barada FA (1983) Anticentromere antibody: clinical correlations and association with favorable prognosis in patients with scleroderma variants. Arthritis Rheum 26: 1–7

McWhorter JE IV, Leroy EC (1974) Pericardial disease in scleroderma (systemic sclerosis). Am J Med 57: 566–575

Medsger TA, Masi AT (1979) Epidemiology of progressive systemic sclerosis. Clin Rheum Dis 5: 15–25

Medsger TA, Masi AT, Rodnan GP, Benedek TG, Robinson H (1971) Survival with systemic sclerosis. Ann Intern Med 75: 369–376

Michet CJ, Hunder GG (1984) The pericardium in rheumatic diseases. In: Ansell BM, Simkin PA (eds) The heart and rheumatic disease. Butterworths, London, pp 14–15

Miller MH, Littlejohn GO, Davidson A, Jones B, Topliss DJ (1987) The clinical significance of the anticentromere antibody. Br J Rheumatol 26: 17–21

Muers M, Stokes W (1976) Treatment of scleroderma heart by D-penicillamine. Br Heart J 38: 864–867

Nasser WK, Mishkin ME, Rosenbaum D, Genovese PD (1968) Pericardial and myocardial disease in progressive systemic sclerosis. Am J Cardiol 22: 538–542

Norton WL, Nardo JM (1970) Vascular disease in progressive systemic sclerosis (scleroderma). Ann Intern Med 73: 317–324

Oetgen WJ, Mutter ML, Lawless OJ, Davia JE (1983) Cardiac abnormalities in mixed connective tissue disease. Chest 82: 185–188

Oram S, Stokes W (1961) The heart in scleroderma. Br Heart J 23: 243–259

Peters-Golden M, Wise RA, Hochberg MC, Stevens MB, Wigley FM (1984) Carbon monoxide diffusing capacity as predictor of outcome in systemic sclerosis. Am J Med 77: 1027–1034

Pisko E, Gallup K, Turner R et al. (1979) Cardiopulmonary manifestations of progressive systemic sclerosis. Arthritis Rheum 22: 518–523

Ridolfi RL, Bulkley BH, Hutchins GM (1976) The cardiac conduction system in progressive systemic sclerosis. Am J Med 61: 361–366

Roberts NK, Cabeen WR, Moss J, Clements PJ, Furst DE (1981) The prevalence of conduction defects and cardiac arrhythmias in progressive systemic sclerosis. Ann Intern Med 94: 38–40

Rodnan GP, Schreiner GP, Black RL (1957) Renal involvement in progressive systemic sclerosis (generalised scleroderma). Am J Med 23: 445–462

Rodnan GP, Myerowitz RL, Justh GO (1980) Morphologic changes in the digital arteries of patients with progressive systemic sclerosis (scleroderma) and Raynaud phenomenon. Medicine (Baltimore) 59: 393–408

Sackner MA, Heinz RA, Steinberg AJ (1966) The heart in scleroderma. Am J Cardiol 17: 542–559

Salerni R, Rodnan GP, Leon DF, Shaver JA (1977) Pulmonary hypertension in the CREST syndrome variant of progressive systemic sclerosis (scleroderma). Ann Intern Med 86: 394–399

Schneider PD, Wise RA, Hochberg MC, Wigley FM (1982) Serial pulmonary function in systemic sclerosis. Am J Med 73: 385–394

Sharp GC (1974) Mixed connective tissue disease. Bull Rheum Dis 25: 828–831

Sharp GC (1975) Mixed connective tissue disease – Overlap syndromes. Clin Rheum Dis 1: 561–572

Silver RM, Metcalf JM, Leroy EC (1986) Interstitial lung disease in scleroderma. Immune complexes in sera and broncho-alveolar lavage fluid. Arthritis Rheum 29: 525–531

Singh A, Singh TP, Saxena MB (1974) Ventricular tachycardia – an unusual presenting symptom of scleroderma. Br Heart J 36: 107–110

Singsen BH, Bernstein BH, Kornreich HK, King KK, Hanson V, Tan EM (1977) Mixed connective tissue disease in childhood. J Pediatr 90: 893–900

Smith JW, Clements PJ, Levisman J, Furst D, Ross M (1979) Echocardiographic features of progressive systemic sclerosis. Am J Med 66: 28–33

Steen VD, Owens GR, Fino GJ, Rodnan GP, Medsger TA (1985) Pulmonary involvement in systemic sclerosis (scleroderma). Arthritis Rheum 28: 759–767

Summerfield BJ (1975) Progressive systemic sclerosis with complete heart block. Br Heart J 37: 1308–1310

Tan EM, Rodnan GP, Garcia I, Moroi Y, Fritzler MJ, Peebles CA (1980) Diversity of antinuclear antibodies in progressive systemic sclerosis. Arthritis Rheum 23: 617–625

Thurm RH, Alexander JC (1984) Captopril in the treatment of scleroderma renal crisis. Arch Intern Med 144: 733–735

Traub YM, Shapiro AP, Rodnan GP et al. (1983) Hypertension and renal failure (scleroderma renal crisis) in progressive systemic sclerosis. Medicine (Baltimore) 62: 335–352

Trell E, Lindstrom C (1971) Pulmonary hypertension in systemic sclerosis. Ann Rheum Dis 30: 390–400

Uhl GS, Koppes GM (1979) Pericardial tamponade in systemic sclerosis (scleroderma). Br Heart J 42: 345–348

Ungerer RG, Tashkin DP, Furst D et al. (1983) Prevalence and clinical correlates of pulmonary arterial hypertension in progressive systemic sclerosis. Am J Med 75: 65–74

Wade G (1984) Pulmonary hypertension in rheumatic heart disease. In: Ansell BM, Simkin PA (eds) The heart and rheumatic disease. Butterworths, London, pp 151–185

Whitlow PL, Gilliam JN, Chubick A, Ziff M (1980) Myocarditis in mixed connective tissue disease. Arthritis Rheum 23: 808–815

Whitman HH, Case DB, Laragh JH et al. (1982) Variable response to oral angiotensin-converting enzyme blockade in hypertensive scleroderma patients. Arthritis Rheum 28: 241–248

Wood PHN (1977) The challenge of arthritis and rheumatism. British League against Rheumatism, London

Young RH, Mark GJ (1978) Pulmonary vascular changes in scleroderma. Am J Med 64: 998–1004

Yunus MB, Radford CM, Masi AT, Zimmerman TJ, Calabro JJ, Miller KA (1984) Aortic regurgitation in scleroderma. J Rheumatol 11: 384–386

Chapter 10

Miscellaneous Conditions

Giant Cell Arteritis and Polymyalgia Rheumatica

These two conditions are now seen as being different manifestations of the same disease process. The difference between them is mainly one of degree (Hamrin 1972). Giant cell arteritis is the more severe, presenting with arteritis which is usually clinically obvious, while polymyalgia is essentially a symptom complex in which evidence of arteritis is found in a minority. The difference between them is somewhat artificial, as the two conditions may overlap. Their cause is unknown but the basis for each appears to be an arteritis of an autoimmune nature developing in older adults.

In giant cell arteritis there is occasional involvement of the aorta, main arteries and heart.

Giant Cell Arteritis (GCA)

Giant cell arteritis (GCA, temporal arteritis, cranial arteritis) presents most often as temporal arteritis; the combination of tender, thickened and inflamed temporal arteries with systemic illness and rheumatic symptoms is characteristic. Other cranial arteries may be affected instead of, or as well as, the temporals, the most serious being involvement of the retinal arteries causing blindness. Systemic symptoms can be severe; they include temporal headache. fever, malaise and weight loss and the symptom complex of polymyalgia in two-thirds of cases (Healey and Wilske 1978; Olhagen 1986).

Investigations show a normochromic anaemia, elevated ESR and C-reactive protein, increased serum globulin and abnormal liver function tests. Temporal artery biopsy clinches the diagnosis, and may prove positive even if taken from an apparently normal section of artery. But biopsy should be carried out before corticosteroid therapy is started, as the histology returns to normal within a matter of days. The rate of positive biopsy in GCA was 68% before treatment, falling to 10% one week after starting treatment (Allison and Gallagher 1984).

Polymyalgia Rheumatica (PMR)

In a multicentre review of 236 patients with PMR Bird and colleagues (1979) found that the seven most characteristic features of the disorder were as listed in Table 10.1. They proposed that the diagnosis of "probable PMR" should be based on the presence of any three of the seven features, or on any one in combination with clinical or biopsy evidence of temporal arteritis. A positive biopsy is found in about 20% of patients with PMR (Healey 1984). Some patients also develop synovitis in one or more joints, most often the shoulder or knee; this subsides promptly with the start of corticosteroid treatment and there is no lasting joint damage.

Table 10.1. Polymyalgia rheumatica: clinical features, listed in diminishing order of their discriminatory value in diagnosis. From Bird et al. (1979)

1. Bilateral shoulder pain or stiffness
2. Evolution from onset to peak of symptoms within 2 weeks
3. Initial ESR over 40 mm/h
4. Patient's age over 65 years
5. Depression or weight loss
6. Bilateral tenderness in upper arms
7. Morning stiffness over 1 hour

A striking feature of PMR is the rapid disappearance of all symptoms within a day or two of starting corticosteroids.

Aetiology

GCA and PMR mainly affect patients over 60 years of age and are rarely seen under the age of 50. Women are affected twice or three times as often as men. The disease is mainly seen in Caucasians, and is rare in Orientals. A family history has been observed (Liang et al. 1974).

The incidence of the disease (GCA and PMR being considered together) has been estimated in Sweden as 9.3/100 000 population per annum, or 16.8/100 000 per annum among adults over 50 years of age (Bengtsson and Malmvall 1981). A similar figure for patients aged over 50 was found by Huston et al. (1978), namely 17.4/100 000.

GCA and PMR are essentially benign conditions and run a self-limiting course. The majority are able to withdraw corticosteroid treatment within 4–5 years, and a few within one year, although relapses occur (Ayoub et al. 1985; Healey 1984).

Pathology

The most significant finding is the inflammatory process in the wall of affected arteries, with infiltration by lymphocytes and plasma cells, a patchy destruction of muscle cells, and swelling of the media with an inflammatory exudate. The internal elastic lamina is fragmented and it is here that histiocytes and giant cells are mainly seen (Figs. 10.1, 10.2). The intima is thickened and swollen without much cellular infiltration. As a result the arterial lumen is greatly narrowed, sometimes to the point of obliteration, or is filled with thrombus. In the adventitia there is also a cellular infiltrate with mononuclear cells and polymorphs, but it is less intensely affected than the media.

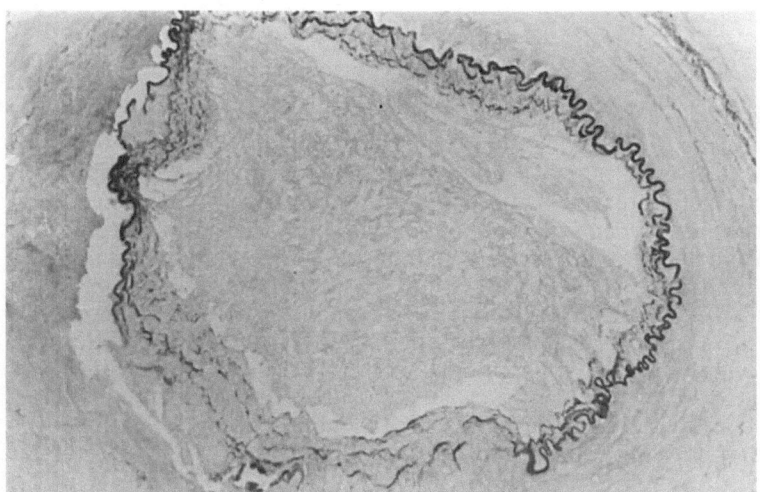

Fig. 10.1. Giant cell arteritis. Cross-section of temporal artery stained to show fragmentation of internal elastic lamina. The lumen is filled with thrombus. (Elastin stain × 40.)

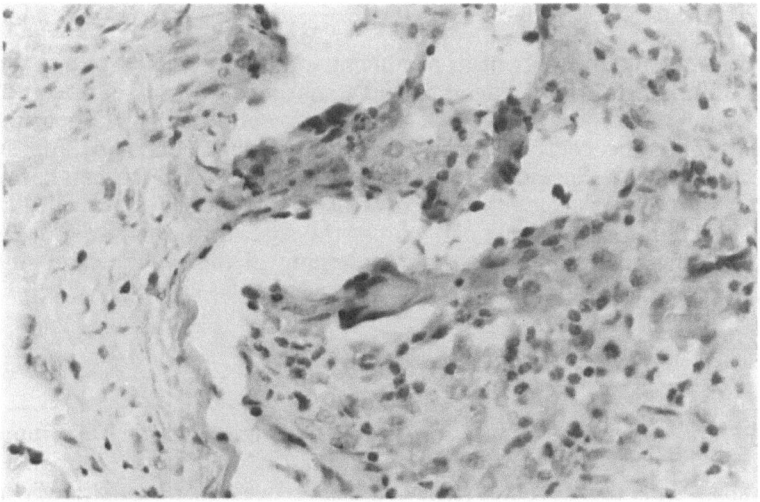

Fig. 10.2. Giant cell arteritis. Enlargement of an area of fragmented elastic lamina from the previous figure, showing giant cells (× 160).

These pathological changes are irregularly distributed in smaller arteries such as the temporal, retinal, occipital and other branches of the external carotid, with occasional involvement of bigger arteries or even the aorta. These are all arteries with a significant component of elastic tissue in their walls. In the cases in which the aorta is affected, weakening of the media leads to sufficient stretching of the aortic valve ring for aortic incompetence to occur, and rupture with dissection of the aortic wall has resulted on occasion.

Immunology

An immunological cause for GCA/PMR is highly likely in view of the nature of the arteritis. Deposits of immunoglobulin and complement have been found in the region of the arterial elastic lamina, suggesting a possible autoimmune reaction directed against elastic tissue (Park and Hazleman 1978). Circulating immune complexes have been found in patients with active arteritis, but there is no close correlation between the levels of circulating complexes and the severity of the systemic illness (Park et al. 1981; Smith et al. 1987).

Patients with GCA/PMR have an increased frequency of the histocompatibility antigens DR4 and, to a lesser extent CW6. There is little difference between the antigens carried by patients with GCA and those with PMR (Armstrong et al. 1983).

There is thus considerable evidence pointing to an immunological basis for the disease, but the underlying cause remains unknown.

Cardiovascular Lesions

Aortitis

Giant cell arteritis may involve the aorta, producing inflammatory changes in the wall of the ascending aorta, the aortic arch and sometimes beyond. It does not usually cause pain. Unlike the aortitis of ankylosing spondylitis, it does not spread proximally into the central fibrous body of the heart (Fig. 8.6) and so does not cause heart block. Serious results are uncommon, but GCA can cause the aortic arch syndrome, in which there is obstruction to the main branches of the aorta at their origin, or the weakened wall of the ascending aorta may split, producing a dissecting aneurysm, or simple stretching of the aortic valve ring may cause aortic valve incompetence.

Aortic Arch Syndrome

In a series of 248 histologically proven cases of GCA Klein et al. (1975) found signs of aortic involvement that they classed as "definite" in 23 and "probable" in 11. The physical signs of arterial obstruction were of vascular insufficiency or claudication in the arms or legs, or the presence of an arterial bruit, supported by the evidence of aortograms or arteriograms. If only their definite cases are accepted, this gives an incidence of nearly 10% of aortitis with signs of the aortic arch syndrome in GCA. Three of the affected patients, all over 65 years of age, died as a result of dissection of the proximal aorta after a history of up to 6 years of GCA treated by corticosteroids. Patients who developed aortitis had no particular clinical features distinguishing them from the remainder of the patients with GCA.

The pathology and extent of aortitis in GCA was recorded by Ostberg (1971). Among over one thousand autopsies performed in the course of a year aortitis was found in 12 and in 6 of these there were pathological changes throughout the whole aorta involving the origins of the subclavian, carotid and iliac arteries.

Other accounts of the aortic arch syndrome in GCA were given by Hamrin (1972) and Perruquet et al. (1986).

Dissecting Aneurysm

Among reported series of patients with dissecting aortic aneurysm a few were noted to be due to GCA. Harris (1968) found two examples in a series of 77; one had been under treatment with corticosteroids for temporal arteritis, but in the other the pathology was only recognised at autopsy. Similarly Leonard and Hasleton (1979) found two cases in a series of 171, one of whom had had a positive temporal artery biopsy 14 months before death. A combination of these figures indicates that 2% of dissecting aneurysms may be due to GCA and that this is sometimes unrecognised in life.

Another report (Salisbury and Hazleman 1981) describes successful surgical treatment for aortic dissection in a woman aged 72 years with known GCA and hypertension, who had been under corticosteroid treatment. The resected portion of ascending aorta showed the histological changes of giant cell arteritis.

Aortic Incompetence

Aortic incompetence developed in 3 of a series of 35 patients being treated and followed up with GCA (Fauchald et al. 1972). The degree of aortic regurgitation was not severe, but one of the three, and one other among the 35 died subsequently as a result of aortic dissection. How and Strachan (1978) also report a case of aortic incompetence developing in a normotensive woman who had been under treatment for GCA for 2 years.

It appears that aortic incompetence in this condition is not in itself a serious problem, but the pathological change in the aortic wall is a potential threat to life through aortic dissection which is not necessarily prevented by corticosteroid treatment.

Coronary Arteritis

Cornonary arteritis was a cause of fatal myocardial infarction in one patient with known temporal arteritis (Martin et al. 1980) and in another among the series of

25 cases of GCA reported by Hamilton et al. (1971). In each case the arteritis was in the coronary artery wall itself and was not an extension of aortitis.

Diagnosis

Giant cell arteritis can usually be recognised without difficulty on the basis of the local signs of temporal arteritis, symptoms such as scalp tenderness, bitemporal headache, claudication of the temporal muscles on chewing, the patient's age and the combination of rheumatic and systemic symptoms. If arteritis seems likely a temporal artery biopsy should be made, even if the artery feels normal. A fairly generous strip of artery should be removed, e.g. 4 or 5 cm (Hall et al. 1983). As well as giving the diagnosis, temporal artery biopsy usually relieves local pain and tenderness.

Clinical examination should include palpation of peripheral pulses, seeking any suggestion of pulse deficit, and cardiac auscultation for possible aortic incompetence. Chest X-ray and echocardiography are advisable if aortitis is a possibility.

Polymyalgia rheumatica can be recognised clinically by the constitutional symptoms and the severity of the morning stiffness, mainly affecting the shoulder and hip girdle muscles in an older adult patient. The early stages of rheumatoid arthritis may be very similar to PMR, and a period of observation while giving symptomatic treatment may be necessary until the diagnosis is clarified. Similarly, systemic lupus may present in an older person with symptoms very like PMR (Hutton and Maddison 1986).

In suspected cases of PMR it is common practice to make a therapeutic trial with prednisone 10 mg daily. Prompt remission of symptoms within 48 hours is then accepted as confirming the diagnosis. However, it must be borne in mind that this is not a true diagnostic test, and if there is a possibility of another diagnosis such as rheumatoid arthritis or SLE it is safer to treat symptomatically with non-steroid drugs for the time being and arrange for a temporal artery biopsy.

Treatment

The risk of possible future retinal artery involvement and blindness requires that giant cell arteritis should be treated with corticosteroid. An initial dose of 30–60 mg prednisone daily is advisable with gradual reduction subsequently according to the response. It is usually necessary for corticosteroid to be continued for 4–5 years keeping the dose as low as possible, e.g. 5–10 mg daily, to avoid complications; in some patients it is possible to withdraw corticosteroids within 1–2 years.

Polymyalgia rheumatica can as a rule be treated successfully with a dose of not more than 10 mg prednisone daily, reducing gradually when possible. However, it is usually necessary to continue prednisone for 1–2 years or more. Some clinicians give non-steroidal anti-inflammatory drugs also as "steroid sparers" or even as substitutes for corticosteroids, but at any sign of relapse or of new signs suggesting arteritis, corticosteroid treatment becomes necessary, or the dose should be increased until the polymyalgia is under control.

Polyarteritis Nodosa

Polyarteritis nodosa is a multi-system disease in which a necrotising arteritis affects medium-sized and small arteries in any part or system of the body. Among its manifestations are musculoskeletal symptoms, polyarteritis and lesions of the heart.

Aetiology

Polyarteritis nodosa mainly affects young or middle-aged adults and is seen in men more than women in a ratio of about 3:1. Its cause is not known, but in common with other vasculitides, circulating immune complexes probably have a significant role. In 25% to 40% of cases the hepatitis B surface antigen (HBsAg or Australia antigen) is present and has been identified in immune complexes. Deposition of complexes on vascular endothelium, and combination with complement is the probable initiating event in the development of a local arteritic lesion (Duffy et al. 1976; Sergent et al. 1976; Trepo et al. 1972).

Pathology

In affected vessels, all coats are infiltrated with inflammatory cells, mainly polymorphs, and there is fibrinoid necrosis in the media (Figs. 10.3, 10.4). Swelling of the vessel wall may reduce the lumen, which is sometimes occluded by thrombosis. Alternatively, focal stretching of the wall may lead to aneurysm formation, sometimes with rupture. The lesions heal in due course, leaving the affected vessels distorted, narrowed or occluded.

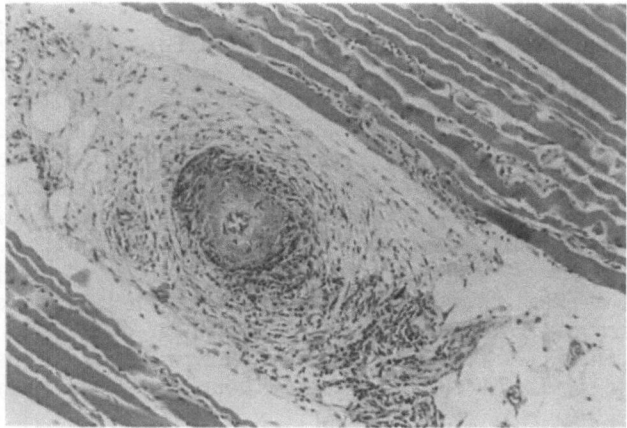

Fig. 10.3. Polyarteritis nodosa. Cross-section of small artery in voluntary muscle showing necrotising vasculitis, with inflammatory exudate spreading from the vessel wall into the adventitia (× 30).

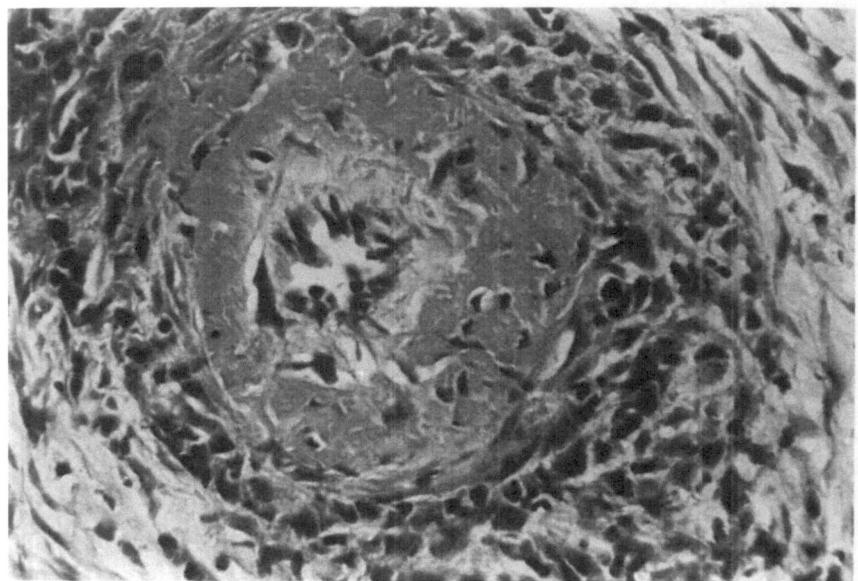

Fig. 10.4. Polyarteritis nodosa. High-power view of the artery seen in the previous figure, showing the fibrinoid necrosis in the vessel wall and the cellular infiltrate consisting of polymorphs, lymphoid cells and macrophages (× 180).

Clinical Features

Systemic symptoms often develop acutely, with fever, tachycardia, weight loss and prostration. There is a polymorph leucocytosis, and about one-third of patients have eosinophilia, especially if there are pulmonary lesions. The systems most often involved are, in descending order, musculoskeletal, neurological, renal, pulmonary and cardiac (Fan et al. 1980). There is striking tenderness, aching and weakness of muscles, and there may be arthralgia or frank polyarteritis. Polyneuritis and mononeuritis multiplex result from vasculitis of the vasa nervorum. In about two-thirds of patients vascular lesions in the kidneys lead to renal functional impairment and hypertension, and death may be due to renal failure. Abdominal pain is common, with liver damage, pancreatitis or cholecystitis and infarction of viscera. Case History 10.1 illustrates many of these features, and unsuspected pericarditis was found at autopsy.

The heart may be affected as a secondary result of hypertension of renal origin, but it may also be affected directly by coronary arteritis, presenting as angina or as cardiac infarction (Ettlinger et al. 1979; Holsinger et al. 1962; Parrillo and Fauci 1984). There may be pericarditis. Involvement of the vessels supplying the AV node and conducting system may cause heart block (Thiene et al. 1978).

The peripheral circulation may also be affected, producing symptoms such as Raynaud's phenomenon, claudication, and sometimes gangrene in the lower limb.

Diagnosis

Diagnosis is made on the evidence of a multisystem disease with fever and leucocytosis. Proof of arteritis may be sought on biopsy of muscle, liver or kidney as appropriate. An arteriogram may be more informative than a biopsy, particularly for visceral lesions, and may reveal arterial narrowing, distortion, aneurysm or occlusion (Travers et al. 1979).

Treatment

Treatment with high dose corticosteroid should start without delay as soon as the diagnosis is made, e.g. prednisone 60–100 mg daily. The addition of immunosuppressive drugs such as cyclophosphamide or azathioprine have been shown to improve the outcome. Leib et al. (1979) achieved a 5-year survival rate of 80% with combined corticosteroid and immunosuppressive therapy, compared with 53% with corticosteroids alone. The prognosis is determined particularly by the degree of renal damage, and by polyneuritis (Sack et al. 1975).

Case History 10.1
Polyarteritis nodosa
Polyneuritis
Renal failure

Mrs. D.B., Housewife, born 1910

1965	Mild osteoarthritis knees and toes
1978	Onset of weakness in legs and numbness in feet
January	Mild synovitis in hands, wrists and knees
March	Sensory polyneuritis advancing in legs and starting in hands
	Mononeuritis with R foot-drop
	WBC 21 000 (N 90%) Hb 10.1
April	Abnormal liver function tests
	Liver biopsy: small granulomas
	Started ACTH with some benefit
July	Renal function impaired
	Renal biopsy: polyarteritis
August	Deteriorating
September	Died in renal failure
Autopsy	Kidneys small with adherent capsules
	Vessels show necrotising polyarteritis
	Heart: signs of old pericarditis
Comment	Rapid progression of the disease over 8 months, presenting with polyneuritis and dying in renal failure. The pericarditis was an unexpected autopsy finding

---

Takayasu's Disease

Takayasu's disease (pulseless disease) is a rare disorder of unknown cause in which there is aortitis and an arteritis of major branches of the aorta, liable to progress to arterial obstruction (Marquis et al. 1968). Unlike giant cell arteritis, it affects younger adults, including Orientals and blacks; it is commoner in women.

Clinical Features

Takayasu's disease presents as a systemic illness, initially resembling rheumatic fever, with a high incidence of arthralgia or frank synovitis (Schrire and Asherson 1964; Strachan 1964). In the 32 cases described by Hall et al. (1985) 26 were women, 18 suffered joint pain, 14 were febrile and many lost weight. After a course of weeks or months signs of arterial obstruction develop, with arterial bruits and reduction in or disappearance of pulsation in major arteries such as the femorals, brachials or carotids.

The distribution of the aortitis and arteritis is variable, but there are two main patterns. In one the aortic arch and its branches are involved, and in the other the disease affects the lower aorta and its branches, including the renal and iliac arteries. The latter is the more serious pattern as it may prove fatal through renal failure or malignant hypertension (Danaraj et al. 1963; Fraga et al. 1972). Other serious consequences include major reduction in cerebral blood flow, sometimes with hemiparesis, and blindness, which led to the original description by Takayasu in 1908. Vision is lost through obstruction to the internal carotids, and not the retinal arteries, as in giant cell arteritis.

The heart may be involved as a result of hypertension and also, more directly, by pericarditis in the early stages of the illness. Aortic valve incompetence may develop as part of the aortic arch syndrome due to dilatation of the aortic valve ring and proximal aorta.

Case History 10.2 and Fig. 10.5 describe a patient with the aortic arch syndrome. Among other lesions she had an obstruction to the subclavian artery at its origin from the aorta. This was compensated for by secondary filling of the subclavian artery via the vertebral artery ("subclavian steal") which contributed to the impairment of cerebral blood flow and cerebral atrophy.

Pathology

Inflammatory changes in the aortic or arterial walls may be focal or diffuse. There is round cell infiltration of the media and adventitia with disruption of the elastic fibres in the media and the internal elastic lamina, where occasional giant cells may be seen in a picture resembling giant cell arteritis. The intima becomes thickened and sclerosed, obstructing the lumen; calcification may follow in the later stages (Schrire and Asherson 1964). While the disease is active blood changes include anaemia, raised ESR, increased immunoglobulin and occasionally antinuclear antibodies.

Management

An aortogram or arteriogram is necessary to determine the extent of the disease. Echocardiography is valuable in assessing and following changes in aortic diameter, and Doppler studies of the blood flow in main arteries are helpful in monitoring progress and the response to treatment. While the disease is active, corticosteroids in relatively high doses are indicated, e.g. prednisone 40–60 mg daily, reducing to a lower maintenance dose as the disease responds and deficient pulses improve. Hypertension requires treatment, probably with an angiotensin-converting enzyme inhibitor, i.e. captopril or enalapril, combined if necessary with other anti-hypertensive drugs such as beta blockers, hydralazine or diuretics. Residual arterial obstructive lesions which have not responded to corticosteroid treatment may require restoration by vascular surgery. In the series of Hall et al. (1985) 3 patients ultimately needed resection of aortic aneurysms and one needed an aortic valve replacement for valvular incompetence.

Case History 10.2
Takayasu's Disease
Aortic arch syndrome
Aortic valve incompetence

Ms. J.J., Factory hand, born 1922

1953	Presented with fever, ESR 100, Aortic incompetence 2 year history of limb and back pain BP: R arm 210/80, L arm 140/90 Infective endocarditis excluded
1967	Returned with headache and dyspnoea ESR 85 BP: still reduced in L arm *Aortogram*: dilated aortic arch Narrowed origin L subclavian artery Localised narrowing lower aorta
1978	Depression and mild dementia Aortic incompetence. ESR 115 BP: R arm 220/70, L arm 150/115 ECG: LV hypertrophy, PR 0.24 s *Repeat aortogram*: Widening of proximal aorta Occlusion of origin of L subclavian A (Fig. 10.5) Reversal of flow in left vertebral artery *Brain scan*: cerebral atrophy
Comment	Probable aortitis in 1953: ? still active Progressive occlusion of the origin of the L subclavian artery led to "subclavian steal" via vertebral artery possibly contributing to cerebral atrophy

With acknowledgement to Dr. Graham Wakefield

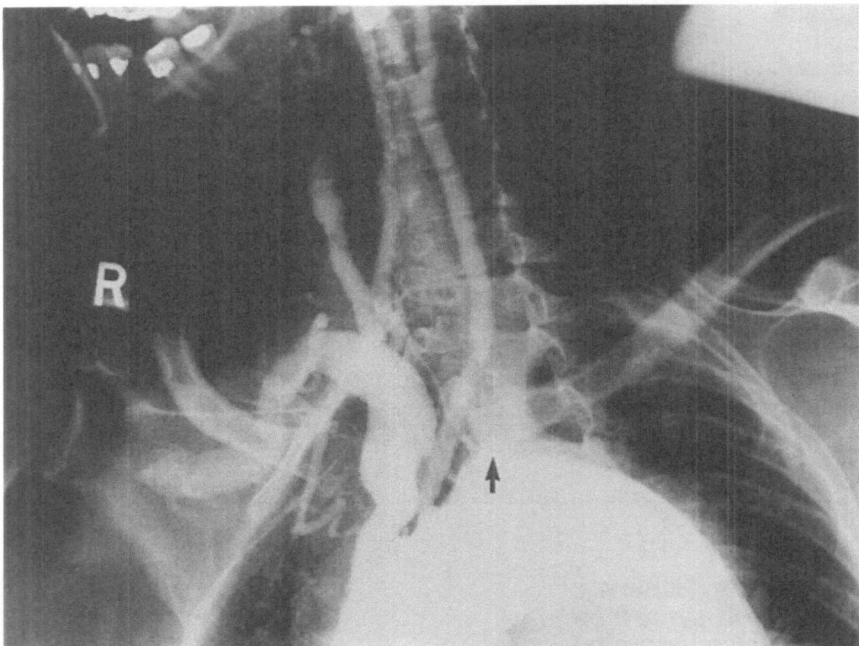

Fig. 10.5. Arch aortogram of the patient with Takayasu's disease in Case History 10.2. The left subclavian artery is obstructed near its origin from the aorta (*arrow*). There is also widening and irregularity of the innominate artery and the carotids.

Polymyositis and Dermatomyositis

Polymyositis

Polymyositis is an inflammatory disease of muscle, of unknown cause; it runs a progressive course over a period of weeks or months, and occurs in patients of all age groups with a female to male ratio of 2:1. It causes weakness and wasting of proximal limb muscles at first, later spreading to spinal and trunk muscles; it may affect swallowing and the muscles of respiration. Heart muscle is frequently affected as well as skeletal muscle, mainly in the chronic rather than the acute forms of the disease.

Dermatomyositis

In dermatomyositis, polymyositis is combined with skin lesions; typical findings are a lilac discoloration of the eyelids with oedema, and erythema with scaling and patchy dermal atrophy on the limbs and upper trunk. Children with the condition may also have a digital vasculitis, and subsequent widespread calcinosis.

Some 20% of adult patients are found to have malignant disease, with the poly.nyositis usually appearing in advance and receding, at least for a time, if the malignant disease is successfully treated.

In the "overlap" conditions polymyositis occurs in combination with manifestations of connective tissue diseases, usually with features of systemic lupus and of systemic sclerosis as in mixed connective tissue disease (Chap. 7, p. 140 and Chap. 9, p. 195).

Characteristic abnormalities are found on electromyography: fibrillation, polyphasic action potentials and repetitive high frequency discharges.

Table 10.2 shows a classification of the various clinical patterns which polymyositis may take.

Table 10.2. Clinical patterns of polymyositis. From Bohan et al. (1977)

I	Primary polymyositis
II	Primary dermatomyositis
III	Myositis associated with malignancy
IV	Childhood polymyositis/dermatomyositis
V	Myositis associated with connective tissue diseases e.g. MCTD

Immunopathology

The fundamental cause of polymyositis is not known, but the serological findings clearly indicate an autoimmune basis. A number of antibodies have been identified in the sera of polymyositis patients, in particular antibodies against nRNP, against the antigens La and Sm and, less often, antinuclear antibodies. However, a significant frequency has now been reported of antibody to the soluble ribosomal nucleoprotein antigen Ro. Behan et al. (1987) have found this antibody to be present in 60% of a series of 33 patients with polymyositis, and more frequently still (69%) in those patients who had cardiac involvement. The antigen Ro has already been shown to be associated with cardiac damage and heart block in neonatal SLE, and it is suggested that it is a marker specifically identified with damage to myocardium and conducting tissue.

The pathological changes in skeletal muscle are of necrosis of muscle fibres associated with perivascular collections of lymphocytes and plasma cells. In some areas necrosis is followed by atrophy and in others by regeneration. Muscle necrosis causes the release of muscle enzymes into the serum, particularly creatine phosphokinase and glutamic oxalic transaminase. The finding of the creatine phosphokinase MB isoenzyme in the serum is an indicator of myocardial damage (Strongwater et al. 1983).

In the myocardium the pathological changes are similar to those in skeletal muscle: there is a diffuse interstitial and perivascular infiltration with mononuclear cells and an irregular replacement of necrotic myocardial cells by fibrous tissue. These changes have been found on endomyocardial biopsy as well as at autopsy (Behan et al. 1986; Denbow et al. 1979; Weiss et al. 1982).

Atrial as well as ventricular myocardium is affected, also nodal and conducting tissue, associated with heart block (Lynch 1971). Pericarditis too has been reported and in one case appeared to result in subsequent constriction (R. Tamir, I. A. Pick and E. Theodor, personal communication).

The Heart

The heart is now known to be affected in some 70% of patients with polymyositis and the conducting system is involved in one-third of these (Askari and Huettner 1982). The commonest clinical effects are of arrhythmias, conduction disturbances and cardiac failure (Denbow et al. 1979; Sharratt et al. 1977; Stern et al. 1984). The electrocardiogram may show various arrhythmias, forms of heart block, or changes in the ST–T segment indicating myocardial damage (Table 10.3). Myocarditis may cause congestive failure and this, or heart block, may be the cause of death.

Table 10.3.   ECG findings in polymyositis. From Sharratt et al. (1977)

Arrhythmias	Atrial fibrillation
	Atrial paroxysmal tachycardia
	Ventricular paroxysmal tachycardia
Conduction defects	Bundle branch block
	Complete heart block
Ventricular dysfunction	ST depression
	T flattening or inversion

Treatment

Polymyositis is usually treated with corticosteroids in large doses e.g. prednisone 60 mg daily. An alternate-day regime may be used to reduce steroid side-effects. However, the benefits are uncertain (Bohan and Peter 1975). Immunosuppressive drugs have also been given, e.g. azathioprine, cyclophosphamide or methotrexate, with apparent benefit. For heart failure diuretics are needed, but digoxin should be used with caution in view of the risk of promoting arrhythmias. Complete heart block has been successfully treated with permanent pacing (Reid and Murdoch 1979).

Behçet's Syndrome

The Syndrome

As originally described by Behçet in 1937 the syndrome consisted of a triad of persistent mouth ulceration, genital ulceration and relapsing iritis. Since then it has been proposed that skin lesions should be accepted as an additional major manifestation of the syndrome and a number of other, minor manifestations have also been designated (Mason and Barnes 1969). These include gastrointestinal lesions, thrombophlebitis, cardiovascular lesions, arthritis, neurological lesions and a positive family history (Chajek and Fainaru 1975; Wright and Chamberlain 1978). As there is no single criterion for identifying Behçet's syndrome, diagnosis is at present an empirical matter based on the presence of three major criteria or two major with two minor criteria for "definite" cases.

Behçet's syndrome has been proposed as a member of the group of spondylarthropathies, but it has only a limited number of features in common with other conditions in the group (Chap. 8). Polyarthritis is commonly seen, mainly affecting knees and ankles, and less often the upper limb joints. It is a relatively mild arthritis, non-erosive and not progressive. Sacro-iliitis is infrequent and mild, and spondylitis is rare: in a group of 11 patients with the syndrome, three had spondylitis, of whom two were B27-positive (Dubost et al. 1985). There is an increasing incidence of two histocompatibility antigens, HLA–B27 being found in 25%, and HLA–B5 being somewhat increased in male patients (Wright and Chamberlain 1978).

The cause of Behçet's syndrome is unknown. Some studies have suggested the presence of a virus in lympho-reticular cells, but none has been definitely identified. Circulating immune complexes have been found in patients with the syndrome and there is evidence for an underlying vasculitis in the ulcerative and synovial lesions which could be the result of deposition of complexes.

Cardiovascular Lesions

Thrombophlebitis is a feature of the syndrome, in peripheral veins or in the venae cavae, which may be partially or totally occluded with thrombus (Kansu et al. 1972; Roguin et al. 1978; Shimizu et al. 1979). Probably these thromboses are initiated by a localised vasculitis in the vessel wall and are an integral part of the syndrome.

The heart is not often affected, but there are reports of pericarditis and of myocarditis. Pericardial effusion has been found during an active febrile phase of the syndrome, responding promptly to indomethacin (Scarlett et al. 1979). Myocarditis has been observed, causing cardiac enlargement and congestive failure with gallop rhythm and tachycardia. Higashihara et al. (1982) and Lewis (1964) have both recorded such cases; there may be accompanying ECG changes, with the appearance of Q waves and T inversions and atrial fibrillation. Both of the reported cases recovered after conventional treatment for congestive heart failure.

Aortic valve incompetence has been reported, developing rapidly 18 months after the onset of Behçet's syndrome in a woman aged 31 years. She had become urgently breathless as a result of gross aortic regurgitation. Surgical valve replacement was necessary after which she did well; it was found that a large deficit, or fenestration, had developed in one cusp, causing the sudden deterioration. There was a small aneurysmal dilatation of one of the sinuses of Valsalva and she also had first degree heart block (Comess et al. 1983).

Relapsing Polychondritis

Description

Relapsing polychondritis is a rare disease in which locally destructive inflammation develops in cartilage at various sites. The cartilage most often affected is in the external ear, the nose, larynx, trachea, bronchi and costo-chondral junctions. Connective tissue may also be involved in the sclera of the eye, joint synovium, the aortic wall and the heart valves. The disease runs an episodic and unpredictable course. It is potentially fatal in its effects on the lung and the aorta, and lesions in the ear and eye may threaten hearing and sight (Arkin and Masi 1975; Dolan et al. 1966).

Pathology

The underlying pathology appears to be a cell-mediated immunological reaction against the mucopolysaccharide content of cartilage, the sclera and the aorta (Rajapakse and Bywaters 1974). The inflammatory process tends to run a self-limiting course at each site, giving rise to local pain and swelling and finally healing by fibrosis. It produces characteristic deformities such as saddle nose and cauliflower ear.

Heart and Aorta

Lesions in the aorta may cause aneurysmal dilatation and lead to dissection or rupture (Hainer and Hamilton 1969). Lesser degrees of dilatation in the proximal aorta and aortic valve ring can cause aortic valve incompetence (Owen et al. 1970). Direct involvement of the valve cusps themselves may lead to aortic or mitral incompetence requiring surgical valve replacement. Arteritis, phlebitis and pericarditis have also been found. McAdam et al. (1976) described 23 cases and reviewed a further 136 in the literature. In the combined total of 159 cases there were 9 examples of aortic incompetence (6%) and an equal number of instances of arteritis and of aneurysm of a major artery; there were 5 examples each (3%) of mitral incompetence, intracranial arteritis and phlebitis.

Treatment

Corticosteroids promptly suppress the inflammatory process and arrest tissue damage, bringing the disease under control. Immunosuppressive drugs may also be used, either alone or in combination with corticosteroids. In remission drug treatment can be withdrawn, but relapses are characteristic, requiring re-commencement of treatment.

Inherited Disorders of Connective Tissue

The inherited connective tissue disorders are known to be associated with abnormalities in the structure, synthesis and metabolism of collagen (Beighton 1972; Jiminez and Lally 1979). A clinical feature of some of these disorders is increased joint laxity or hypermobility which frequently are the cause of musculoskeletal symptoms. They are also associated with certain cardiovascular abnormalities, notably faults in the aortic and mitral valves, and of the aorta and the main pulmonary artery. Mitral valve prolapse is a common finding. If surgical valve replacement is required, the fragile nature of connective tissue in the great vessels and the valve rings presents a problem to the surgeon.

Some examples of the major cardiovascular abnormalities in these conditions are as follows.

Marfan's syndrome: aneurysmal dilatation of the aorta or of the main pulmonary artery, atrial or ventricular septal defects, coarctation of aorta, patent ductus arteriosus, mitral valve prolapse (Brown et al. 1975; McKusick 1974; Pyeritz and Wappel 1983).

Ehlers–Danlos syndrome: aneurysms of the sinuses of Valsalva or of the aorta, aortic valve incompetence, aortic dissection (Beighton et al. 1969; Cupo et al. 1981; Edmondson et al. 1979).

Osteogenesis imperfecta: stretching of the aortic or mitral valve rings with valvular incompetence (Criscitiello et al. 1965; Stein and Kloster 1977; Weisinger et al. 1975; White et al. 1983).

A variant of the Marfan syndrome is the "Marfanoid hypermobility syndrome", in which the patient has the characteristic lanky bodily habitus of Marfan's syndrome with hyperextensile skin and hypermobile joints, but without the gross deformities of the thorax and spine of the full Marfan's syndrome. Cardiovascular abnormalities include mitral valve prolapse and aortic coarctation or aneurysm (Cotton and Brandt 1976; Daneshwar et al. 1979; Walker et al. 1969).

The Hypermobility Syndrome and Mitral Valve Prolapse

The Hypermobility Syndrome

The hypermobility syndrome was originally described by Kirk et al. (1967), who proposed the name. It consists of a definable degree of hyperextensibility of limb joints and spine which give rise, over the course of time, to musculoskeletal symptoms and arthralgia, but not necessarily to a frank arthritis or osteo-arthritis. There is some evidence, however, that the syndrome may be a predisposing factor in the later development of osteoarthritis (Scott et al. 1979).

The syndrome of joint hypermobility, or increased joint laxity, exists in various degrees which can be graded (Bird et al. 1979). These grades form a spectrum which ranges from normal individuals who are unusually mobile, perhaps with a familial trait, to examples of the major connective tissue disorders. Comparison of hypermobile subjects with normal controls shows that those with the higher grades of hypermobility have an increased incidence of mitral valve prolapse (Grahame et al. 1981). An increased aortic wall compliance, measured by a Doppler technique, has been found in such patients as well as mitral valve prolapse and an abnormality of collagen studied by skin biopsy (Child 1986; Handler et al. 1985).

Mitral Valve Prolapse

Mitral valve prolapse has been described under a variety of names, beginning with the "billowing leaflet" of Barlow et al. (1963) and including floppy mitral valve, balloon cusp, parachute valve, myxomatous degeneration of valve or "the syndrome of mid-systolic click with late systolic murmur".

The pathological basis is a myxomatous change in the spongiosa layer with a weakening of the central fibrous layer, affecting the posterior rather than the anterior mitral cusp (Rippe et al. 1980b). This, with elongation of the chordae, allows the cusp, or part of it, to billow back into the left atrium during systole (Davies et al. 1978; Hammer et al. 1979). Regurgitation at the valve is usually slight, but accounts for the systolic murmur. In some cases there is a family history of a similar inherited defect (Rizzon et al. 1973; Strahan et al. 1983) and, in a few, similar "floppy" changes in the aortic or tricuspid valve have been identified on echocardiography (Rippe et al. 1980a; Rodger and Morley 1982).

The typical auscultatory finding is of a late systolic murmur, heard at or medial to the cardiac apex accompanied by a mid-systolic click, with some variability in these signs induced by changes in posture. This finding is commonest in middle-aged or older adults, men more than women. It is usually symptomless but may be associated with left-sided chest pain and arrhythmia. It is known also to carry a risk of complications: chordal rupture, worsening regurgitation, infective endocarditis, platelet emboli, transient cerebral ischaemic attacks, serious arrhythmias and even sudden death (Beton et al. 1983; Kouvaras and Bacoulas 1985).

On echocardiography the abnormal prolapsing movement of the posterior cusp is well shown (Fig. 10.6). Oakley (1984, 1985) has drawn attention to the frequency of the echocardiographic finding, sometimes without a murmur, and its overall benign nature, contrasting this with the many reports of complications, usually in middle-aged or older adults. In the Framingham survey echocardiographic prolapse was seen in 5% of 5000 subjects, yet only 5 of them had clinical features of prolapse. Oakley therefore sees a difference between the benign "echo only" lesion, commonly seen in younger women and liable to disappear after some years, and the "auscultatory" prolapse of older adults with its possible complications.

It is likely, therefore, that the syndrome of mitral valve prolapse is a heterogenous one. It includes some who may have an inherited abnormality which is a minor variant of the major defects of connective tissue, manifesting as the hypermobility syndrome: also many younger adults with a harmless finding on echocardiography: and many older adults with what is probably a degenerative changes at the valve, carrying some risk of complications.

Treatment

In the majority no treatment is required. The patient with hypermobility syndrome needs to be reassured that his aches and pains are real and not neurotic, but that they do not mark the beginning of serious rheumatic disease. Reassurance may be given about the condition of the heart. But prophylaxis should be given where appropriate against infective endocarditis and anti-platelet agents, disopyramide or aspirin offered if there have been signs of platelet emboli.

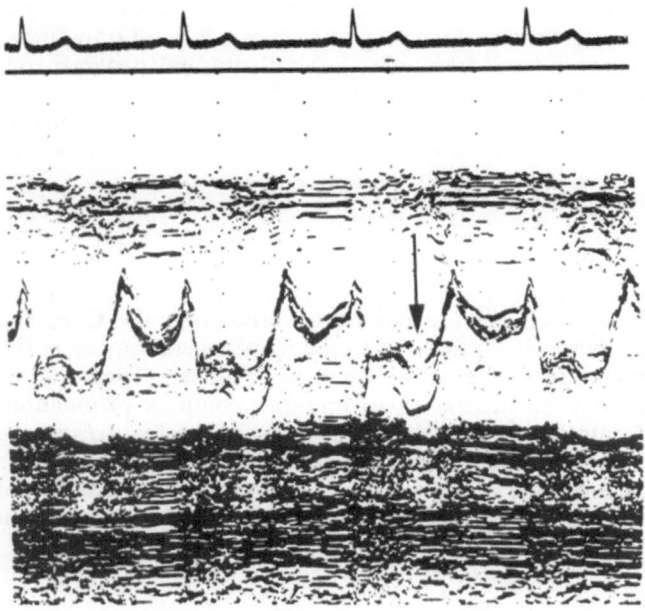

Fig. 10.6. Mitral valve prolapse. The echocardiogram shows the abnormal movement of the posterior valve cusp in systole (*arrow*). With acknowledgement to Dr. FGM Ross.

Lyme Disease

Description

Lyme disease is a seasonal infection caused by the spirochaete *Borrelia bergdorfi*, transmitted to man by the bite of a tick of the genus Ixodes. The disease was first recognised in 1975 following a local epidemic in Connecticut of what appeared to be juvenile polyarthritis. It was later recognised as being the consequence of infection by the spirochaete. Sporadic cases have been seen in Britain, Europe and Australia, but the greatest number continues to appear in the United States.

The first stage of the illness is the skin lesion, erythema chronicum migrans, usually centring on the site of the tick bite, sometimes with secondary lesions elsewhere. There are systemic symptoms such as headache, fever, myalgia and lymphadenopathy.

After a variable interval of up to a few weeks about 15% of patients develop neurological symptoms. These include meningitis, with a lymphocyte pleocytosis in the spinal fluid and cranial neuropathies such as facial palsy, and radiculitis. Some 8% in the American series have cardiac symptoms due to myocarditis with heart block of various grades.

Approximately half the patients with Lyme disease develop arthritis, occasionally soon after the onset but more usually after an interval of weeks or months. There is a true inflammatory arthritis which may affect a single joint only, most often the knee, or other joints in the lower limbs. The arthritis may progress to a chronic synovitis with cartilage erosion (Parke 1987).

In the smaller numbers of cases reported from Britain, Ireland and Europe cardiac involvement appears to be rare (Huaux et al. 1988; Muhlemann and Wright 1987).

Pathology

In a number of cases the spirochaete has been recovered from the CSF, the myocardium and the joint synovia. Antibodies to the spirochaete appear in the blood within a few weeks and form the main diagnostic evidence. The systemic nature of the symptoms may be attributed to immune complex production. Alternatively, or as well, interleukin I, mediator of many of the features of the inflammatory reaction, may be produced in response to the liposaccharide component of the spirochaete. This would explain the temporary reactivation of symptoms, the Herxheimer reaction, which may follow antibiotic treatment (Habicht 1987).

The Heart

The signs of cardiac involvement appear at a variable interval, usually of a few weeks, after the skin lesion of the first stage. Symptoms of dyspnoea, fatigue, dizziness or syncope are found to be due to carditis and heart block. Steere et al. (1980) reported 18 patients with fluctuating degrees of heart block, 13 with cardiac enlargement. The patient described by Vlay (1986) was already ill with fever and lethargy when he developed bradycardia due to complete block. After treatment with a temporary pacemaker and antibiotics he recovered within a few days, passing through a phase of second degree block with Wenckebach periods before normal conduction returned.

The patient of Resnick et al. (1986) was found to have second degree block with 2:1 AV conduction, and cardiomegaly, following illness caused by a tick bite. Echocardiography showed some dilatation of the left ventricle and radionuclide studies showed a reduced ejection fraction. On the third hospital day heart block became complete. A temporary pacemaker was introduced, and with antibiotic treatment he recovered normal conduction in a week. Endo-myocardial biopsy was performed, revealing focal myocarditis and a spirochaete was actually seen in the specimen (Figs. 10.7, 10.8).

Treatment

The illness responds promptly to antibiotics – tetracycline, penicillin or erythromycin. In adults the best results have followed tetracycline 250 mg four times daily for 10 days, and in children oral phenoxymethyl penicillin 50 mg/kg/ day. Freedom from later manifestations such as synovitis was best achieved with tetracycline (Parke 1987).

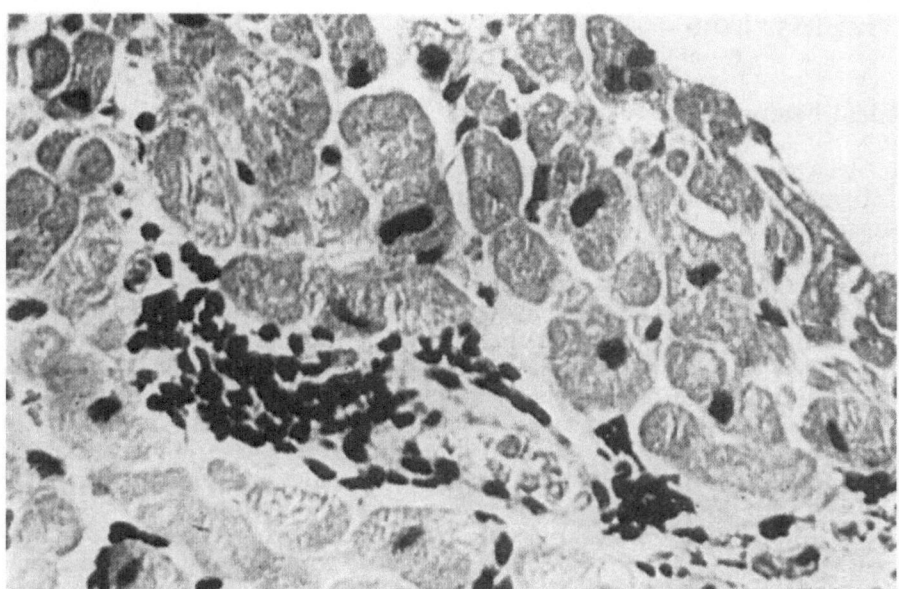

Fig. 10.7. Lyme carditis. Endomyocardial biopsy specimen showing perivascular lymphocyte infiltration and myocyte necrosis (× 800). (Reproduced from Resnick et al. (1986) Am J Med 81: 925, by kind permission of the editor and of the author.)

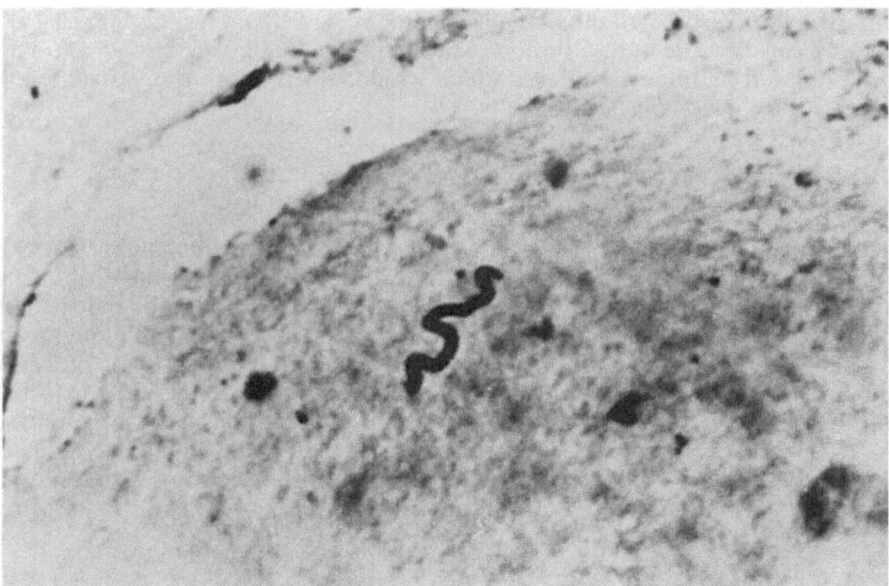

Fig. 10.8. Lyme carditis. Endomyocardial biopsy showing a loosely coiled spirochaete within a recess in the endocardial cavity (× 1280). (Reproduced from Resnick et al. (1986) Am J Med 81: 925, by kind permission of the editor and of the author.)

Atrial Myxoma

Clinical Features

Left atrial myxoma is an uncommon benign tumour which grows slowly to a considerable size. It occupies the cavity of the atrium progressively until it produces signs of mitral valve obstruction which may mimic mitral stenosis with pulmonary venous congestion and pulmonary hypertension. There is an inconstant mitral diastolic murmur, but not the typical opening snap of mitral stenosis. Obstruction at the valve may be sufficient to produce syncope due to a reduction in cardiac output, but the obstruction and the mitral murmur are influenced by the patient's posture. On leaning forward the signs of obstruction and of reduction in cardiac output are enhanced, while when the patient is lying back these signs diminish or disappear. Thrombi may form in the left atrium with a risk of systemic embolism. A similar tumour in the right atrium is much less common, and is less liable to obstruct the cardiac output; however, it may be associated with thrombus formation and pulmonary embolism.

Atrial myxomas are unusual in that they give rise to well-marked constitutional symptoms (Goodwin 1963). These include fever, weight loss, anaemia, arthralgia and sometimes a frank polyarthritis suggestive of rheumatoid arthritis (Currey et al. 1967; Dixon 1965).

There is an increase in serum globulin and the ESR is raised. Rheumatoid factor and antinuclear antibodies are not found, but in some cases there is a systemic vasculitis. Vascular changes resembling polyarteritis nodosa have been seen (Thomas 1981) and in some cases there has been evidence of circulating immune complexes (Byrd et al. 1980; Huston et al. 1978). It is thought that the myxoma cells may secrete a protein which is antigenic, giving rise to antibody formation and immune complexes which would explain both the vasculitic and the constitutional changes.

Management

Atrial myxomas are well shown on echocardiography, as the tumour forms a solid echo-producing mass behind the mitral or the tricuspid valve. Alternatively, and less satisfactorily, cardioangiography shows the tumour as a filling defect within the atrium. The main difficulty in diagnosis lies in thinking of the possibility of an atrial tumour in the first place, as the physical signs are often indefinite or variable, sometimes with no auscultatory signs or else an inconstant mitral diastolic murmur. Often the diagnosis is not considered until the patient has an attack of syncope. Once recognised, the tumour should be removed without delay. The response to surgery is very satisfactory, with relief of obstructive symptoms and the prompt disappearance of constitutional symptoms. Recurrences are uncommon.

References

Giant Cell Arteritis and Polymyalgia Rheumatica

Allison MC, Gallagher PJ (1984) Temporal artery biopsy and corticosteroid treatment. Ann Rheum Dis 43: 416–417

Armstrong RD, Behn A, Myles A, Panayi GS, Welsh KL (1983) Histocompatibility antigens in polymyalgia rheumatica and giant cell arteritis. J Rheumatol 10: 659–661

Ayoub WT, Franklin CM, Torretti D (1985) Polymyalgia rheumatica. Duration of therapy and long term outcome. Am J Med 79: 309–315

Bengtsson BA, Malmvall BE (1981) The epidemiology of giant cell arteritis and polymyalgia rheumatica. Incidences of different clinical presentations and eye complication. Arthritis Rheum 24: 899–904

Bird HA, Esselinckx W, Dixon AS, Mowat AG, Wood PHN (1979) An evaluation of criteria for polymyalgia rheumatica. Ann Rheum Dis 38: 434–439

Fauchald P, Rygvold O, Oystese B (1972) Temporal arteritis and polymyalgia rheumatica. Clinical and biopsy findings. Ann Intern Med 77: 845–852

Hall S, Lie JT, Kurland LT, Persellin S, O'Brien PC, Hunder GG (1983) The therapeutic impact of temporal artery biopsy. Lancet II: 1217–1220

Hamilton CR, Shelley WM, Tumulty PA (1971) Giant cell arteritis, including temporal arteritis and polymyalgia rheumatica. Medicine (Baltimore) 50: 1–27

Hamrin B (1972) Polymyalgia arteritica. Acta Med Scand (Suppl) 533: 1–131

Harris M (1968) Dissecting aneurysm of aorta due to giant cell arteritis. Br Heart J 30: 840–844

Healey LA (1984) Long term follow up of polymyalgia rheumatica: evidence for synovitis. Semin Arthritis Rheum 13: 322–328

Healey LA, Wilske KR (1978) The systemic manifestations of temporal arteritis. Grune and Stratton, New York

How J, Strachan RW (1978) Aortic regurgitation as a manifestation of giant cell arteritis. Br Heart J 40: 1052–1054

Huston KA, Hunder GG, Lie JJ et al. (1978) Temporal arteritis: a 25 year epidemiologic, clinical and pathologic study. Ann Intern Med 88: 162–167

Hutton CW, Maddison PJ (1986) Systemic lupus erythematosus presenting as polymyalgia rheumatica in the elderly. Ann Rheum Dis 45: 641–644

Klein RG, Hunder GG, Stanson AW, Sheps SG (1975) Large artery involvement in giant cell (temporal) arteritis. Ann Intern Med 83: 806–812

Leonard JC, Hasleton PS (1979) Dissecting aortic aneurysms: a clinical-pathological study. Q J Med 48: 55–76

Liang GG, Simkin PA, Hunder GG, Wilske KR, Healey LA (1974) Familial aggregation of polymyalgia and giant cell arteritis. Arthritis Rheum 17: 19–24

Martin JF, Kittas C, Triger DR (1980) Giant cell arteritis of coronary arteries causing myocardial infarction. Br Heart J 43: 487–489

Olhagen B (1986) Polymyalgia rheumatica. Clin Rheum Dis 12: 33–47

Ostberg G (1971) Temporal arteritis in a large autopsy series. Ann Rheum Dis 30: 224–235

Park JR, Hazleman BL (1978) Immunological and histological studies of temporal arteritis. Ann Rheum Dis 37: 238–243

Park JR, Jones JG, Harkiss GD, Hazleman BL (1981) Circulating immune complexes in polymyalgia rheumatica and giant cell arteritis. Ann Rheum Dis 49: 360–365

Perruquet JL, Davis DE, Harrington TM (1986) Aortic arch arteritis in the elderly. An important manifestation of giant cell arteritis. Arch Intern Med 146: 289–291

Salisbury RS, Hazleman BL (1981) Successful treatment of dissecting aortic aneurysm due to giant cell arteritis. Ann Rheum Dis 40: 507–508

Smith AJ, Kyle V, Cawston TE, Hazleman BL (1987) Isolation and analysis of immune complexes from sera of patients with polymyalgia rheumatica and giant cell arteritis. Ann Rheum Dis 46: 468–474

Polyarteritis Nodosa

Duffy J, Lidsky MD, Sharp TJ et al. (1976) Polyarthritis, polyarteritis and hepatitis B. Medicine (Baltimore) 55: 19–37

Ettlinger RE, Nelson AM, Burke EC (1979) Polyarteritis in childhood. A clinical pathologic study. Arthritis Rheum 22: 820–825

Fan PT, Davis JA, Somer T, Kaplan L, Bluestone R (1980) A clinical approach to systemic vasculitis. Semin Arthritis Rheum 9: 248–304

Holsinger DR, Osmundson PJ, Edwards JE (1962) The heart in periarteritis nodosa. Circulation 25: 610–617

Leib ES, Restivo C, Paulus H (1979) Immunosuppressive and corticosteroid therapy of polyarteritis nodosa. Am J Med 67: 941–947

Parrillo JE, Fauci AS (1984) Coronary vasculitis. In: Ansell BM, Simkin PA (eds) The heart and rheumatic disease. Butterworths, London, pp 213–233

Sack M, Cassidy JT, Bole GG (1975) Prognostic factors in polyarteritis. J Rheumatol 2: 411–420

Sergent JS, Lockshin MD, Christian CZ, Gocke DJ (1976) Vasculitis with hepatitis B antigenemia: long term observations in 9 patients. Medicine (Baltimore) 55: 1–18

Thiene G, Valente M, Rossi L (1978) Involvement of the cardiac conducting system in panarteritis nodosa. Am Heart J 95: 716–724

Travers RL, Allison DJ, Brettle RP, Hughes JRV (1979) Polyarteritis nodosa: a clinical and angiographic analysis of 17 cases. Semin Arthritis Rheum 8: 184–199

Trepo CG, Thivolet J, Prince AM (1972) Australia antigen and polyarteritis nodosa. Am J Dis Childh 123: 390–392

Takayasu's Disease

Danaraj TJ, Wong HO, Thomas MA (1963) Primary arteritis of aorta causing renal artery stenosis and hypertension. Br Heart J 25: 153–165

Fraga A, Mintz F, Valle L, Flores-Izguierdo G (1972) Takayasu's arteritis: frequency of systemic manifestations (study of 22 patients) and favorable response to maintenance therapy with adrenocorticosteroids (12 patients). Arthritis Rheum 15: 617–624

Hall S, Barr W, Lie JT, Stanson AW, Kazmier FJ, Hunder GG (1985) Takayasu arteritis. A study of 32 N American patients. Medicine (Baltimore) 64: 89–99

Marquis Y, Richardson JB, Ritchie AC, Wigle ED (1968) Idiopathic medial aortopathy and arteriopathy. Am J Med 44: 939–954

Schrire V, Asherson RA (1964) Arteritis of the aorta and its major branches. Q J Med 33: 439–463

Strachan RW (1964) The natural history of Takayasu's arteriopathy. Q J Med 33: 57–69

Takayasu M (1908) A case with peculiar changes of the central retinal vessels. Acta Soc Ophth Jap 12: 554

Polymyositis and Dermatomyositis

Askari AD, Huettner TL (1982) Cardiac abnormalities in polymyositis/dermatomyositis. Semin Arthritis Rheum 12: 208–219

Behan WMH, Aitchison M, Behan PO (1986) Pathogenesis of heart block in a fatal case of dermatomyositis. Br Heart J 56: 479–482

Behan WMH, Behan PO, Gairns J (1987) Cardiac damage in polymyositis associated with antibodies to tissue ribonucleoproteins. Br Heart J 57: 176–180

Bohan A, Peter JB (1975) Polymyositis and dermatomyositis. N Engl J Med 292: 344–347, 403–407

Bohan A, Peter JB, Bowman RL, Pearson CM (1977) A computer assisted survey of 153 patients with polymyositis and dermatomyositis. Medicine (Baltimore) 56: 255–286

Denbow CE, Lie JT, Tancredi RG, Bunch TW (1979) Cardiac involvement in polymyositis. Arthritis Rheum 22: 1088–1092

Lynch PG (1971) Cardiac involvement in chronic polymyositis. Br Heart J 33: 416–419

Reid JM, Murdoch R (1979) Polymyositis and complete heart block. Br Heart J 41: 628–629

Sharratt GP, Danta G, Carson PHM (1977) Cardiac abnormalities in polymyositis. Ann Rheum Dis 36: 575–578

Stern R, Godbold JH, Chess Q, Kagen LJ (1984) ECG abnormalities in polymyositis. Arch Intern Med 144: 2185–2189
Strongwater SL, Annesley T, Schnitzer TJ (1983) Myocardial involvement in polymyositis. J Rheumatol 10: 459–463
Weiss J, Shark W. Fishbein M et al. (1982) The use of endomyocardial biopsy in a serious cardiac abnormality associated with polymyositis: a case report. J Rheumatol 9: 299–302

Behçet's Syndrome

Chajek T, Fainaru M (1975) Behçet's disease. Report of 41 cases and review of the literature. Medicine (Baltimore) 54: 179–196
Comess KA, Zibelli LR, Gordon D, Fredrickson SR (1983) Acute severe aortic regurgitation in Behçet's syndrome. Ann Intern Med 99: 639–640
Dubost JJ, Sauvezie B, Galtier B et al. (1985) Behçet's syndrome and ankylosing spondylitis. Rev Rhum Mal Osteoartic 52: 457–461
Higashihara M, Mori M, Takeuchi A et al. (1982) Myocarditis in Behçet's disease – a case report and review of the literature. J Rheumatol 9: 630–633
Kansu E, Ozer FL, Akalin E et al. (1972) Behçet's syndrome with obstruction of the venae cavae. Q J Med 41: 151–168
Lewis PE (1964) Behçet's disease and carditis. Br Med J i: 1026–1027
Mason RM, Barnes CG (1969) Behçet's syndrome with arthritis. Ann Rheum Dis 28: 95–103
Roguin N, Haim S, Reshe FR, Peleg E, Riss E (1978) Cardiac involvement and superior vena cava obstruction in Behçet's disease. Thorax 33: 375–377
Scarlett JA, Kistner ML, Yang LC (1979) Behçet's syndrome: report of a case associated with pericardial effusion and cryoglobulinaemia treated with indomethacin. Am J Med 66: 146–148
Shimizu T, Ehrlich GE, Inaba G, Hayashi K (1979) Behçet disease (Behçet syndrome). Semin Arthritis Rheum 8: 223–260
Wright V, Chamberlain A (1978) Behçet's syndrome. Bull Rheum Dis 29: 972–977

Relapsing Polychondritis

Arkin CR, Masi AT (1975) Relapsing polychondritis: review of current status and case report. Arthritis Rheum 5: 41–62
Dolan DL, Lemmon GB, Teitelbaum SL (1966) Relapsing polychondritis: analytical literature review and studies on pathogenesis. Am J Med 41: 285–299
Hainer JW, Hamilton GW (1969) Aortic abnormalities in relapsing polychondritis. Report of a case with dissecting aneurysm. N Engl J Med 280: 1166–1168
McAdam LP, O'Hanlan MA, Bluestone R, Pearson CM (1976) Relapsing polychondritis. Prospective study of 23 patients and review of the literature. Medicine (Baltimore) 55: 193–215
Owen DS, Irby R, Toone E (1970) Relapsing polychondritis with aortic involvement. Arthritis Rheum 13: 877–881
Rajapakse DA, Bywaters EGL (1974) Cell mediated immunity to cartilage proteoglycan in relapsing polychondritis. Clin Exp Immunol 16: 497–502

Inherited Disorders of Connective Tissue

Beighton P (1972) The inherited disorders of connective tissue. Bull Rheum Dis 23: 696–707
Beighton P, Price A, Lord J, Dickson E (1969) Variants of the Ehlers-Danlos syndrome. Clinical, biochemical, haematological and chromosomal features of 100 patients. Ann Rheum Dis 28: 228–245
Brown OR, DeMots H, Kloster FE, Roberts A, Menashe VD, Beals RK (1975) Aortic root dilatation and mitral valve prolapse in Marfan's syndrome. Circulation 52: 651–657
Cotton DJ, Brandt KD (1976) Cardiovascular abnormalities in the Marfanoid hypermobility syndrome. Arthritis Rheum 19: 763–768

Criscitiello MG, Ronan JA, Besterman EMM, Schoenwetter W (1965) Cardiovascular abnormalities in osteogenesis imperfecta. Circulation 31: 255–262

Cupo LN, Pyeritz R, Olson JL, McPhee SJ, Hutchins GM, McKusick VA (1981) Ehlers–Danlos syndrome with abnormal collagen fibrils, sinus of Valsalva aneurysms, myocardial infarction, panacinar emphysema and cerebral heterotopias. Am J Med 71: 1051–1058

Daneshwar A, Tavakoli D, Nazarian J (1979) Marfanoid hypermobility syndrome associated with coarctation of aorta. Br Heart J 41: 621–623

Edmondson P, Nellen M, Ross DN (1979) Aortic valve replacement in a case of Ehlers-Danlos syndrome. Br Heart J 42: 103–105

Jiminez SA, Lally EV (1979) Disorders of collagen structure and metabolism. Bull Rheum Dis 30: 1016–1022

McKusick VA (1974) Heritable disorders of connective tissue, 4th edition, C V Mosby, St Louis

Pyeritz RE, Wappel MA (1983) Mitral valve dysfunction in the Marfan syndrome. Am J Med 74: 797–807

Stein D, Kloster FE (1977) Valvular heart disease in osteogenesis imperfecta. Am Heart J 94: 637–641

Walker BA, Beighton PH, Murdoch JL (1969) The Marfanoid hypermobility syndrome. Ann Intern Med 71: 349–352

Weisinger B, Glassman E, Spencer FC, Berger A (1975) Successful aortic valve replacement for aortic regurgitation associated with osteogenesis imperfecta. Br Heart J 37: 475–477

White NJ, Winearls CG, Smith R (1983) Cardiovascular abnormalities in osteogenesis imperfecta. Am Heart J 106: 1416–1421

Hypermobility Syndrome and Mitral Valve Prolapse

Barlow JB, Pocock WA, Marchand P, Denny M (1963) The significant late systolic murmurs. Am Heart J 66: 443–452

Beton DC, Brear SG, Edwards JD, Leonard JC (1983) Mitral valve prolapse: an assessment of clinical features, associated conditions and prognosis. Q J Med 52: 150–164

Bird HA, Brodie DA, Wright V (1979) Quantification of joint laxity. Rheumatol Rehabil 18: 161–166

Child A (1986) Joint hypermobility syndrome: inherited disorders of collagen synthesis. (Editorial.) J Rheumatol 13: 239–243

Davies MJ, Moore BP, Braimbridge MV (1978) The floppy mitral valve. Study of incidence, pathology and complications in surgical, necropsy and forensic material. Br Heart J 40: 468–481

Grahame R, Edwards JC, Pitcher V, Gabell A, Harvey W (1981) A clinical and echocardiographic study of patients with hypermobility syndrome. Ann Rheum Dis 40: 541–546

Hammer D, Leier CV, Baba N, Vasko JS, Wooley CF, Pinnel SR (1979) Altered collagen composition in a prolapsing mitral valve with ruptured chordae tendinae. Am J Med 67: 863–866

Handler CE, Child A, Light ND, Dorrance DE (1985) Mitral valve prolapse, aortic compliance and skin collagen in joint hypermobility syndrome. Br Heart J 54: 501–508

Kirk JA, Ansell BM, Bywaters EGL (1967) The hypermobility syndrome. Musculoskeletal complaints associated with generalised joint hypermobility. Ann Rheum Dis 26: 419–425

Kouvaras G, Bacoulas G (1985) Association of mitral valve leaflet prolapse with cerebral ischaemic events in the young and early middle aged patient. Q J Med 55: 387–392

Oakley CM (1984) Mitral valve prolapse: harbinger of death or variant of normal? (Editorial.) Br Med J 288: 1853–1854

Oakley CM (1985) Mitral valve prolapse. (Editorial.) Q J Med 55: 317–320

Rippe JM, Angoff G, Sloss LJ, Wynne J, Alpert JS (1980a) Multiple floppy valves: an echocardiographic syndrome. Am J Med 66: 817–824

Rippe JM, Fishbein MC, Carabello B et al. (1980b) Primary myxomatous degeneration of cardiac valves; clinical, pathological, haemodynamic and echocardiographic profile. Br Heart J 44: 621–629

Rizzon P, Biasco G, Brindicci G, Mauro F (1973) Familial syndrome of mid-systolic click and late systolic murmur. Br Heart J 35: 245–259

Rodger JC, Morley P (1982) Abnormal aortic valve echoes in mitral prolapse. Echocardiographic features of floppy aortic valve. Br Heart J 47: 337–343

Scott D, Bird H, Wright V (1979) Joint laxity leading to osteoarthrosis. Rheumatol Rehabil 18: 167–169

Strahan NV, Murphy EA, Fortuin NJ, Come PC, Humphries JO (1983) Inheritance of the mitral valve prolapse syndrome. Am J Med 74: 967–972

Lyme Disease

Habicht GS, Beck G, Benach JL (1987) Lyme disease. Sci Am 257: 60–65

Huaux JP, Bigaignon G, Stadtsbaeder S, Zangerle PF, Deuxchaisnes CN (1988) Pattern of Lyme disease in Europe: report of 14 cases. Ann Rheum Dis 47: 164–165

Muhlemann MF, Wright DJM (1987) Emerging pattern of Lyme disease in the United Kingdom and the Irish republic. Lancet I: 260–262

Parke A (1987) From New to Old England: the progress of Lyme disease. (Editorial.) Br Med J 294: 525–526

Resnick JW, Braunstein DB, Walsh RL et al. (1986) Lyme carditis. Electrophysiologic and histopathologic study. Am J Med 81: 923–927

Steere AC, Batsford WP, Weinberg M (1980) Lyme carditis: cardiac abnormalities of Lyme disease. Ann Intern Med 93: 8–16

Vlay SC (1986) Complete heart block due to Lyme disease. N Engl J Med 315: 1418

Atrial Myxoma

Byrd WE, Matthews OP, Hunt RE (1980) Left atrial myxoma presenting as a systemic vasculitis. Arthritis Rheum 23: 240–243

Currey HFL, Mathews JA, Robinson J (1967) Right atrial myxoma mimicking a rheumatic disorder. Br Med J i: 547–548

Dixon AS (1965) Left atrial myxoma. In: Dixon AS (ed) Progress in clinical rheumatology. Churchill, London, p 362

Goodwin JF (1963) Diagnosis of left atrial myxoma. Lancet I: 464–466

Huston KA, Combs JJ, Lie JT, Giuliani ER (1978) Left atrial myxoma simulating peripheral vasculitis. Mayo Clin Proc 53: 752–756

Thomas MH (1981) Myxoma masquerading as polyarteritis nodosa. J Rheumatol 8: 133–137

Subject Index